Paediatric Neuropsychology Within the Multidisciplinary Context

Paediatric Neuropsychology Within the Multidisciplinary Context

Rhonda Booth
Lecturer (Teaching), Cognitive Neuroscience and Neuropsychiatry Section,
UCL Great Ormond Street Institute of Child Health, London, UK

Tara Murphy
Consultant Paediatric Neuropsychologist and
Co-lead of the Paediatric Neuropsychology Team,
Psychological and Mental Health Services,
Great Ormond Street Hospital NHS Foundation Trust, London, UK

Kathy Zebracki
Chief of Psychology, Shriners Children's Chicago and
Adjunct Professor of Psychiatry and Behavioral Sciences,
Northwestern University Feinberg School of Medicine, Chicago, IL, USA

2022
Mac Keith Press

© 2022 Mac Keith Press

Managing Director: Ann-Marie Halligan
Senior Publishing Manager: Sally Wilkinson
Publishing and Marketing Co-ordinator: Paul Grossman
Production Manager: Andy Booth

First published in this edition in 2022 by Mac Keith Press
2nd Floor, Rankin Building, 139–143 Bermondsey Street, London, SE1 3UW

British Library Cataloguing-in-Publication data
A catalogue record for this book is available from the British Library

Cover artist: Suzanne McCoy
Cover designer: Marten Sealby

ISBN: 978-1-911612-57-5

Typeset by Riverside Publishing Solutions Ltd
Printed by Hobbs the Printers Ltd, Totton, Hampshire, UK

Contents

Author Appointments ix

Foreword xv

Preface xix

PART 1: SENSORY AND COGNITIVE PROCESSES

1 Vision 3
Rebecca Greenaway and Naomi Dale

2 Hearing 19
Fionna Bathgate and Lindsey Edwards

3 Sensory Integration and Processing 31
Sarah A Schoen, Virginia Spielmann, and Cristin M Holland

4 Motor Coordination 43
Dido Green and Elisabeth L Hill

5 Language 57
Anne Hoffmann, Karen Riley, and Christina Hawkins

6 Speech 71
Frédérique Liégeois and Angela Morgan

7 Visuo-Spatial Processing 81
Katie A Gilligan-Lee, Elizabeth Roberts, and Emily Farran

8 Attention 93
Megan N Scott and Tom Manly

9   **Memory**   105
    Rachael Elward, Patricia Martin-Sanfilippo, and Faraneh Vargha-Khadem

10 **Auditory Processing**   119
    Teresa Bailey

11 **Executive Function**   131
    Deborah Budding and Laura Flores Shaw

12 **Social Functioning**   143
    Miriam Bindman, Sarah Cole, and Rhonda Booth

13 **Disruptive Behaviour**   159
    Alice Jones Bartoli and Stuart F White

14 **Literacy**   171
    Valerie Muter and Margaret Snowling

15 **Handwriting**   183
    Mellissa Prunty and Emma Sumner

PART 2: FACTORS INFLUENCING CLINICAL FORMULATION

16 **Prenatal Exposure to Medicines and Chemicals**   195
    Rebecca Bromley and Jennifer Shields

17 **Early Adversity**   209
    Bettina Hohnen and Jane Gilmour

18 **School and Education**   219
    Rebecca Ashton and Helen Jackson

19 **Mental Health**   233
    Megan Eve and Fiona McFarlane

20 **Intellectual Disability**   245
    Kyle Deane, Lindsay Katz, and Scott Hunter

21 **Speech, Motor Impairments, and Physical Limitations**   261
    Seth A Warschausky

PART 3: FACTORS INFLUENCING ASSESSMENT AND FEEDBACK

22 Culture   277
Daniel Stark

23 Validity Testing in Paediatric Neuropsychology   289
Brian L Brooks and William MacAllister

24 Paediatric Teleneuropsychology   301
Elizabeth Roberts, Rosie Brett, and Tara Murphy

25 Feedback   319
Karen Postal

Measure Index   331

Index   349

Author Appointments

Rebecca Ashton
Consultant Associate and Supervisor, Recolo UK Ltd, London; Freelance Educational Psychologist, Ashton Psychology Ltd, Preston, UK.

Teresa Bailey
Neuropsychologist and Independent Scholar, California, USA.

Fionna Bathgate
Clinical Psychologist, Great Ormond Street Hospital, London, UK.

Miriam Bindman
Principal Clinical Psychologist, Social Communication & Autism Spectrum Service, Great Ormond Street Hospital for Children NHS Trust, London, UK.

Rose Brett
PhD Student, University of Surrey, Guildford, UK.

Rebecca Bromley
Research Fellow, Child Neuropsychologist, Division of Neuroscience & Experimental Psychology, The University of Manchester, Manchester, UK.

Brian L Brooks
Pediatric Neuropsychologist, Neurosciences Program, Alberta Children's Hospital, Calgary; Adjunct Associate Professor, Departments of Pediatrics, Clinical Neurosciences, and Psychology, University of Calgary, Calgary, Canada.

Deborah Budding
Psychology Division, Department of Psychiatry, Harbor–UCLA Medical Center, Torrance, California, USA.

Sarah Cole
Senior Clinical Psychologist, Social Communication & Autism Spectrum Service, Great Ormond Street Hospital for Children NHS Trust, London, UK.

Naomi Dale
Consultant Clinical Psychologist and Paediatric Neuropsychologist, Great Ormond Street Hospital for Children; Professor of Paediatric Neurodisability, UCL Great Ormond Street Institute of Child Health, London, UK.

Kyle Deane
Pediatric Psychologist, Shriners Children's Chicago; Clinical Assistant Professor, Psychology Faculty, Rosalind Franklin University of Medicine and Science, Chicago, Illinois, USA.

Lindsey Edwards
Honorary Consultant Clinical Psychologist, Great Ormond Street Hospital for Children NHS Foundation Trust, London, UK.

Rachael Elward
Senior Lecturer, School of Applied Sciences, London South Bank University, London; Honorary Lecturer, UCL Great Ormond Street Institute of Child Health, London, UK.

Megan Eve
Paediatric Clinical Neuropsychologist, Psychological Health Services, Bristol Royal Hospital for Children, Bristol, UK.

Emily Farran
Professor of Cognitive Development, School of Psychology, University of Surrey, Guildford, UK.

Katie A Gilligan-Lee
Lecturer of Developmental Psychology, School of Psychology, University of Surrey, Guildford, UK.

Jane Gilmour
Honorary Consultant Clinical Psychologist, Great Ormond Street Hospital; Course Director, Infancy and Early Childhood Development, University College London, London, UK.

Dido Green
Professor in Occupational Therapy, Jönköping University, Jönköping, Sweden; Honorary Professor in Occupational Therapy, College of Health, Medicine and Life Sciences, Brunel University, London, UK.

Rebecca Greenaway
Consultant Clinical Psychologist and Paediatric Neuropsychologist, Great Ormond Street Hospital NHS Foundation Trust, London, UK.

Christina Hawkins
Independent Speech and Language Therapist, London, UK.

Elisabeth L Hill
Professor of Neurodevelopmental Disorders, Goldsmiths, University of London, London, UK.

Anne Hoffmann
Assistant Professor, Department of Communication Disorders and Sciences, Department of Pediatrics, Rush University, Chicago, Illinois, USA.

Bettina Hohnen
Consultant Clinical Psychologist, Honorary Senior Teaching Fellow, University College London, London, UK.

Cristin M Holland
Postdoctoral Research Fellow, Department of Psychiatry, Columbia University Irving Medical Center, New York, New York, USA.

Scott Hunter
Senior Scientific Expert, Neurodevelopment, WCG MedAvante-ProPhase; Clinical Professor, Psychiatry & Behavioral Neuroscience, The University of Chicago, Chicago, Illinois, USA.

Helen Jackson
Educational Psychologist, Brainwise Educational Services Ltd, Cambridge, UK.

Alice Jones Bartoli
Professor of Psychology of Education, Goldsmiths, University of London, London, UK.

Lindsay Katz
Postdoctoral Fellow, Pediatric Neuropsychology, Neuropsychology Section, Department of Psychiatry, University of Michigan, Ann Arbor, Michigan, USA.

Frédérique Liégeois
Associate Professor, Developmental Neurosciences Department, UCL Great Ormond Street Institute of Child Health, London; Section Head, Clinical Systems Neuroscience; Co-Director, MSc/PGDip Paediatric Neuropsychology, UCL Great Ormond Street Institute of Child Health, London, UK.

William MacAllister
Pediatric Neuropsychologist, Neurosciences Program, Alberta Children's Hospital, Calgary; Adjunct Associate Professor, Departments of Pediatrics, Clinical Neurosciences, and Psychology, University of Calgary, Calgary, Canada.

Tom Manly
Programme Leader, MRC Cognition and Brain Sciences Unit, University of Cambridge, Cambridge, UK.

Patricia Martin-Sanfilippo
Clinical Psychologist, Neuropsychology Service, Great Ormond Street Hospital NHS Foundation Trust, London; Honorary Senior Research Associate, UCL Great Ormond Street Institute of Child Health, London, UK.

Fiona McFarlane
Clinical Psychologist and Course Tutor, The Oxford Institute of Clinical Psychology Training and Research, Oxford; Clinical Psychologist, Oxford Health Specialist Psychological Intervention Centre, Oxford, UK.

Angela Morgan
Head of Speech and Language, Murdoch Children's Research Institute; Professor of Speech Pathology, University of Melbourne; Speech Pathologist, Royal Children's Hospital, Melbourne, Australia.

Valerie Muter
Honorary Research Associate, Neuroscience, Institute of Child Health, University College London, London, UK.

Karen Postal
Clinical Instructor in Psychology, Department of Psychiatry, Harvard Medical School, Boston, Massachusetts, USA.

Mellissa Prunty
Senior Lecturer in Occupational Therapy, Department of Health Sciences, Brunel University, London, UK.

Karen Riley
Provost and Chief Academic Officer, Regis University, Denver, Colorado, USA.

Elizabeth Roberts
Specialist Educational Psychologist in Paediatric Neuropsychology, The Children's Trust, Surrey, UK.

Sarah A Schoen
Director of Research, STAR Institute, Centennial, Colorado; Associate Professor, Rocky Mountain University of Health Professions, Provo, Utah, USA.

Megan N Scott
Pediatric Neuropsychologist, Pritzker Department of Psychiatry and Behavioral Health, Ann & Robert H. Lurie Children's Hospital of Chicago; Associate Professor of Psychiatry and Behavioral Science, Northwestern University Feinberg School of Medicine, Chicago, Illinois, USA.

Laura Flores Shaw
Assistant Professor, School of Education, Johns Hopkins University, Baltimore, Maryland, USA.

Jennifer Shields
Principal Clinical Psychologist and Lecturer, University of Edinburgh, Edinburgh, UK.

Margaret Snowling
President and Honorary Professor, Department of Experimental Psychology, St John's College, Oxford, UK.

Virginia Spielmann
Executive Director of STAR Institute, Centennial, Colorado, USA.

Daniel Stark
Clinical Psychologist and Paediatric Neuropsychologist, Department of Neuropsychology, Great Ormond Street Hospital NHS Foundation Trust; University College London, London, UK.

Emma Sumner
Associate Professor of Psychology and Special Educational Needs, University College London; Associate Professor, Psychology and Human Development Department, Institute of Education, London, UK.

Faraneh Vargha-Khadem
Professor of Developmental Cognitive Neuroscience, Developmental Neuroscience Research and Teaching Department, UCL Great Ormond Street Institute of Child Health, Great Ormond Street Hospital for Children NHS Trust, London, UK.

Seth A Warschausky
Professor, Department of Physical Medicine and Rehabilitation, University of Michigan, Ann Arbor, Michigan, USA.

Stuart F White
Director, Developmental Clinical Neuroscience Lab, Institute for Human Neuroscience, Boys Town National Research Hospital, Boys Town, Nebraska, USA.

Foreword

My career as a paediatric neuropsychologist has included a faculty position at an academic medical centre, a stint in the test publishing industry, and most recently, serving as a consultant and advocate for the international Montessori education movement.

I love being a paediatric neuropsychologist. I love that our work requires a blend of knowledge, curiosity, experience, interpersonal skills, and (sometimes) persuasiveness, all of which we apply toward the goal of making a difference in the life of a child (and family) that, in some way, is struggling. I enjoy 'talking shop' with colleagues at conferences or online, learning about the latest research and new tests, and value that there is always more to know about brain–behaviour relationships in the context of human development. I cannot think of a more satisfying profession, at least for me.

Of course, I also love books about neuropsychology (especially paediatric neuropsychology), and every year, my bookcase gets a little more crowded. At every conference, I approach the publishers' tables with interest, hoping that I'll find something that will stand out and maybe even make a difference in my work. This is one of those books.

I first learned about *Paediatric Neuropsychology Within the Multidisciplinary Context* in March 2017, while it was still in its planning stages. I was in the planning stages of an international move from my home in Minneapolis, Minnesota, USA to London, England. This was a big step, both personally and professionally, and among the many thoughts swimming around in my head was the question of how practising paediatric neuropsychology in the UK might be different from what I'd known in the USA. I decided it might be a good idea to get in touch with some London-based contacts that I have made over the years.

Tara Murphy, one of the editors of this book, was one of them. I wrote to her asking if she would mind answering a few questions. In fact, she didn't mind at all, and I soon met Tara at her office at Great Ormond Street Hospital for Children (GOSH) in London. As co-leader of the Paediatric Neuropsychology Service at GOSH, Tara is well-connected in London and offered many useful tips that helped get me grounded, ranging from London office real estate to the process of getting registered as a psychologist in the UK.

Somewhere in all the excitement, I heard about a book that Tara and her colleagues were putting together: a paediatric neuropsychology textbook. They had in mind to do something a little different from the usual. Tara talked about a real-world, applied approach that connected theory and research with the practicalities of assessment and intervention through illustrative examples. It sounded interesting, and I looked forward to hearing more about the project as it took shape.

While I was planning my international move, Tara was also planning one of her own – to Kampala, Uganda, where she was spending a year volunteering at a psychiatric hospital. I learned later that, after her year in Uganda, Tara accepted a job on the Island of St. Helena, where she worked as the sole psychologist serving the island's population of 4,500, finally returning to London (and GOSH) after 2 years in this remarkable, remote setting.

I wonder what she gained through those remarkable sets of experiences. I imagine they would deepen anyone's understanding of neurological and psychiatric illness, and enrich their understanding of the effects of culture on disorders and their treatment. I believe I could learn a lot from someone whose perspective on our profession has been seasoned in such a way, and I am happy that I can through this lovely book.

Tara's collaborators in editing *Paediatric Neuropsychology Within the Multidisciplinary Context* are two other outstanding scientist-practitioner-educators. One is Dr Rhonda Booth, a lecturer at Great Ormond Street Institute of Child Health and a leading expert on agenesis of the corpus callosum. Dr Booth serves on the Governance Board of the International Research Consortium for the Corpus Callosum and Cerebral Connectivity, and she brings her own international experiences to this work, having trained and worked in her native New Zealand before relocating to the UK.

We also benefit from the expertise of Dr Kathy Zebracki, Chief of Psychology at Shriners Children's Chicago and an Adjunct Professor of Psychiatry and Behavioral Sciences at Northwestern University Feinberg School of Medicine. A Fellow of the American Psychological Association (Division 54 Pediatric Psychology and Division 22 Rehabilitation Psychology), she is on the Board of Directors of the American Spinal Injury Association and the Steel Assembly for Pediatric Spinal Cord Injury and Dysfunction, and formerly on the Board of the American Academy of Cerebral Palsy and Developmental Medicine. Dr Zebracki is an active clinician and researcher serving as a mentor for clinical psychology doctoral students and postdoctoral fellows.

Together, Booth, Murphy, and Zebracki represent decades of experience gained in teaching, training, research, and clinical practice, which they have used to create a book that can serve as both an applied textbook to help prepare upcoming clinicians, and as a 'go-to' reference for more seasoned clinicians.

After general clinical training, internship, and fellowship years, an early-career paediatric neuropsychologist should know enough about child development, developmental disorders, neuroanatomical systems, and therapeutic interventions to be able to competently evaluate and make a difference in the lives of almost any child in need of their services. As a textbook, *Paediatric Neuropsychology Within the Multidisciplinary Context* will help ensure that early-career clinicians are getting off on the right foot.

As we advance in our careers, many paediatric neuropsychologists develop unique expertise around particular disorders or types of disorders (there is just no substitute for seeing many cases of, say, 22q11.2 detection syndrome to develop a rich understanding of its varied clinical presentation). Sometimes, it's best to refer a new patient to someone in the community who has such expertise. Other times, that more-experienced colleague is unavailable or does not exist, so it is up to you to do the evaluation. How will you proceed? Maybe you can drop an email to a more knowledgeable friend, dash off a message to a Listserv, or perform a quick literature review? All that would help, but not as much as the relevant chapter from *Paediatric Neuropsychology Within the Multidisciplinary Context*. This is where this book shines as a reference for more experienced clinicians.

I cannot think of the last time I evaluated a child with a significant visual impairment, but if I was in such a situation, I know I would do a better job of it after reviewing Chapter 1. The same would be true for a child with a significant hearing impairment thanks to Chapter 2. In fact, looking at the comprehensive range of topics addressed, it is hard to see how I could not do at least a *somewhat* better job on nearly any case with its help. Each chapter is a mini-seminar, offering anatomical and theoretical background, prior research, and practical test applications, all with a clinical case forming the backdrop.

Booth, Murphy, and Zebracki have organised the book logically, with the first section dealing with many of the sensory and cognitive processing issues that lead to referral, such as language or speech impairment (Chapters 5 and 6), problems with attention (Chapter 8), auditory processing (Chapter 10), executive functioning (Chapter 11), and social functioning (Chapter 12).

This is followed by a section devoted to factors that influence clinical formulation. How has early adversity affected this child's functioning (Chapter 17)? Is their performance affected by prenatal exposure to medications or chemicals (Chapter 16)? Or, is this child affected by wider intellectual disability, perhaps (Chapter 20)?

The book concludes with chapters on factors that influence the process of assessment and feedback, including cultural differences between examiner and patient (Chapter 22), response validity (Chapter 23), and nicely wraps up with an overview on the process of effective feedback (Chapter 25). I'm just hitting some of the highlights here, but I think you get the picture. If you are still in training, you will get an excellent overview of paediatric neuropsychology. If you are well into your career, you will get a nice update and overview for what might be your next case.

Many chapters are written or co-written by recognised experts from the UK and the USA. It's nice to see these international collaborations – they help us learn from those outside of our own spheres (and would have been particularly useful to me as I moved across the Atlantic).

Finally – and I don't want to leave this out – they have thoughtfully included a handy index of measures mentioned in the text, which I think is just icing on the cake.

Should this book become part of your collection? Well, certainly an important reflection of a book's usefulness is the impact it makes on one's work. While I've only had *Paediatric Neuropsychology Within the Multidisciplinary Context* for a few weeks, since reading it, I have ordered a new performance validity test, reviewed my language measures, and begun preparing to offer teleassessment services. I expect it will continue to affect my work in the months ahead, and I am sure this excellent book will have an impact on your practice too.

Steven J. Hughes
Psychotherapist and pediatric neuropsychologist,
Prague English Psychology Services,
Prague, Czechia

Preface

Paediatric Neuropsychology Within the Multidisciplinary Context is a practical guide written for early career paediatric neuropsychologists to hone their skills as well as seasoned clinicians looking for a go-to guide. This book provides a wide breadth of clinically relevant knowledge that will also be valuable to a diverse range of professionals including clinical and educational psychologists, speech and language therapists, occupational therapists, paediatric neurologists, and paediatricians working with children with neurodevelopmental and health conditions. We hope this book will be an essential text for use in a variety of paediatric multidisciplinary settings and will inspire future research.

Our inspiration for this practical guide emanated from over 20 years of providing clinical services, educating trainees, and conducting research at specialist hospitals and institutions. We noted a divide between academic and clinical ways of working, despite opportunities for collaboration and reciprocal learning. The field of paediatric neuropsychology is exciting, dynamic, and expanding; new technologies have allowed researchers to explore the development of brain–behaviour relationships with ever-increasing visual detail, alongside discovering new findings on the interacting contributions of genes and environment on the developing brain. While there is an abundance of studies on developmental cognitive neuroscience now in existence, applying these data to the clinic setting and personalising them to the individual child remains a challenge.

Our vision for *Paediatric Neuropsychology Within the Multidisciplinary Context* is to create a platform where research, theory, and clinical practice are integrated in an accessible and meaningful format. Renowned experts across multiple disciplines were invited to co-author chapters that detail the complex journey from referral and assessment through formulation to intervention and outcome. Consequently, the book offers a fresh perspective on neuropsychological theory and its influence on clinical practice. This, however, is not solely a unidirectional influence from lab to clinic. We were interested in drawing on evidence-based practice and also practice-based evidence drawn from clinical experience and teaching.

This project allowed us the privilege of collaborating with experts from across the world, which has resulted in a diversity of application across countries and cultures. We hope this melding of approaches and models will inspire the development/adoption of new approaches and cross-culture applicability. What is unique about this work is that many of our authors collaborated for the first time, brought together by this book, finding new perspectives and approaches. The focus on the multidisciplinary and interdisciplinary team and neuropsychology's pivotal role in drawing distinct roles and practices together, was particularly important in our design. This rewarding experience occurred during a challenging time in our world's history as the majority of the chapters were written and reviewed between 2019 and 2021, when the world was united in responding to and coping with the COVID-19 pandemic.

This practical guide consists of three parts, with each focusing on process rather than pathology. Part 1 details sensory and cognitive processes important for learning. Each chapter begins with a brief overview of current understanding of typical development of the process in question, before detailing how this may go awry in development or following injury. Much of the information may apply to any typically developing child but also serves to advise readers on assessment and intervention for children with commonly occurring as well as rare conditions that require detailed neuropsychological and multidisciplinary contact. Chapters emphasise the importance of formulation in understanding the presenting challenges to the child, so that a holistic viewpoint is taken, which drives a comprehensive and hopefully effective intervention. Case studies are used to illustrate these complex processes.

Part 2 covers important factors that influence clinical formulation. Chapters cover a number of extrinsic factors that impact development such as prenatal exposure to medicines and chemicals, early adversity, culture, and the school and educational environment. Intrinsic factors to the child include mental health, intellectual disability, and speech, motor, and physical limitations. The process of assessment and feedback are addressed in Part 3: how we can ensure our assessments and interviews are valid both in face-to-face and online (i.e. teleneuropsychology) settings, the cultural-specific factors that we need to consider, and important ingredients we need to think about when providing feedback to the referrer, the family, and the child. As in Part 1, case studies are described alongside research and theory to demonstrate how these factors play out in real-life situations.

Readers may find the overlap between the chapters and the cases used to illustrate the book particularly interesting. The importance of acknowledging the co-occurrence of challenges and strengths that children and families experience is evident between the chapters. In order to describe what is seen in clinical and research practice, many of the cases demonstrate the complexity of real-life neuropsychological needs, in which co-occurrence of several deficits is central. We hope that this enables readers to consider this point but be well informed in making decisions around prioritisation in assessment, formulation, and treatment.

The development and editing of this book was also part of a personal journey for us involving liaison, introductions, and collaborations with longstanding colleagues as well as new. Our skills of negotiation, encouragement, and organisation have certainly been honed. The journey of pulling many linked but disparate areas and styles together into one volume has been filled with joys and challenges with much growth and self-reflection along the process. This final product is the result of a supportive and driven collegiate team. We are very appreciative to the stalwart support from Mac Keith Press in believing in our vision and mission and helping us reach this goal and disseminating the knowledge.

We are extremely grateful to our academic and clinical colleagues from all over the world who worked together, combining their expertise, to produce chapters that met our vision. They willingly took on the challenge to integrate neuroscience into the assessment and formulation of the clinical case and furthermore, shared practical advice on intervention and management strategies. In particular we thank Maja Palmquist, MA, Laura Nicholson, PhD, and Laura Distel, PhD for their contributions to the development of the book. We are also blessed to have loving and supportive families who provided opportunities for us to schedule international Zoom calls as well as to quietly write and reflect upon our book. This book, however, could not have been completed without our paediatric patients and families who continuously inspire and amaze us with their genuineness, strength, and resiliency. Thank you for welcoming us into your lives (and bookshelves), trusting our knowledge, and challenging us to continued growth.

Rhonda Booth, Tara Murphy, and Kathy Zebracki

PART 1

Sensory and Cognitive Processes

CHAPTER 1

Vision

Rebecca Greenaway and Naomi Dale

Presenting Concern

William, a 12-year-old boy with optic nerve hypoplasia and vision impairment, was referred for neuropsychological assessment owing to concerns about slow academic progress. He had a vision level of logMAR 1.2 (severe range) and used a combination of braille, enlarged print, and a video magnifier. William's support included weekly visits from a specialist teacher for vision impairment and a full-time learning support assistant. William could express ideas during informal discussion but had difficulty applying and demonstrating his knowledge in classwork. He lacked motivation for learning, was distractible, and frequently went off task. His teachers expressed that he forgot instructions and had difficulty with planning and organisation. Academically, he was performing at the lower end of the class. Moreover, William struggled to develop independence skills. He was the only student with vision impairment in his school and found it difficult to make friends. He was active and enjoyed outside play but disliked ball games and team sports.

THEORY

Development of Vision

Vision is the sense of processing visual information from the environment and interpreting it as conscious visual stimuli. The visual pathways from the eye and within the brain are complex and extensive (see Fig. 1.1). They are divided into subcortical networks (from the eye to the posterior of the brain) and cortical networks (linking different regions within the brain). The eye and brain pathways and regions work together to reproduce and interpret a dynamic visual scene.

The ocular system is a complex optical system that collects light from the surrounding environment and converts this into chemico-electrical signals transmitted to neurons. It includes the iris, which regulates light intensity, and an adjustable system of lens for

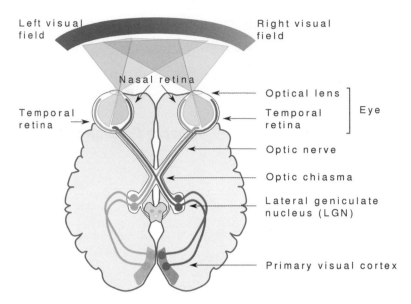

Figure 1.1 The visual pathways from eye to visual cortex. Reused from Miquel Perello Nieto (Wikimedia Commons). This figure is licensed under the Creative Commons Attribution-Share Alike 4.0 International license (https://creativecommons.org/licenses/by-sa/4.0/deed.en). (A colour version of this figure can be seen in the colour plate section)

focusing light into an image (see Fig. 1.2). The lens and eye globe refract or bend light rays to achieve focus on the retina where the rod and cone cells respond differently to light of different wavelengths. When visual information leaves the retina, it travels via the optic nerve, which becomes the optic tract, to a nucleus of the thalamus called the lateral geniculate nucleus (see Fig. 1.1). This main subcortical pathway progresses along a tract called the optic radiation. The axons of the optic radiation curve around the wall of the lateral ventricle in each cerebral hemisphere to reach the visual striate cortex (V1) in the occipital lobe. The magnocellular pathway is specialised to detect movement (e.g. location, speed, and direction), whilst the parvocellular pathway is important for spatial resolution (e.g. shape, colour, and size of object). There are two other subcortical routes via the superior colliculus or via the lateral geniculate that bypass V1 and go straight to the cortical area called V5/MT, which is important for motion detection. V1 is essential for the conscious processing of visual stimuli, including visual perception. The areas around the visual cortex (known as the visual association areas or extra-striate cortex) are involved in complex visual processing. Information from the visual cortex travels to the posterior parietal lobe and this 'dorsal stream' (also known as the 'where' pathway) is believed to be involved in perception of motion and spatial relationships in the visual world. Information travelling to the inferior temporal lobe from the visual cortex is known as the 'ventral stream' (or 'what' pathway) and believed to carry information involved with object form and recognition (Mishkin, Ungerleider, and Macko 1983; Milner and Goodale 1995) (see Fig. 1.3).

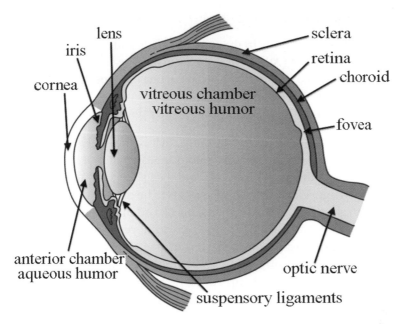

Figure 1.2 The eye structure. Reused from Holly Fischer (Wikimedia Commons). This file is licensed under the Creative Commons Attribution 3.0 Unported license. (https://creativecommons.org/licenses/by/3.0/deed.en). (A colour version of this figure can be seen in the colour plate section)

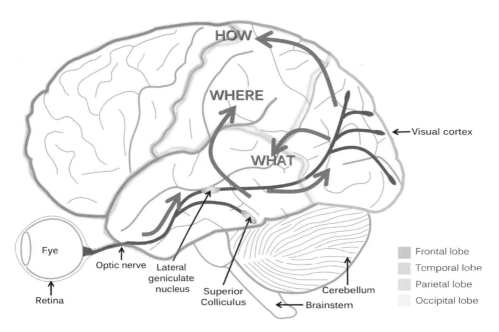

Figure 1.3 Dorsal and ventral pathways of the visual system. (A colour version of this figure can be seen in the colour plate section)

The visual system develops rapidly in the first year of life and continues to develop during the early years of childhood (Atkinson 2017). There appear to be 'sensitive periods' of neuroplasticity of the visual system. For example if one eye is deprived of a normal visual input in early life because of strabismus or very blurred vision (e.g. due to cataract or severe long or short sightedness) that eye may never develop normal vision.

A basic measure of vision is called 'visual acuity', that is, the level at which fine detail can be resolved. At birth, visual acuity is very poor (approximately 1/30th of adult acuity). It improves rapidly over the first year of life, and then slowly improves up to adult levels by around 7 years of age. Visual attention appears to be limited to near distances for the first months of life, but by 1 year of age infants can attend to visual objects at 1.5m or more. As vision maturation advances in the preschool years, higher-order visuo-motor and visuo-cognitive abilities progress, underpinning construction play, drawing, and recognising pictures of increasing detail and complexity. Gross and fine motor actions advance such as walking, climbing up stairs, pouring water into a cup, or catching a ball. Distant vision progresses; the child can point out a bird in a tree or recognise their parent arriving in the playground. By 4 to 5 years, the child can copy patterns and learn to recognise letters.

Childhood Vision Impairment

Almost all aspects of everyday function rely on vision. Learning through observation, whether of physical properties and relationships or social behaviour of others, depends on vision, visual perception, and visuocognition.

Childhood vision impairment is relatively rare, but major disability can arise from disorders of the anterior (peripheral) eye system or disorders of the brain. The majority are congenital, though some occur later in childhood through late-onset genetic disorders, infection, brain injury, or tumour. For children with vision impairment arising from the peripheral visual system, the aetiology involves damage to the eye globe, retina, or anterior optic nerve (see Fig. 1.2) leading to various different congenital developmental eye disorders (see Table 1.1). Over 400 genes have been identified so far causing these developmental eye disorders (Patel et al. 2019). In congenital cerebral visual impairment, visual dysfunction occurs due to damage to areas of the brain involved in processing visual stimuli.

This chapter focuses primarily on children with congenital vision impairment and, in particular, those with severe to profound vision impairment. Severe vision impairment is acuity of 1.0 logMAR (6/60 meaning seeing at 6m what a typically sighted person can see at 60m) or worse. Children at this level of vision will need additional low vision aids to help enlarge print or bring distant images to close vision (Barker et al. 2015). Those who are within the very severe vision impairment or blind range will rely on

Table 1.1 Examples of congenital disorders of the peripheral visual system (optic nerve, retina, and eye globe)

Optic nerve	Retina	Globe
Optic nerve hypoplasia	Cone dystrophy	Anophthalmia
Congenital optic atrophy	Norrie disease	Microphthalmia
	Leber amaurosis	
Disc coloboma	Aniridia	Coloboma
Chiasmal lesions	Albinism	Glaucoma
Tumours	Buphthalmos	Opacities

haptic or tactile means of learning and braille (see Table 1.2). Children with cerebral visual impairment may have acuity reduction ranging from near-normal to severe or profound, with those with near-normal acuity having difficulties in visual processing and visuocognitive abilities (for further reading of visual perceptual and visuo-motor neuropsychological assessments, see Sakki et al. 2021, Dale et al. 2022).

Table 1.2 Levels of visual acuity ranges and educational implications

Category	Presenting distance visual acuity	
	Worse than:	**Equal to or better than:**
0 Mild or no visual impairment		6/18
		3/10 (0.3)
		20/70
1 Moderate visual impairment	6/18	6/60
	3/10 (0.3)	1/10 (0.1)
	20/70	20/200
2 Severe visual impairment	6/60	3/60
	1/10 (0.1)	1/20 (0.05)
	20/200	20/400
3 Blindness	3/60	1/60*
	1/20 (0.05)	1/50 (0.02)
	20/400	5/300 (20/1200)
4 Blindness	1/60*	Light perception
	1/50 (0.02)	
	5/300 (20/1200)	
5 Blindness	No light perception	
9	Undetermined or unspecified	
	*or counts fingers (CF) at 1 metre	

International Statistical Classification of Diseases and Related Health Problems, 10th Revision (ICD-10) Version for 2010.

EARLY DEVELOPMENT

In the months following birth, early learning with limited vision creates a major developmental challenge. Infants with severe or profound vision impairment may not be able to see their parent's face or fixate on near objects. Even if there is improvement in the infant's vision, this severe reduction still impacts on the infant's opportunity to learn in a social or sensorimotor way from their environment. Whilst the infant with typical sight will reach for objects before they develop an understanding of object permanence, reaching happens later in the infant with vision impairment who cannot see that there is an object to reach for. Learning about object relationships is also more challenging in the absence of vision. On the Reynell-Zinkin Developmental Scales for young children with vision impairment, children under 5 years are slower to reach developmental milestones across all domains compared with children with typical vision (Reynell 1978). Thus, it is important that norms for children with typical vision are not used in developmental assessments in the preschool years, as there is a risk of diagnosing developmental delay in a child who is developing at the expected rate for their level of vision. The greatest delays are apparent in young children with profound vision impairment who have light perception at best and these children are particularly vulnerable (Dale et al. 2017; Dale et al. 2019).

INTELLECTUAL AND LEARNING PROFILES

Children with vision impairment are at high risk of intellectual disability, as there is a high co-occurrence of vision and neurological differences (Rahi, Cable, and British Childhood Visual Impairment Study Group 2003). Nevertheless, across the full spectrum of vision impairment there are children and young people who excel intellectually and progress to higher education and successful employment. For those without additional needs, early delays in cognition may be overcome in the school years, as they compensate by using auditory and haptic modalities as well as the considerable benefit derived from their developing language skills (Tadić, Pring, and Dale 2010). These children, however, remain vulnerable in the classroom. An additional or expanded core curriculum defines skills beyond core subjects that students with vision impairment have limited opportunity to acquire through observation but can learn via direct and specialist instruction in the school setting.

ATTENTION, EXECUTIVE FUNCTIONS, AND MEMORY

In an observational study, preschool children with profound vision impairment were found to be weaker in their response to adults' attempts to establish and maintain their attention and also in flexibly shifting attention from one object to another (Tadić, Pring, and Dale 2009). In two small-scale studies, children and adolescents with vision impairment with verbal cognition in the average range performed similarly on average to peers with typical vision on measures of sustained auditory attention, divided attention, and verbal fluency (Greenaway et al. 2017; Bathelt et al. 2018). In both studies, parent responses on questionnaires assessing everyday executive function indicated more difficulties for children with vision impairment, particularly those with more severe–profound vision impairment. Bathelt et al. suggested that lack of environmental visual feedback during everyday executive function tasks may increase the cognitive load and disrupt dynamic executive performance. Studies have typically shown that verbal short-term and working memory, as measured by digit span tasks, are either in line with or in advance of age-matched typically sighted peers (e.g. Withagen et al. 2013). Of the limited studies in children, there is evidence that episodic verbal memory is either similar or superior to typically sighted comparison groups (Pring 1988; Greenaway et al. 2017).

LANGUAGE AND SOCIAL COMMUNICATION

Language holds a particular significance for children with vision impairment; it is primarily through verbal descriptions from parents, educators, and others that the child receives information about their environment. Of the limited research in this area, there is some evidence for relative weakness in pragmatic compared to structural language, which for some may be related to social communication weaknesses (for an overview, see Greenaway and Dale 2017). The rate of autism spectrum disorder is estimated to be 31 times that of peers who are typically sighted (Do et al. 2017). Social communication may be more vulnerable because of the role of vision in the precursors of social communication development including gaze following, joint attention, and the difficulties for parent and young child in achieving joint referencing using coordinated vision and gesture (Dale, Tadić, and Sonksen 2014). Social interactions are affected by the child's difficulties in seeing the other person's eyes or facial expressions, or challenges for others in understanding what the child is attending to. Even if the child has some vision, abnormal feedback in terms of eye gaze may arise from nystagmus, strabismus, and abnormal eye movements.

ADAPTIVE BEHAVIOUR

There are no up-to-date and widely available measures of adaptive behaviour normed on children with vision impairment. Where measures from the general population have been used with samples of children with vision impairment, they typically score lower than their peers with typical vision (Bathelt et al. 2019). This is unsurprising given the importance of mobility and navigational skills in accessing community life and the visuo-motor aspects of many everyday practical tasks. Bathelt et al. found a relationship between adaptive behaviour and quality of life among school-aged children with vision impairment, suggesting the potential value of specialist habilitation training.

Results from recent studies indicated that there is a cluster of visuocognitive deficits in visual attention, visuomotor skills, motion sensitivity, and spatial cognition that are common across many disorders, including children with vision impairment. This has been called 'dorsal stream vulnerability' as these deficits relate largely to development of different neural networks within the dorsal stream (see Fig. 1.3) (Atkinson 2017).

ASSESSMENT AND FORMULATION

It is vital that the neuropsychologist does not administer assessments in a way that penalises the child because of their vision impairment, such as using nonverbal pictorial material with a child who is severely vision impaired and cannot fully access the stimuli. Supporting the child to have fair access to an assessment will help to identify strengths and learning needs so that appropriate support can be put in place.

Preparation of the Assessment

Given the paucity of measures for assessing individuals with vision impairment, taking a careful history interview is very important. This should include developmental questions adapted to consider the child's vision, alongside observation and information from the child, parent, and other relevant professionals working with the child including the ophthalmologist, paediatrician, and specialist teacher for vision impairment. For a practice guide for professionals working with children with vision impairment see Dale et al. (2022). Degrees of vision impairment vary widely; it is important to understand the child's visual acuity. A child with moderate vision impairment may be able to access some pictorial and visual materials, whilst those with severe or profound vision impairment should not be administered assessments involving visual stimuli. For children with moderate vision impairment, it is important to consider the suitability of each subtest involving visual content and use clinical judgement based on the size, detail, and contrast of the test materials. Test materials that require the ability to resolve fine visual detail may be unsuitable, especially on timed subtests (see Hunt and Bassi 2010). It is important to know the child's usual way of working in school and whether they are using braille, enlarged print, and/or low vision aids and to find out about other visual deficits that may affect the assessment, including adaptability to light, eye movement disorders, and visual field loss. Prior visual experience in a child who has subsequently lost vision capability is also highly relevant as differing neuropsychological profiles are associated with congenital as against acquired vision impairment (see Dekker et al. 1989).

Behaviour, Social Relating, and Adaptive Skills

Questionnaire measures to provide standard information on the child's current behaviour, social relating, and adaptive skills can be helpful. These need to be interpreted with caution by the clinician, as there are very few measures that have been validated for children with vision impairment. Questionnaires need to be chosen carefully and any items drawing entirely on vision capacity (such as eye contact) should be excluded and scores prorated as appropriate. Measures that lead to more than a couple of items being excluded should be used very cautiously and as indicated in the manual. This is particularly relevant for measures of adaptive function and social communication, as the development and assessment of these skills may be particularly impacted by vision impairment.

There are challenges in assessing children with vision impairment for social communicative and autism spectrum disorder difficulties as many of the items in parent interviews (or observational schedules) rely on vision (e.g. eye contact, gestural communication). A preliminary version of an observational schedule for preschoolers with severe-profound vision impairment has been developed (Absoud et al. 2011). A modified version of the Autism Diagnostic Observation Schedule (ADOS-2®) for the selective assessment of social communication difficulties in 4- to 7-year-old children with vision impairment (fluent language level) is being validated in consultation with the original author and test publishers; a new diagnostic algorithm is undergoing feasibility tests (Dale et al. forthcoming).

Issues of Cognitive and Attainment Testing

For a comprehensive assessment of intellectual abilities, both verbal and nonverbal domains should be assessed using normative standardised assessment tools. Where standardised haptic non-verbal assessment is not possible, the neuropsychologist needs to restrict their assessment to the verbal domain and be aware of the limitations of this.

Allowances need to be made for the preschool child underperforming on a normative developmental test (Reynell 1978). By the time the child is at school they are beginning to learn at a roughly similar rate to the peers with typical sight if they do not have additional learning needs. Their concepts may be less well developed and need compensatory support through haptic/tactile and experiential teaching. Nevertheless, the possibility of general intellectual and specific learning disabilities should be given consideration if a child is having sustained and significant difficulties with learning in the classroom environment and they continue to score significantly below normative expectations. Assuming that all problems are related to the child's vision impairment can lead to missed opportunities for greater understanding of the child's needs and to implementing more targeted habilitation and support.

Further considerations are required for attainment testing. For children who access enlarged print, it may be possible to adapt attainment assessments to the child's mode of access (e.g. enlarged print or use of a magnifier for reading, using the child's usual writing equipment for spelling). Braille reading skills can be assessed via the braille version of the Neale Analysis of Reading Ability (Greaney, Hill, and Tobin 1998), although braille teaching approaches have changed since this measure was normed. Braille is not directly comparable with print; it is typically slower to learn and associated with slower reading speed. Specific learning disorders in reading are recognised in a proportion of braille readers and higher processing demands have been linked to the strictly sequential nature of braille, which place high demands on phonological skills (Veispak et al. 2013).

Assessment Measures

The majority of subtests used in any standard neuropsychological battery for all ages involve visual presentation such as pictorial materials or blocks. Alternative tests have therefore been developed for children with vision impairment, though these are rarely fully standardised or widely available. The Reynell-Zinkin Developmental Scales (Reynell 1978) are semistandardised and provide assessment of sensorimotor understanding, response to sound and verbal comprehension, and expressive language from birth to 5 years, with age related equivalents for vision impairment and typical vision normative groups. The strengths and limitations of these scales are discussed in Vervloed et al. (2000), Dale et al. (2017); and Dale et al. (2019). The Comprehensive Vocational Evaluation System (CVES), a neuropsychological battery, is probably the most comprehensive to date but is designed for use with adults (Dial et al. 1990). For children aged 5 to 16 years, the Intelligence Test for Visually Impaired Children (ITVIC); (Dekker 1993) combines haptic and verbal subtests and is normed on 156 Dutch-speaking, braille-educated children. The ITVIC nonverbal reasoning subtests are a haptic approach to measuring non-verbal cognitive abilities; however, whether these subtests are tapping the same underlying processes as visually presented nonverbal reasoning subtests is not conclusive. Furthermore, as the ITVIC is normed on braille-educated children, the norms are not generalisable to children with severe vision impairment who read enlarged print rather than braille and are less experienced in tactile discrimination. The standardisation of vision impairment-specific measures or norms is hampered by the rare heterogeneous and complex nature of vision disorders. For example in the data collection for the CVES norms, three quarters of individuals sampled for the norms had at least one known additional disability or medical condition (Dial et al. 1990). Factors leading to heterogeneity include variation in vision level, intellectual and other comorbidities, aetiology (such as congenital or acquired through head injury or tumour), and age of onset. Where standardisation is achieved, these challenges mean that norms are rarely updated and are at risk of becoming obsolete and need interpreting with caution (e.g. the Flynn effect, which describes the tendency for increased scores at population level over time).

Given the limited availability of vision impairment-specific tests or norms, traditional neuropsychological measures involving verbal/auditory presentation (e.g. verbal reasoning subscales and auditory working memory subscales of the Wechsler Intelligence Scales) normed on sighted populations can be cautiously used in individuals with vision impairment as they do not involve much adaptation for this population. Even in verbal subtests, items that are vision related (e.g. pictures in the early items or questions including visual concepts like 'colour' or 'smoke') may need to be omitted or changed to a similar element ('smelling burning' instead of 'seeing smoke') when administered and scored and interpreted with greater caution.

Some colleagues argue that cognitive assessments normed on typically sighted children should not be used to assess children with vision impairment. However, in the absence of widely available vision impairment-specific standardised assessments or norms, it is our stance that when interpreted cautiously and with expertise this can be beneficial for the child in order to highlight strengths and needs, to ensure the child is meeting their potential and inform support needs and intervention. Using such measures, our clinical and research experience with smaller samples of children and young adolescents of average to superior verbal skills revealed intra-individual variation and a subgroup with uneven neuropsychological profiles, including in auditory attention, executive function, and memory (Greenaway et al. 2017; Bathelt et al. 2018). It is important to consider the individual developmental trajectories of these children with vision impairment and ecological evidence from school progress. Cautionary statements in one's reporting and being transparent about any 'unknowns', the appropriacy of normative data, and any accommodations or modifications made will support the clinical formulations reached and recommendations provided.

INTERVENTION AND MANAGEMENT

Given the impact of severe vision impairment on early development and the importance of parental guidance and support, there has been a growing practical focus on home-based, parent-mediated early intervention. Specialist (vision impairment) peripatetic education staff often provide the delivery. A national initiative (Early Support) in the UK led to development and widespread usage of the vision impairment-specific structured developmental materials: Developmental Journal for babies and young children with vision impairment (DJVI; Salt and Dale 2017). A recent national cohort observational study has shown that home-based early intervention using the DJVI led to clinically relevant advances in cognition and language, reduction in behaviour difficulties, and enhanced support for parents (including reduced parenting stress) compared to home-based 'other support' (Dale et al. 2019).

To our knowledge, there are no scientifically reported evidence-based neuropsychological intervention studies for older children with vision impairment. A current pragmatic approach is to use existing research evidence to inform the results and formulation arising from the child's neuropsychological assessment. The final formulation should be used to guide appropriate recommendations and intervention. Multisensory and experiential learning approaches are beneficial for learning, attention, and concept development. Reduced opportunities for multisensory learning during didactic classroom teaching, due to no or limited access to visual information and nonverbal communication, have been highlighted as a barrier to engagement for the child with vision impairment in the classroom (Bardin and Lewis 2008). Bardin and Lewis highlighted the importance of creating multiple opportunities to increase active participation and engagement in learning. Creating alternative opportunities for accessible multisensory learning for children with vision impairment include tactile graphics, hands-on-learning, and audio supports. A commonly used classroom strategy for managing attention difficulties is to reduce auditory distractors. As information received by the non-visual senses may be more salient for children with vision impairment, understanding the nature and impact of stimuli that are distracting for the individual is important when making recommendations regarding environmental modifications; for example it may be important to consider the classroom acoustical environment.

The importance of executive functions, such as flexibility, goal-setting, and problem-solving, in academic success and adaptive behaviour is increasingly recognised and there is recent interest in the direct teaching of executive function strategies in the classroom (Meltzer 2018). Executive function development is hardly understood in children with vision impairment, in part due to the visual nature of most executive function standardised measures. Verbal mediation strategies, which draw on strengths in verbal and sequential processing, may be particularly beneficial in promoting self-regulation via language and developing metacognitive strategies. Self-determination has been reported to be weaker among children and adolescents with vision impairment, whilst higher self-determination is associated with better employment outcomes (McDonnall and Crudden 2009). These authors suggest providing the young person with opportunities for decision-making and active participation in education planning and vocational choices to promote self-determination.

It has been suggested that technology holds promise in developing spatial ability, orientation, and mobility amongst children with vision impairment. Cuturi et al. (2016) highlight the potential habilitative impact of technology for children with vision impairment, particularly if used in early development. They discuss developments that would help achieve this potential, including technologies designed specifically for children with vision impairment and driven by neuroscientific knowledge. A key area is consideration of the learning media for the child and how this is impacting on learning, such as use of larger computer screens and keyboards or computer software linking with the teacher's whiteboard or electronic braille notetakers.

Outcome

The neuropsychological assessment indicated that William's verbal and non-verbal (haptic) reasoning abilities were at age-expected levels. The assessment highlighted weaknesses in auditory attention, phonological working memory, and braille (both accuracy and speed). Selective vulnerabilities have been shown in some children with severe vision impairment (see Veispak et al. 2013; Bathelt et al. 2018). William's lower academic progress, including in executive written organisation of ideas and spelling, reflected difficulties in these aspects of his profile. This combination of difficulties is likely to be particularly challenging for William in the context of severe vision impairment given the greater dependence on the auditory environment. Parental responses on standardised questionnaires highlighted difficulties in executive functioning and adaptive behaviour (as highlighted in research by Bathelt et al. 2018; 2019). The intervention focused on helping William, his parents, teachers, and habilitation specialist understand his potential and profile of academic and adaptive behavioural strengths and weaknesses as well as implementing strategies for supporting him. This included enabling him to show his greater verbal comprehension strengths through verbal recounting rather than written reporting, which helped to engage him more in the classroom topic work. A scribe was used in certain academic tasks such as essay and test situations. Once there was greater understanding about working within William's attention span, providing him with rest and movement breaks and not expecting him to stay with the same activity for too long, William was more engaged with classroom learning and able to demonstrate his ability. Use of braille schedules and checklists helped provide structure, support executive functioning, and improved William's understanding of what was expected in terms of timetabling and goals and increased his confidence in learning.

SUMMARY

In summary, research with children with vision impairment highlights that differing perceptual experience leads to a unique developmental trajectory and therefore full synchrony between the developmental trajectories of children with and without vision cannot be assumed. There are significant challenges in valid neuropsychological assessment and caution is required when using standardised assessments with this population. It is important to triangulate information from different sources and to understand the diversity of vision impairment-related neuropsychological presentations and implications of vision impairment for the child in everyday settings. It is important to understand how vision impairment may interact with the child's neuropsychological, emotional, and social needs. Given the significant limitations of the available assessments, transparency is required in acknowledging this and being clear about what we do not know. It is of utmost importance that the neuropsychologist understands the risks of underestimating a child's potential and careful consideration is given to formulating and sharing information in a way that optimises the child's potential and quality of life.

REFERENCES

Absoud M, Parr JR, Salt A, Dale N (2011) Developing a schedule to identify social communication difficulties and autism spectrum disorder in young children with visual impairment. *Developmental Medicine & Child Neurology* **53**(3): 285–288.

Atkinson J (2017) Visual development. In *Oxford Research Encyclopedia of Psychology*. [online] Available at: https://oxfordre.com/psychology/view/10.1093/acrefore/9780190236557.001.0001/acrefore-9780190236557-e-65 [Accessed 29 December 2021].

Barker L, Thomas R, Rubin G, Dahlmann-Noor A (2015) Optical reading aids for children and young people with low vision. *Cochrane Database Systematic Review* **2015**(3): CD010987. doi: 10.1002/14651858.CD010987.pub2.

Bardin JA, Lewis S (2008) A survey of the academic engagement of students with visual impairments in general education classes. *Journal of Visual Impairment & Blindness* **102**: 472–483.

Bathelt J, de Haan M, Salt A, Dale NJ (2018) Executive abilities in children with congenital visual impairment in mid-childhood. *Child Neuropsychology* **24**(2): 184–202.

Bathelt J, de Haan M, Dale NJ (2019) Adaptive behaviour and quality of life in school-age children with congenital visual disorders and different levels of visual impairment. *Research in Developmental Disabilities* **85**: 154–162.

Cuturi LF, Aggius-Vella E, Campus C, Parmiggiani A, Gori M (2016) From science to technology: Orientation and mobility in blind children and adults. *Neuroscience & Biobehavioral Reviews* **71**: 240–251.

Dale N, Sakkalou E, O'Reilly M, Springall C, De Haan M, Salt A (2017) Functional vision and cognition in infants with congenital disorders of the peripheral visual system. *Developmental Medicine & Child Neurology* **59**(7): 725–731.

Dale NJ, Sakkalou E, O'Reilly MA et al. (2019) Home-based early intervention in infants and young children with visual impairment using the Developmental Journal: Longitudinal cohort study. *Developmental Medicine & Child Neurology* **61**(6): 697–709.

Dale N, Salt A, Sargent J, Greenaway R, editors (2022) *Children with Vision Impairment: Assessment, Development, and Management.* London: Mac Keith Press Practical Guides.

Dale NJ, Tadić V, Sonksen P (2014) Social communicative variation in 1–3-year-olds with severe visual impairment. *Child: Care, Health and Development* **40**(2): 158–164.

Dekker R (1989) Cognitive development of visually handicapped children. In Dekker R, Drenth PJD, Zaal JN, editors, *Intelligence Test for Visually Impaired Children Aged, 6 to 15.* The Netherlands: Bartimeus Zeist, pp. 1–21.

Dekker R (1993) Visually impaired children and haptic intelligence test scores: Intelligence Test for Visually Impaired Children (ITVIC). *Developmental Medicine & Child Neurology* **35**(6): 478–489.

Do B, Lynch P, Macris EM et al. (2017) Systematic review and meta-analysis of the association of Autism Spectrum Disorder in visually or hearing impaired children. *Ophthalmic Physiology* **37**(2): 212–224.

Greaney J, Hill E, Tobin MJ (1998) *Neale Analysis of Reading Ability: University of Birmingham Braille Version.* London: London Royal National Institute for the Blind.

Greenaway R, Dale NJ (2017) Congenital visual impairment. In *Research in Clinical Pragmatics.* Cham: Springer, pp. 441–469.

Greenaway R, Pring L, Schepers A, Isaacs DP, Dale NJ (2017) Neuropsychological presentation and adaptive skills in high-functioning adolescents with visual impairment: A preliminary investigation. *Applied Neuropsychology: Child* **6**(2): 145–157.

Hunt, LA, Bassi CJ (2010) Near-vision acuity levels and performance on neuropsychological assessments used in occupational therapy. *American Journal of Occupational Therapy* **64**(1): 105–113.

McDonnall MC, Crudden A (2009) Factors affecting the successful employment of transition-age youths with visual impairments. *Journal of Visual Impairment & Blindness* **103**(6): 329–341.

Meltzer L, editor (2018) *Executive Function in Education: From Theory to Practice.* New York: Guilford Publications.

Milner AD, Goodale MA (1995) *The Visual Brain in Action.* Oxford, UK: Oxford University Press.

Mishkin M, Ungerleider L, Macko KA (1983) Object vision and spatial vision: Two critical pathways. *Trends in Neuroscience* **6**: 414–417.

Patel A, Hayward JD, Tailor V et al. (2019) The Oculome panel test: Next-generation sequencing to diagnose a diverse range of genetic developmental eye disorders. *Ophthalmology* **126**(6): 888–907.

Pring L (1988) The 'reverse-generation' effect: A comparison of memory performance between blind and sighted children. *British Journal of Psychology* **79**(3): 387–400.

Rahi JS, Cable N, British Childhood Visual Impairment Study Group (2003) Severe visual impairment and blindness in children in the UK. *The Lancet* **362**(9393): 1359–1365.

Reynell J (1978) Developmental patterns of visually handicapped children. *Child: Care, Health and Development* **4**(5): 291–303.

Sakki H, Bowman R, Sargent J, Kukadia R, Dale N (2021) Visual function subtyping in children with early-onset cerebral visual impairment. *Developmental Medicine & Child Neurology* **63**: 303–312. https://doi.org/10.1111/dmcn.14710.

Salt A, Dale N (2017) *Developmental Journal for Babies and Young Children with Visual Impairment*, 2nd edition (DJVI). London: Great Ormond Street Hospital for Children. Available from: https://xip.uclb.com/i/healthcare_tools/DJVI_professional.html.

Tadić V, Pring L, Dale N (2009) Attentional processes in young children with congenital visual impairment. *British Journal of Developmental Psychology* **27**(2): 311–330.

Tadić V, Pring L, Dale N (2010) Are language and social communication intact in children with congenital visual impairment at school age? *Journal of Child Psychology and Psychiatry* **51**(6): 696–705.

Veispak A, Boets B, Ghesquière P (2013) Differential cognitive and perceptual correlates of print reading versus braille reading. *Research in Developmental Disabilities* **34**(1): 372–385. doi: 10.1016/j.ridd.2012.08.012.

Vervloed MP, Hamers JH, van Mens-Weisz MM, Timmer-Van de Vosse H (2000) New age levels of the Reynell-Zinkin developmental scales for young children with visual impairments. *Journal of Visual Impairment & Blindness* **94**(10): 613–624.

Withagen A, Kappers AM, Vervloed MP, Knoors H, Verhoeven L (2013) Short term memory and working memory in blind versus sighted children. *Research in Developmental Disabilities* **34**(7): 2161–2172.

CHAPTER 2

Hearing

Fionna Bathgate and Lindsey Edwards

Presenting Concern

Referral for assessment was made as Zainab, an 8-year-old child with hearing loss, was not making expected progress in developing spoken language following cochlear implantation. Although we are describing a child with cochlear implants, much of what we discuss will also be relevant to a child with hearing loss using other devices such as hearing aids or bone-anchored hearing aids.

Zainab has bilateral sensorineural hearing loss of unknown aetiology but likely due to being born early at 30 weeks and having a stormy neonatal journey. She spent 2 months in a special care baby unit and was treated with gentamicin, which can be ototoxic (toxic to the hair cells of the inner ears).

Zainab failed her newborn hearing screen and was fitted with hearing aids at 4 months of age. Audiological testing first indicated a moderate hearing loss, but assessment at age 3 years noted a severe loss. She was reported to be a consistent user of her hearing aids, but there were concerns that she was not developing language in line with her aided levels. She was referred for assessment for cochlear implants and received implants at age 4 years. Cognitive assessment at that time indicated that she had nonverbal skills that fell in the average to high average range.

Motor milestones were slightly delayed: she sat unsupported at 9 months and walked at 18 months. Balance problems are often seen in children with hearing impairment, which slows the development of their gross motor skills but tends not to impact on their fine motor skill development (Bathgate et al. 2014).

Zainab made good progress in the initial stages post-implant in terms of her speech sounds detection and discrimination, with a good level of input from speech and language therapy. Having reached age-appropriate language levels at 2 years post-implant, she was discharged from local speech and language services. However, later assessments by the cochlear implant team highlighted that the gap between her and her hearing peers was widening.

Zainab attends a mainstream primary school where she does not receive any additional support. Her parents notice that she struggles to retain spellings and times tables. Her school reports concerns about attention and learning, but they have no concerns about her behaviour. They feel she is about 2 years behind her hearing peers academically.

Zainab lives with her parents, who are hearing. The family speaks English as a first language but speaks to extended family on the phone in Urdu. Zainab does not use sign, although she was taught some by local professionals when she was younger. She enjoys art-based activities and watching football on TV.

THEORY

Permanent sensorineural hearing loss is considered a low-incidence disability/disorder, with a prevalence of approximately 0.3% of school-age children (www.patient.co.uk). Genetic anomalies are the primary cause, accounting for around 60% of cases, 30% of which are syndromic, for example CHARGE, Pendred, Waardenburg, Treacher Collins, and Usher syndromes. Less frequently, permanent sensorineural hearing loss is the result of infections such as rubella, cytomegalovirus, or bacterial meningitis, severely preterm birth, or other neonatal complications. More than 95% of deaf children are born to two hearing parents, frequently compounding the language delays associated with significant hearing loss, as these children do not generally have access to a full, natural language such as sign language from birth (Knoors and Marschark 2014). The impact of hearing loss is not confined to delays in language development but is also apparent in a variety of other domains, including cognitive, behavioural, social, and emotional (Dale and Edwards 2017).

Interventions for severe to profound hearing loss, such as cochlear implants, whilst giving access to speech sounds and therefore enhancing spoken language and literacy development, do not restore normal hearing. In addition, although ideally children will receive cochlear implants at around their first birthday in order to achieve the most favourable outcomes (Dettman et al. 2016), for many children it is considerably later, resulting in an extended period of auditory and therefore typical language deprivation. Thus, deficits in cognitive functions and their behavioural sequelae are apparent in deaf children with or without cochlear implants.

The audiogram in Figure 2.1 illustrates the levels of hearing needed to perceive a variety of environmental and speech sounds at different volumes and frequencies. Table 2.1 describes the different types of hearing loss and associated difficulties. The auditory neural pathway, comprising the hair cells of the cochlea, auditory (VIIIth) nerve, brain stem, thalamus, and auditory cortex in the temporal lobe, decodes sounds in terms of their duration, intensity, frequency, and location, followed by integration with other sensory input, and finally recognises and processes them in the context of previously learnt information. Congenital or prelingual sensorineural hearing loss results from early damage to, or absence of, the hair cells in the cochlea. This disrupts the development of the auditory neural pathway at the earliest stage and, therefore, has a profound impact on the child's ability to decode speech and develop spoken language skills. Auditory

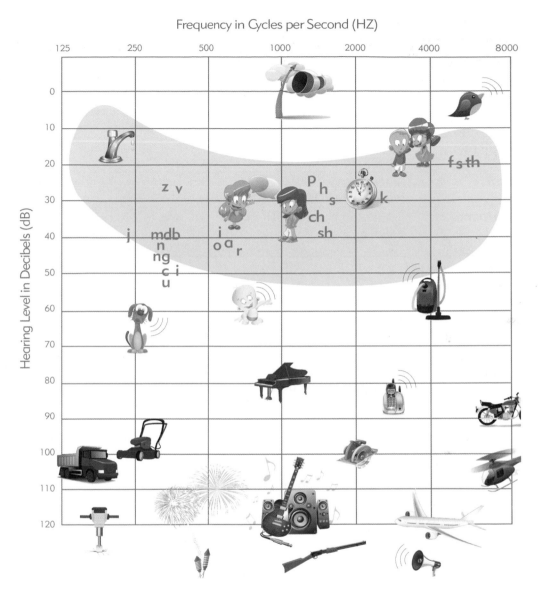

Figure 2.1 Tools for Schools: audiogram of familiar sounds. ©2015 Advanced Bionics AG and affiliates. All rights reserved. (A colour version of this figure can be seen in the colour plate section)

deprivation of this nature has been shown to result in reorganisation of the function of the central auditory pathways, such that higher order areas of the auditory cortex become recruited by vision, and the frontal and prefrontal areas become more active as auditory input is attenuated (Glick and Sharma 2017). In recent years the idea of a connectome, a comprehensive map or 'wiring diagram' of neural connections in the human brain, has become a useful model for understanding how functional brain states

Table 2.1 Types of hearing loss and associated difficulties

Level of hearing loss	Audiology	Practical
Normal hearing	You can hear quiet sounds down to 20dBHL (hearing loss in decibels)	No difficulties
Mild	Hearing loss in your better ear between 25 and 39dBHL	You have difficulty following speech in noisy situations
Moderate	Hearing loss in your better ear between 40 and 69dBHL	You have difficulty following speech without a hearing aid
Severe	Hearing loss in your better ear between 70 and 89dBHL	You require powerful hearing aids or a cochlear implant
Profound	Hearing loss in your better ear from 90dBHL	You need to rely mainly on lip-reading and/or sign language, or a cochlear implant

relate to their underlying structural substrate, and how brain function is affected if this substrate is disrupted (Sporns, Tononi, and Kötter 2005). Kral et al. (2016) apply this connectome model to the case of auditory processing and auditory deprivation (and neurosensory restoration with cochlear implants). In humans, the development of cortical connections starts in utero, accelerates after birth, and continues into adolescence, with the number of synaptic connections peaking between 1 and 4 years of age, and maturation of myelin sheaths continuing into adulthood. Therefore, Kral et al. argue that the absence of stimulation of the auditory nervous system early in life prevents typical functional maturation, with implications for the development not only of language but also visual processing, sequential processing, executive function, and concept formation.

Research suggests that deaf children do not generally differ from their hearing counterparts in their general intellectual ability when measured using visual/nonverbal tasks and controlling for medical and other relevant factors (Edwards and Isquith 2020). In contrast, deaf children, including those with cochlear implants, have been found to have specific deficits or delays, particularly in attention, memory, and reasoning/problem-solving, as well as social cognition (Marschark et al. 2019; Edwards and Isquith 2020). The ability to sustain visual attention, as measured in neuropsychological tests, is poorer in deaf children, and although cochlear implants may result in some 'catch-up' with hearing peers, difficulties often remain into adolescence. Problems with attention skills are also evidenced on behavioural assessments using standardised rating scales. Short-term and working memory deficits are particularly strongly associated with hearing loss, most notably when the materials to be memorised can be verbally encoded. Unsurprisingly, deaf children are also disadvantaged compared with their hearing peers on tests of verbal reasoning abilities, but there is also some evidence that they have difficulty on tests of analogical and sequential reasoning as well, even when the stimuli are not so readily encoded verbally (see Edwards and Isquith 2020, for a review).

Around 40% of deaf children are known to have cognitive, behavioural, or learning difficulties in addition to their deafness (Dale and Edwards 2017), either as a direct result of shared aetiology or coincidentally. Children with certain aetiologies of deafness, for example bacterial meningitis or preterm birth, are at increased risk of neuropsychological deficits and often exhibit predictable cognitive profiles.

ASSESSMENT AND FORMULATION

The aim of the assessment is potentially multifaceted depending upon the reason for referral: (1) to establish learning potential; (2) to identify ability–achievement discrepancy (nonverbal ability); (3) to diagnose coincidental learning disability or disorder (e.g. specific reading disability, possible developmental coordination disorder), and (d) to describe a cognitive profile with hypothesis-led testing based on referral information and information from other sources.

A comprehensive history was taken from Zainab's parents, as well as a clear description of the current concerns and reported areas of strength. Questionnaires such as the Strengths and Difficulties Questionnaire, and the Behavior Rating Inventory for Executive Functioning, Second Edition are sent out for completion to gather a general picture from multiple informants (i.e. parents and teachers). The picture painted by the history-taking and information from school is not suggestive of a global learning problem but potentially a specific one. Reported difficulties with memory indicate that the Working Memory Rating Scale (Alloway, Gathercole, and Kirkwood 2008) might also be helpful. Feedback from school staff states that although she is making progress with her literacy, she struggles with higher language level skills such as inference and deduction. It is noted that her concentration is much better when she is working in a quiet environment.

Recent assessment by our speech and language therapy colleagues indicated that she has good aural discrimination, gaining 20/20 on minimal word groups. For example she can correctly choose 'bear' from a target of three pictures with 'pear' and 'chair' as distractors, without lip-reading. Additionally, she can repeat back short sentences correctly (known as open-set listening).

This is supported by audiological assessment, which shows that she can hear down to 20 to 25 decibels, which is the equivalent of 'normal' hearing. However, she demonstrated difficulty in listening when there is background noise. Data-logging of the processors showed an average 11 to 12 hours a day of usage, which indicates that she is probably wearing them all of her waking hours.

To assess Zainab's nonverbal skills, and to compare performance pre-implant, the Leiter International Performance Scale, Third Edition was administered. Alternative assessments of nonverbal skills are presented in Table 2.2 (for further detail see McCallum

Table 2.2 Examples of nonverbal assessments

Test	Age range (y or y:mo)	Time to administer	Description
Snijders-Oomen Nonverbal Intelligence Test, Revised (SON-R)	2:6–7 6–40	50min 45–60min	Published in 1998. Six subtests. UK norms. Published in 2011. English, Dutch, and German versions. Four subtests. Entirely nonverbal in delivery and response.
Leiter International Performance Scale, Third Edition (Leiter-3)	3–75+	About 30min	Published in 2013. Cognitive battery and Attention/Memory battery. Entirely nonverbal in delivery and response.
Wechsler Nonverbal Scale of Ability (WNV)	4–21:11 (4–7:11) (8–21:11)	Brief version 15–20min Full version 45min	Published in 2006. Full battery of six subtests. Brief battery of two subtests. Can be compared to Wechsler Individual Achievement Test, Second Edition. Verbal and pictorial instructions. Minimal verbal instructions are also available in French, Spanish, Chinese, German, and Dutch.
Comprehensive Test of Nonverbal Intelligence, Second Edition (CTONI-2)	6–89:11	60min	Second edition published in 2009. Six subtests: Pictorial Nonverbal IQ (three subtests) and Geometric Nonverbal IQ (three subtests). Pictorial Nonverbal IQ correlated with language ability. Geometric Nonverbal IQ correlated with nonverbal IQ and fluid intelligence.
Test of Nonverbal Intelligence, Fourth Edition (TONI-4)	6–89	15–20min	Published in 2010. Available in seven languages. Caution re: use for under 9 years – poorer norms?
Universal Nonverbal Intelligence Test, Second Edition (UNIT-2)	5–21	10–15min for Abbreviated Battery 30min for Standard Battery 45–60min for Extended Battery	Second edition published in 2016. Offers Abbreviated Battery, Standard Battery With Memory, Standard Battery Without Memory, Full Scale (Extended) Battery. Gives seven composite scores including a Full Scale IQ. Entirely nonverbal in delivery and response.

(Continued)

Test	Age range (y or y:mo)	Time to administer	Description
Naglieri Nonverbal Ability Test, Third Edition (NNAT3)	5–17:11	30min	3rd edition published in 2016. 4 subtests. Verbal instructions are given. Online and paper versions available. Earlier versions were criticised for significant score variability.

2017). Depending upon the referral and the background of the child, an assessment with a high verbal component may also be appropriate (e.g. Wechsler Intelligence Scale for Children, Fifth Edition).

Zainab was assessed in a well-lit, sound-treated room at the cochlear implant clinic. In less well set up environments, there are a number of factors to take into consideration (see Table 2.3). Zainab presented as a lively, energetic child, who needed some refocusing to the task at hand but otherwise demonstrated good attention during tasks. She gained scores on the Leiter International Performance Scale, Third Edition that fell broadly in the Average Range, including on a cancellation task of visual sustained attention, with a slightly lower score on the subtests that assessed sequential processing.

On subtests selected from the Developmental Neuropsychological Assessment, Second Edition, Zainab demonstrated good immediate recall in both the auditory and visual domains but was poorer at retaining the information after a delay, and this was more evident in the auditory than in the visual domain. This suggests that she was able to encode the presented information but struggled with retention and/or recall. Repetition did not seem to enhance her performance.

Table 2.3 Testing considerations for the hearing impaired

Limit background noise, if possible.   You want a quiet room, with little reverberation – background noise makes it much harder for the child to focus on what you are saying. An echoey room also makes it harder for the child to hear what you are saying.
Lighting – do not sit with your back against the window.   If you sit with your back to a light source, then the child cannot gain the benefit of lip-reading.
Sit opposite the child so they can lip-read if needed.
Use a frequency modulation system if the child uses one.
Changes to administration – how far can you go before you invalidate the assessment?
Be flexible! It is okay to change your mind.   In order to be flexible, you will need to have different assessment tools available.

She scored as High on the Hyperactivity/Inattention subscale on both the parent and teacher versions of the Strengths and Difficulties Questionnaire but close to Average (i.e. no concern) on all other subscales. On the Behavior Rating Inventory for Executive Functioning, Second Edition, her mother and her teacher rated her as having difficulties in the areas of shifting attention, initiating tasks, working memory, planning and organisation, and ratings by her teacher on the Working Memory Rating Scale suggested she has a marked deficit in this area.

The results of the assessment highlight a number of areas of difficulty for Zainab in terms of her cognitive abilities and their impact on 'real-world' behaviours in the context of learning, particularly in the classroom environment but also at home. First, she did not appear to be able to learn from repeated presentations of the same information, which will have very significant implications across all areas of the curriculum but may be most obviously seen in tasks such as learning spellings or her times tables. She would therefore need significantly more 'overlearning' than other children. Second, she has significant difficulties in almost all areas of executive functioning but mostly working memory. She would need a substantial amount of individual support in the classroom in order for her to engage in, and learn from, teaching activities and interactions with her peers. Currently, her ability to regulate her own behaviour and organise herself are significant barriers to her progress.

Audiological assessment indicates that there is no problem with Zainab's listening per se; she can detect and discriminate speech sounds. However, her executive functioning difficulties are impacting upon her ability to progress with learning language as well as all areas of the curriculum. She has difficulties with working memory that are most evident in the auditory domain. In terms of strengths, her visual problem-solving is age appropriate, and she enjoys art-based activities. She is a cheerful and resilient child. Although she is becoming aware that she is behind in some areas compared to her peers, she also recognises that she has strengths in other domains. Her parents and the school staff are keen to find out how best to support her to reach her potential.

INTERVENTION AND MANAGEMENT

General Educational Strategies

There are a number of accommodations that can be made to support a child with hearing loss in their learning in the classroom, along with general strategies that will enable them to access the curriculum to the greatest extent possible. De Raeve (2015) provides numerous suggestions for ways in which this can be achieved. Ensuring that all the staff who interact with the child receive deaf awareness training and use good communication techniques, seating the child at the front of the class with a clear view of the teacher, and optimising the acoustics of the classroom are all important first-line interventions.

Increasing the visual cues and support available to children with a hearing loss will help them understand materials better, maintain attention on tasks, and retain information (De Raeve 2015). Providing written summaries of videos or films, written instructions for tasks rather than only speaking them, and pictures, diagrams, and graphs where possible will all be beneficial. Beyond this, allowing extra processing time, avoiding multitasking, pre-teaching of new topic vocabulary, and over-learning of essential information, along with 'error-free' learning and regularly checking for comprehension to prevent the child from wasting time completing a task incorrectly, are all helpful strategies (e.g. Hermans et al. 2015). When a deaf or hard-of-hearing child is in a mainstream placement, one-to-one support for at least part of the school day, from someone with congruent communication skills (i.e. including signing if necessary), should provide scaffolding of language and increased attention to tasks.

It may seem intuitive to increase the emphasis on visual aids and approaches to teaching in order to improve deaf children's learning. However, this should not be done in the belief that as a result of the impact of auditory deprivation on the brain and its functional organisation, deaf children have superior ability to process visual information compared with their hearing peers, for example in terms of their performance on visual-spatial tasks (see Marschark, Sarchet, and Trani 2016; Edwards and Isquith 2020). Nor should it be taken to imply that deaf students are 'visual learners' where this refers to a learning style, contrasted with a verbal learning style. Marschark et al. (2017) demonstrated that college-age deaf students are no more likely than their hearing counterparts to be visual learners and are no stronger in their visual skills and preferences than their verbal skills. This, along with the heterogeneity of the deaf population as a result of factors such as degree of hearing loss, communication mode, and language skills, means that classroom interventions need to be individually tailored to maximise learning outcomes.

Intervention Research

Although general classroom interventions and the use of strategies that take into account a child's learning style are crucial in optimising a deaf child's learning and are likely to enhance executive functioning as a result of reducing the load on working memory capacity, there are some specific interventions that are potentially applicable to the executive function deficits or delays experienced by many deaf children. However, empirical evidence for the efficacy and effectiveness of such interventions in children with hearing loss is extremely rare. Although studies have attempted to assess the impact of interventions on abilities such as attention, memory, and executive functioning in hearing children, such approaches have not been systematically applied to children with hearing loss. To date, the only study that has attempted to apply an established intervention for working memory – computer-based Cogmed – to deaf children, was conducted by Kronenberger et al. (2011). They observed improvements in scores in a group of nine children on a range of working memory tasks immediately after training and 3 months later, but these benefits were no longer evident at 6 months. It is also unclear whether any improvements impacted on other cognitive abilities, language, or academic development; trials in hearing children have produced equivocal findings, and such training packages remain controversial (Hulme and Melby-Lervåg 2012; Melby-Lervåg, Redick, and Hulme 2016). Interventions to improve executive function skills such as goal planning, initiating and following through on tasks, and self-regulation have not been the focus of empirical research in deaf children; this is clearly a useful focus for future research.

In terms of specific advice for Zainab, consideration should be given to the acoustics of the classroom (Siebein et al. 2000). Ensuring the class teacher uses a radio aid to minimise the impact of background noise and that staff working with her are trained in deaf awareness to maximise communication and interactions are essential interventions. Further, information for staff to ensure they understand the impact of working memory difficulties on learning, and how these can be supported, is very important (e.g. Gathercole and Alloway 2007). Zainab needs regular and frequent input from teachers of the deaf and speech and language therapists specialised in childhood hearing impairment.

Outcome

A year later, Zainab was reviewed again by the cochlear implant team. Assessment by the speech and language therapists indicated that she was beginning to close the gap between her and her hearing peers in terms of her receptive and expressive vocabulary, as well as her grammar. Feedback from school also indicated that she was making faster progress than she had in the previous year, with pleasing improvement in her development of literacy skills. Continued monitoring by the multidisciplinary cochlear implant team and liaison with her school will ensure that this progress is maintained, and any additional difficulties that may emerge are addressed in a timely fashion.

SUMMARY

There is significant heterogeneity of hearing-impaired children. During assessment, it is important to understand the aetiology of a child's deafness (if it is known) to determine potential association with specific difficulties. Consider the purpose of assessment. Gather information about the child before meeting them (e.g. feedback from school, questionnaires, etc.) as this helps in the choice of the most appropriate assessment tools, in developing hypotheses, and in informing the formulation. Consider the testing environment carefully. If it is less than ideal for a child with a hearing loss, this must be taken into account when interpreting the results of the assessment and included in the report. Similarly, if it has been necessary to adapt or change the administration of the assessment tests, this must also be considered in the interpretation of the results and described in the report.

Although hearing aids or cochlear implants are effective in supporting listening for deaf children, they do not restore normal hearing, and significant challenges remain with background noise and listening effort. Thus, children with hearing loss remain at a disadvantage in noisy environments (e.g. school classrooms) compared to their peers.

Ongoing support for these children from specialists in hearing loss is essential for them to achieve their potential (e.g. Marshark and Knoors 2018).

REFERENCES

Bathgate F, Maltby K, Mahon M, Hilkhuysen G, Rajput K (2014) Do pre-implant motor development and age at switch-on predict speech intelligibility outcomes in a heterogeneous population of children with cochlear implants? *Developmental Medicine & Child Neurology*, Special Issue: Proceedings of the 4th UK Paediatric Neuropsychology Symposium: Atypical Developmental Pathways, 19–23 May 2014, London, UK, Volume 56, Issue Supplement s3, pp. 18–19.

Dale N, Edwards L (2017) Children with specific sensory impairments. In: Thapar A, Pine D, Leckman J et al., editors, *Rutter's Child and Adolescent Psychiatry*, 6th edition. Chichester: Wiley, pp. 612–622.

De Raeve L (2015) Classroom adaptations for effective classroom learning in deaf students. In: Knoors H, Marschark M, editors, *Educating Deaf Learners: Creating a Global Evidence Base*. New York, NY: Oxford University Press, pp. 547–572.

Dettman SJ, Dowell RC, Choo D et al. (2016) Long-term communication outcomes for children receiving cochlear implants younger than 12 months: A multicenter study. *Otology & Neurotology* 37(2): e82–e95.

Edwards L, Isquith P (2020) Cognitive development: The impact of pediatric cochlear implantation. In: Marschark M, Knoors H, editors, *The Oxford Handbook of Deaf Studies in Learning and Cognition*. New York, NY: Oxford University Press, pp. 198–212.

Gathercole SE, Alloway TP (2007) *Understanding Working Memory: A Classroom Guide*. London: Harcourt Assessment. [online] Available at: https://www.mrc-cbu.cam.ac.uk/wp-content/uploads/2013/01/WM-classroom-guide.pdf [Accessed 19 January 2021].

Glick H, Sharma A (2017) Cross-modal plasticity in developmental and age-related hearing loss: Clinical implications. *Hearing Research* 343: 191–201.

Hermans D, Vugs B, van Berkel-van Hoof L, Knoors H (2015) Deaf children's executive functions: From research to practice? In: Knoors H, Marschark M, editors, *Educating Deaf Learners: Creating a Global Evidence Base*. New York, NY: Oxford University Press, pp. 231–260.

Hulme C, Melby-Lervåg M (2012) Current evidence does not support the claims made for CogMed working memory training. *Journal of Applied Research in Memory and Cognition* 1: 197–200.

Knoors H, Marschark M (2014) Deaf learners: An introduction. In: *Teaching Deaf Learners: Psychological and Developmental Foundations*. New York, NY: Oxford University Press, pp. 24–42.

Kral A, Kronenberger WG, Pisoni DB, O'Donoghue GM (2016) Neurocognitive factors in sensory restoration of early deafness: A connectome model. *The Lancet Neurology* 15: 610–621.

Kronenberger WG, Pisoni DB, Henning SC, Colson BG, Hazzard LM (2011) Working memory training for children with cochlear implants: A pilot study. *Journal of Speech, Language, and Hearing Research* 54: 1182–1196.

Marschark M, Edwards L, Peterson C, Crowe K, Walton D (2019) Understanding theory of mind in deaf and hearing college students. *Journal of Deaf Studies and Deaf Education* 24: 104–118.

Marschark M, Knoors H (2018) Sleuthing the 93% solution in deaf education. In: Knoors H, Marschark M, editors, *Evidence-Based Practices in Deaf Education*. New York: Oxford University Press, pp. 1–29. doi: 10.1093/oso/9780190880545.001.0001.

Marschark M, Paivio A, Spencer LJ et al. (2017) Don't assume deaf students are visual learners. *Journal of Developmental and Physical Disabilities* **29**(1): 153–171.

Marschark M, Sarchet T, Trani A (2016) Effects of hearing status and sign language use on working memory. *Journal of Deaf Studies and Deaf Education* **21**: 148–155.

McCallum RS (2017) *Handbook of Nonverbal Assessment*, 2nd edition. Cham, Switzerland: Springer International Publishing.

Melby-Lervåg M, Redick TS, Hulme C (2016) Working memory training does not improve performance on measures of intelligence or other measures of 'far transfer': Evidence from a meta-analytic review. *Perspectives on Psychological Science* **11**: 512–534.

Siebein GW, Gold MA, Siebein GW, Ermann MG (2000) Ten ways to provide a high quality acoustical environment in schools. *Language, Speech, and Hearing Services in Schools* **31**(4): 376–381. https://doi.org/10.1044/0161-1461.3104.376.

Sporns O, Tononi G, Kötter R (2005) The human connectome: A structural description of the human brain. *PLoS Computational Biology* **1**(4): e43. https://doi.org/10.1371/journal.pcbi.0010042.

CHAPTER 3

Sensory Integration and Processing

Sarah A Schoen, Virginia Spielmann, and Cristin M Holland

Presenting Concern

Elijah is a 6-year-old boy who was referred by his paediatrician due to parental concerns regarding daily meltdowns, difficulty with transitions during the day, and need for assistance in activities of daily living, playing with peers, and completing morning/evening routines. Developmentally, speech milestones were met within normal limits, but physical developmental milestones, such as learning to sit, crawl, and walk, were slightly delayed. Elijah was described as a 'difficult baby' who could not be calmed by holding, caressing, or cuddling. His mother reported that Elijah started screaming from the moment he was born. He did not sleep well and appeared uncomfortable and unhappy for the first 6 months of life.

Elijah lives with his mother and three siblings (an older brother and sister, and a younger brother). His parents are separated, but he sees his father weekly. Elijah demonstrates inflexibility, difficulty with pretend play, and a need for control when playing with siblings or at playdates. He has daily meltdowns when he comes home from school, and his mother reports difficulty performing daily routines, such as getting dressed or brushing his teeth. He requires many prompts and often needs his mother's assistance to complete self-care tasks. He has trouble organising his clothing and completing fastenings to dress and frequently forgets to put toothpaste on his toothbrush before beginning to brush his teeth. Elijah is easily bothered by background noise, such as his siblings making noise while he is trying to watch a video, and unexpected touch. His mother worries about a growing tendency toward anxiety and depression.

Elijah attends the local school where he does not receive support services. His teacher describes Elijah as a relatively quiet/passive child who does not have a lot of friends. She has concerns about his inattention and distractibility in the classroom, his isolation from peers, as well as his inability to work independently, though, when given support to stay on task, Elijah's academic abilities appear to be grade appropriate. He has trouble remaining seated for extended periods, and, when walking in the hallways, he frequently bumps into the walls or other students. He tends to get lost in the hallways if not accompanied by an adult or peer, and he takes a long time to descend the stairs. In physical education, he does not appear to listen or follow the instructions of the teacher. During recess, he walks aimlessly at the periphery of the play equipment and often gets in the way of the games of other children.

THEORY

Introduction to Sensory Integration and Processing

Assessment and treatment of sensory integration and processing tends to fall into the domain of occupational therapy, but such functions are likely to be apparent within the context of a neuropsychological formulation, even if they are not formally assessed and often form part of a multidisciplinary team approach.

Social, emotional, and cognitive development is dependent on our sensory experiences and capacity to process, organise, and use sensation for movement and behavioural responses (Diamond 2007). This is especially true in early childhood when the rapid development of physical, social, and emotional aptitude is reliant on our ability to process and integrate internal and external sensory data (Ayres 1979). It is through sensory integration and processing that we learn about ourselves and the world around us (Stein, Stanford, and Rowland 2020). This sense of self continues to mature and strengthen throughout childhood and early adulthood.

Sensory integration and processing refers to how individuals experience and interpret sensations from themselves and the environment for action and activity in daily life (Ayres 1979). If sensory integration/processing becomes disordered/distorted, many aspects of physical, mental, and psychological functioning may be impacted (Cohn et al. 2014). The literature suggests that many of the behavioural manifestations of sensory integration and processing challenges overlap with neurodevelopmental and mental health conditions across a broad range of phenotypes (e.g. learning disabilities, language disorders, bipolar disorder, etc.) (Levit-Binnun, Davidovitch, and Golland 2013). Addressing the sensory and motor impairments of children with psychiatric, developmental differences, or affective disorders is critical to the overall health and well-being of the individual.

Sensory Integration Theory Overview

Sensory integration theory originated from A Jean Ayres (1972) who postulated the theory of a relationship between the processing and integration of sensory input by the central nervous system (CNS) and behavioural outcomes within an environment (Davies and Gavin 2007). The theory has several assumptions: that there is neuroplasticity within the CNS, that the brain functions as an integrated whole, that adaptive interactions are necessary for development, and that children have an inner drive to participate in sensorimotor activities (Bundy and Lane 2020). Sensory integration therapy postulates a relation between deficits in processing and interpreting sensation from the body and the environment and difficulties with motor, academic, or social and emotional behaviour/functioning (Ayres 1979; Schaaf and Mailloux 2015; Bundy and Lane 2020). Meaningful registration (detection), interpretation, and integration of incoming sensory stimuli from the environment or body is required by the CNS for the individual to make an adaptive response within the environment. When this meaningful process is somehow disrupted or impeded, difficulties adapting to the environment can occur, and it can be challenging to complete or even engage in daily routines and roles (Miller et al. 2007). Additionally, the theory proposes that the CNS drives behaviour to seek out organising or beneficial stimulation, and that sensory input may facilitate or inhibit an organism's state (Ayres 1972; Ayres 1979). Under this hypothesis, some behaviour can be interpreted as the nervous system seeking regulation. Thus, change in behaviour is dependent on receiving, interpreting, and integrating incoming sensory input from the body and environment.

The sensory integration frame of reference describes sensory processing in terms of modulation, discrimination, postural-ocular functions, and praxis (Ayres 1972; Bundy and Lane 2020). Sensory modulation refers to how the CNS regulates its activity when encountering incoming stimuli. It encompasses processing and assessing sensory inputs for relevance and the subsequent adjustment of the nervous system to respond to the stimuli in a manner that is appropriate/consistent with the situation. The term is often used in reference with either over- or under-responsiveness to typical levels of sensory input. The second term, 'discrimination', is the ability of the nervous system to identify and interpret the qualities of sensory input, particularly temporal and spatial qualities, and then the use of this information for skill performance. Postural ocular functions refer to underlying motor abilities that support balance, bilateral coordination, and ocular-motor control. The last term, 'praxis', is the ability to conceive, plan, and perform motor action, and, with discrimination of input, is used to produce motor actions and behaviours with specific goals within an environment.

Disruption in Sensory Processing

Individuals with disordered sensory integration/processing may demonstrate a variety of deficits with perceiving, identifying, discriminating, interpreting, and integrating sensory input, which can impact performance of activities that require using more than one sensory system (Schaaf and Mailloux 2015; Bundy and Lane 2020). For example buttoning a shirt requires integration of tactile, proprioceptive, and visual systems. Poor sensory perception (discrimination), particularly tactile input, and motor planning challenges often manifest in difficulties in areas like getting dressed, which requires perception/interpretation of tactile feedback, and playing sports, which relies on a sense of body position (e.g. proprioceptive and vestibular perception/discrimination). Children may show challenges in posture, balance, and ocular control, which may lead to poor performance of integrated activities that require both sides of the body to work together, such as riding a bicycle or swimming. Additionally, challenges with sitting upright for long periods or tracking across a page when reading may be observed. Difficulty with both visual perception and visual-motor planning may manifest as poor performance in drawing, writing, or colouring, and avoidance of visual activities, like puzzles.

Sensory integration and processing challenges may manifest as over- or under-responsivity to sensory input, which can be related to concepts of arousal regulation and sensory modulation (Mailloux et al. 2011; Schaaf and Mailloux 2015). Over-responsivity is an excessive or exaggerated reaction to what would be considered tolerable levels of sensory input encountered throughout daily life and can impact participation in daily activities. For instance tactile hyperreactivity may result in challenges such as brushing teeth, washing the face, or wearing certain textured clothes. People sensitive to movement sensory inputs may avoid play activities like swinging or climbing. Noise, like fire alarms or busy environments, like restaurants, may negatively impact those with auditory over sensitivities. Children with under-responsivity or hyporeactivity is a lack of awareness/detection or registration of stimuli resulting in an absent, delayed, or reduced/muted reaction to everyday sensations. Children with under-responsivity may not display a readiness to respond to touch input, auditory input, or movement as expected.

While these specific patterns of sensory integrative dysfunction have been identified utilising Ayres' sensory integration frame of reference through early research, and remain utilised within clinical reasoning for applied intervention, current research on them is limited, especially outside of reactivity/responsivity challenges (Mailloux et al. 2011; Miller et al. 2017). However, additional models of sensory processing, such as a model proposing an interaction between neuroscience factors and behavioural concepts to provide a more complex view of children's behaviour, have become frequently utilised to describe sensory modulation (Dunn 2001). Additionally, a nosology was published in 2007 that proposed a similar framework to Ayres' (Miller et al. 2007).

ASSESSMENT AND FORMULATION

A comprehensive assessment with a sensory integration focus will likely have an occupational profile of the child obtained through the primary caregiver. It will generally include a developmental, medical, family, and occupational history (e.g. a semi-structured interview to determine a person's roles, approach to tasks, and sense of identity), as well as patterns of daily living, interests, values, and needs of the child and family (AOTA 2020). Practitioners may review records from schools or other services (Schaaf and Mailloux 2015). The profile also includes strengths and concerns, and supports and barriers, in relation to the child or family performing daily occupations (AOTA 2020). The profile may be obtained through questionnaires, formal interview, casual conversation, or a combination of methods.

The analysis of occupational performance (the activities, tasks, and roles of daily life) should consider all aspects of the domain of occupational therapy (skill performance, patterns of performance, context or environment, body structure and functions, and activity demands), though only select aspects may be directly assessed (AOTA 2020). An analysis of occupational performance with a focus on sensory integration and processing aims to specifically identify a child's strengths and difficulties in sensorimotor integration or processing, and will typically assess sensory perception (discrimination) and responsivity/reactivity (modulation) as well as related motor functions like balance, bilateral coordination, and motor planning (praxis).

These information sources used to analyse occupational performance may cover several areas of interest, including sensory integration and processing, adaptive behaviour and function, and participation, and may be dependent on the child's age and presenting concerns. This may include parent-report measures specific to sensory processing, such as the Sensory Profile-2 (Dunn 2014) or the Sensory Processing Measure, Second Edition (Parham et al. 2021). Parent-report measures of adaptive behaviour or participation may be used as a supplement to sensory processing measures to obtain an expanded understanding of a child's current level of functioning. Frequently used measures include the Adaptive Behavior Assessment System, Third Edition (Harrison and Oakland 2015) and Vineland Adaptive Behavior Scales, Third Edition (Sparrow, Cicchetti, and Saulnier 2016) (see Chapter 20 for more detail on adaptive behaviour).

Standardised observational assessments of a child's behaviour should be utilised in comprehensive evaluation. For many years, the Sensory Integration and Praxis Test (Ayres 1989) was the criterion standard for sensory integration assessment for middle childhood-aged children. However, the assessment has not been updated, and it requires substantial time to administer. New standardised assessments of sensory processing are emerging. For instance, the Evaluation in Ayres Sensory Integration® (Mailloux et al. 2018) and the Sensory Processing Three Dimensions Scale (Miller, Schoen, and Mulligan 2020) are currently being validated as assessments of sensory integration and processing. Additionally, the Structured Observations of Sensory Integration-Motor will provide standard scores for aspects of vestibular and proprioceptive discrimination (Blanche, Reinoso, and Kiefer 2021). Occupational therapy practitioners may use other standardised assessments from which to draw sensory integration and processing observations, as well as provide additional information on motor, cognitive, and occupational performance skills. Motor assessments, such as the Movement Assessment Battery for Children (Henderson, Sugden, and Barnett 2007), can provide information about gross and fine motor skills (see Chapter 4 for more detail). Task-based assessments, like the Miller Function and Participation Scales (Miller 2006) and the Goal Oriented Assessment of Life Skills (Miller, Oakland, and Herzberg 2013), can provide information about performance of school-related tasks as well as daily life activities, like writing, feeding, and dressing. Practitioners may use structured and unstructured clinical observations, often in environments

Table 3.1 Commonly used assessments of sensory integration and processing

Assessment	Age range (y or y:mo)	Type	Domains assessed
Sensory processing and integration			
Structured Observations of Sensory Integration – Motor	5–14	Standardised observational	Proprioception Processing Vestibular Processing Motor Planning Postural Control
Sensory Profile-2	Birth–14:11	Caregiver- or teacher-report	Sensory Processing Patterns
Sensory Processing Measure, Second Edition (SPM-2)	0:4–87:0 2–5 (SPM-Preschool)	Caregiver- or teacher-report	Sensory Processing Praxis Social Participation
Sensory Integration and Praxis Test (SIPT)	4:0–8:11	Standardised observational (17 brief tests)	Visual Perception Tactile Perception Kinesthetic Perception Motor Performance
Evaluation in Ayres Sensory Integration® (EASI®)	In collection of normative data for: 3–12	Standardised observational	Sensory Responsiveness Postural/Ocular/Bilateral Integration Praxis
Sensory Processing Three Dimensions Scale (SP3D)	In validation for: 3–adults	Standardised observational Caregiver-report	Sensory Modulation Sensory Discrimination Posture and Praxis

that provide opportunities for rich sensory experiences, to assess particular sensory and motor skills.

At the completion of an occupational therapy evaluation, information is synthesised to make connections between the theory or frame of reference most relevant to the practice setting and challenges in occupational performance (Schaaf and Mailloux 2015). Synthesising assessment information with sensory integration theory allows a practitioner to connect sensory and motor difficulties to challenges in everyday activities. One frequently used tool for identifying outcomes in intervention using a sensory integration frame of reference is Goal Attainment Scaling (Mailloux et al. 2007). This method allows for objective individualised goals that can be quantified, as well as compared for progress across broad goal areas. Setting targeted outcome measures or goals is a collaborative process between the client/family and occupational therapist, should reflect the parent's priorities, and is generally decided upon prior to the start of intervention (AOTA 2020).

> **Case Study – Assessment**
>
> Elijah was seen by an occupational therapist for an evaluation. Prior to attending the evaluation session, Elijah's mother completed a developmental, medical, and occupational performance history for Elijah, as well as the Sensory Processing Measure and the Vineland Adaptive Behavior Scales, Third Edition. The occupational therapist was able to review this information prior to meeting Elijah. At the evaluation, the occupational therapist administered the Sensory Integration and Praxis Test and the Movement Assessment Battery for Children to assess Elijah's visual, tactile, vestibular, proprioceptive, modulation and discrimination, and fine and gross motor performance. Standardised structured clinical observations were also administered by the occupational therapist to provide additional data on tactile, vestibular, and proprioceptive integration and processing, and praxis. Unstructured observations were collected whilst the occupational therapist observed Elijah playing by himself and with his brother and mother in a gym space outfitted with mats, swings, and climbing equipment to observe his sensory preferences, motor performance, play skills, regulation capacities, and social interactions. After the completion of the evaluation, the occupational therapist synthesised the information reported by Elijah's mother and her interpretations from the standardised assessment, the structured clinical observation, and the unstructured observations. She hypothesised that Elijah had difficulty with over-responsivity to tactile and auditory input, which impacted his self-regulation abilities when presented with unexpected stimuli. In addition, she hypothesised Elijah had difficulty with modulation and discrimination of tactile, vestibular, and proprioceptive input, which contributed to poor body awareness and motor performance that made daily activities and routines, such as buttoning, dressing, and walking around others, challenging for him. She also felt that Elijah presented with challenges in ideation and motor planning that were impacting his participation in play and self-care activities. The occupational therapist and Elijah's mother met to discuss the occupational therapist's clinical interpretations, and the therapist also provided intervention recommendations. Prior to the start of intervention, Elijah's mother and the occupational therapist collaborated on the development of targeted, functional, and measurable goals for intervention based on presenting problems and through the Goal Attainment Scaling framework.

INTERVENTION AND MANAGEMENT

Occupational therapy intervention consists of an intervention plan, implementation, and review and is intended to promote health, wellness, and participation (AOTA 2020). The intervention plan selects the theories or frames of reference that will guide the intervention to target the outcomes that will improve performance and participation in everyday life. Common interventions using a sensory integration frame of reference are Ayres Sensory Integration® (Schaaf and Mailloux 2015), or sensory integration therapy (Goin-Kochel, Mackintosh, and Myers 2009) and are considered evidenced-based practices for children with autism spectrum disorders (Schoen et al. 2019; Steinbrenner et al. 2020). The focus of intervention is addressing the child's underlying sensory integration and processing challenges that are leading to participation challenges in daily life activities. Ayres Sensory Integration® is a dynamic well-reasoned clinical process and is not the same as sensory specific strategies or procedures like brushing, weighted vests, sensory rooms, or sensory diets.

Paediatric sensory integration-focused intervention occurs within the context of play, which occupational therapy practitioners with advanced training in sensory integration use to facilitate change (Ayres 1979; Schaaf and Mailloux 2015). This play involves an environment that provides sensory rich experiences, especially in tactile, vestibular (equilibrium and movement acceleration), and proprioceptive (e.g. muscles and joints) domains, through the use of static and dynamic equipment that promotes active participation of the child. During play, the practitioner uses clinical reasoning and incorporates the child's interests and internal drive for play to scaffold the child to experience success with the 'just right challenge'. The just right challenge involves tailoring the demands of the activity to target an adaptive response from the child that demonstrates growth beyond the child's current level of competence (Schaaf and Mailloux 2015). The adaptive response within a 'just right challenge' provides an experience of success and mastery of the environment for the child and reinforces the child's willingness to engage in more frequent and greater challenges throughout the intervention process. Additionally, therapeutic use of self is an integral tool in occupational therapy intervention, and in intervention using a sensory integration framework this is done through therapeutic alliance with the child and parent, as well as therapist–child, and therapist–parent collaboration.

Depending on presenting concerns, intervention using a sensory integration framework may incorporate programs of targeted sensory input, such as auditory, visual-vestibular, or tactile programs, to augment the play-based intervention. Additionally, it is important to consider the use of environmental supports and adaptations as well as the inclusion of parent- or teacher-mediated techniques (Reynolds et al. 2017). For instance, unimodal sensory strategies, like noise-cancelling headphones, tagless clothes, or weighted vests, may be recommended to facilitate regulation and participation in occupations. Families may also be advised to make adaptations to the environment or how an occupation is performed to reduce or increase sensory stimuli and facilitate engagement in occupation. Examples may include removing excess toys from a play area, giving the child control over wiping their face, or providing preparatory activities prior to an activity, such as a social story or specific sensory input.

Sensory integration theory has also been incorporated into the STAR Frame of Reference (Miller, Schoen, and Spielmann 2018; Miller et al. 2020). The STAR Frame of Reference combines Ayres' principles with principles from DIR®/Floortime (Greenspan and Wieder 2009). An added focus is on relationship and regulation challenges that interfere with functioning in daily life. The foundation of this intervention is the integration of sensory, regulation, and relationship strategies in an intentional, ongoing basis throughout intervention within the context of play.

Other complementary approaches to sensory-based intervention will frequently be used within occupational therapy intervention to address sensory-related or other participation challenges (Reynolds et al. 2017). Cognitive approaches may be employed to assist children in developing strategies to meet participation demands of daily life. These types of programs may be task-oriented, such as the Cognitive Orientation to daily Occupational Performance (Polatajko et al. 2001), which can help analyse and problem-solve occupational performance challenges or may connect more to self-regulation strategies to facilitate appropriate arousal level for engagement in occupations, such as The Alert Program® (Williams and Shellenberger 1994) or The Zones of Regulation® (Kuypers 2011).

Outcome

Elijah attended a total of 30 sensory integration intervention sessions over the course of 10 weeks. Intervention focused on activities providing proprioceptive, tactile, and vestibular inputs to improve regulation, body awareness, and motor planning. Elijah's parents were involved in the intervention to aid implementing strategies at home to promote regulation and organisation. Upon completion of intervention, the occupational therapist and Elijah's parents reviewed the goal attainment scaling cowritten at the start of treatment. Progress was noted in all presenting areas of concern, particularly self-care (i.e. dressing and personal hygiene), positive interaction with peers and siblings, and emotional stability (e.g. decreased meltdowns).

Elijah's mother and occupational therapist collaborated on sensory activities for the transition from school to home. At school, Elijah's teacher reports he can remain seated, as well as attend to tasks, for longer periods of time without significant redirections. His teacher also reports that he is able to join structured games with peers at recess. It is suggested that Elijah be re-evaluated for a possible intervention booster in 9 to 12 months to address any remaining areas of concern.

SUMMARY

Within the Ayres Sensory Integration® frame of reference, occupational therapy uses play to address the underlying sensory and motor challenges that impede participation in daily life activities (Schaaf and Mailloux 2015). Targeted therapeutic play and improved capacity to process and integrate sensation with accommodations in the environment and development of a sensory lifestyle supported regulation and mitigated stress and anxiety for Elijah. This enabled improved 'meaning making', decreasing challenging behaviours and supporting psychological well-being. Sensory integration theory provides a valuable framework for considering how individual differences in sensory integration and processing can impact participation in daily life activities (Ayres 1979; Schaaf and Mailloux 2015).

REFERENCES

AOTA (American Occupational Therapy Association) (2020) Occupational therapy practice framework: Domain and process, 4th edition. *American Journal of Occupational Therapy* **74**(Suppl. 2): 7412410010. https://doi.org/10.5014/ajot.2020.74S2001.

Ayres AJ (1972) Types of sensory integrative dysfunction among disabled learners. *American Journal of Occupational Therapy* **26**: 13–18.

Ayres AJ (1979) *Sensory Integration and the Child*, 1st edition. Los Angeles, CA: Western Psychological Services.

Bundy AC, Lane SJ (2020) *Sensory Integration: Theory and Practice.* Philadelphia, PA: FA Davis.

Cohn ES, Kramer J, Schub JA, May-Benson TA (2014) Parents' explanatory models and hopes for outcomes of occupational therapy using a sensory integration approach. *American Journal of Occupational Therapy* **68**(4): 454–462. doi: 10.5014/ajot.2014.010843.

Davies PL, Gavin WJ (2007) Validating the diagnosis of sensory processing disorders using EEG technology. *American Journal of Occupational Therapy* **61**(2): 176–189.

Diamond A (2007) Interrelated and interdependent. *Developmental Science* **10**(1): 152–158. doi: 10.1111/j.1467-7687.2007.00578.x.

Dunn W (2001) The sensations of everyday life: Empirical, theoretical, and pragmatic considerations, 2001 Eleanor Clarke Slagle lecture. *American Journal of Occupational Therapy* **55**: 608–622.

Goin-Kochel RP, Mackintosh VH, Myers BJ (2009) Parental reports on the efficacy of treatments and therapies for their children with autism spectrum disorders. *Research in Autism Spectrum Disorders* **3**(2): 528–537.

Greenspan SI, Wieder S (2009) *Engaging Autism: Using the Floortime Approach to Help Children Relate, Communicate, and Think.* Cambridge, MA: Hachette Books.

Kuypers L (2011) *Zones of Regulation: A Curriculum Designed to Foster Self-Regulation and Emotional Control.* Minneapolis, MN: Kuypers Consulting, Inc.

Levit-Binnun N, Davidovitch M, Golland Y (2013) Sensory and motor secondary symptoms as indicators of brain vulnerability. *Journal of Neurodevelopmental Disorders* **5**(26): 1–21. doi: 10.1186/1866-1955-5-26.

Mailloux Z, May-Benson TA, Summers CA et al. (2007) Goal attainment scaling as a measure of meaningful outcomes for children with sensory integration disorders. *American Journal of Occupational Therapy* **61**: 254–259.

Mailloux Z, Mulligan S, Roley S et al. (2011) Verification and clarification of patterns of sensory integrative dysfunction. *American Journal of Occupational Therapy* **65**: 143–151. https://doi.org/10.5014/ajot.2011.000752.

Mailloux Z, Parham LD, Roley SS, Ruzzano L, Schaaf RC (2018) Introduction to the Evaluation in Ayres Sensory Integration® (EASI). *American Journal of Occupational Therapy* **72**: 7201195030. https://doi.org/10.5014/ajot.2018.028241.

Miller LJ (2006) *The Miller Function and Participation Scales.* San Antonio, TX: Pearson.

Miller LJ, Anzalone ME, Lane SJ, Cermak SA, Osten ET (2007) Concept evolution in sensory integration: A proposed nosology for diagnosis. *American Journal of Occupational Therapy* **61**(2): 135–140. https://doi.org/10.5014/ajot.61.2.135.

Miller LJ, Chu RC, Parkins M, Spielmann V, Schoen SA (2020) In: Bundy AC, Lane SJ, editors, *Sensory Integration Theory and Practice*, 3rd edition. Philadelphia, PA: FA Davis, pp. 578–584.

Miller LJ, Oakland T, Herzberg DS (2013) *Goal-Oriented Assessment of Lifeskills (GOAL).* Torrance, CA: WPS.

Miller LJ, Schoen SA, Mulligan S, Sullivan J (2017) Identification of sensory processing and integration symptom clusters. *Occupational Therapy International* **2017**: 2876080. doi: 10.1155/2017/2876080.

Miller LJ, Schoen SA, Spielmann V (2018) A frame reference for sensory processing difficulties: Sensory therapies and research (STAR). In: Kramer P, Hinojosa J, Howe T, editors, *Frames of Reference in Pediatric Occupational Therapy*, 4th edition. Philadelphia, PA: Wolters Kluwer, pp. 159–202.

Mueller I, Tronick E (2020) Sensory processing and meaning making in autism spectrum disorder. *Autism 360°*. Elsevier Inc., pp. 255–267. [online] Available at: https://doi.org/10.1016/b978-0-12-818466-0.00014-9.

Polatajko HJ, Mandich AD, Miller LT, Macnab JJ (2001) Cognitive orientation to daily occupational performance (CO-OP): Part II – the evidence. *Physical & Occupational Therapy in Pediatrics* **20**(2–3): 83–106.

Reynolds S, Glennon TJ, Ausderau K et al. (2017) Using a multifaceted approach to working with children who have differences in sensory integration and processing. *American Journal of Occupational Therapy* **71**(2). doi: 10.5014/ajot.2017.019281.

Schaaf R, Mailloux Z (2015) *Clinician's Guide for Implementing Ayres Sensory Integration®: Promoting Participation for Children with Autism*. Bethesda, MD: AOTA Press.

Schoen SA, Lane SJ, Mailloux Z et al. (2019) A systematic review of ayres sensory integration intervention for children with autism. *Autism Research* **12**: 6–19. https://doi.org/10.1002/aur.2046.

Stein BE, Stanford TR, Rowland BA (2020) Multisensory integration and the society for neuroscience: Then and now. *Journal of Neuroscience* **40**(1): 3–11. doi: 10.1523/JNEUROSCI.0737-19.2019.

Steinbrenner JR, Hume K, Odom SL et al. (2020) *Evidence-Based Practices for Children, Youth, and Young Adults With Autism*. The University of North Carolina at Chapel Hill, Frank Porter Graham Child Development Institute, National Clearinghouse on Autism Evidence and Practice Review Team.

Williams MS, Shellenberger S (1994) *How Does Your Engine Run?: A Leader's Guide to the Alert Program for Self-Regulation*. Albuquerque, NM: TherapyWorks.

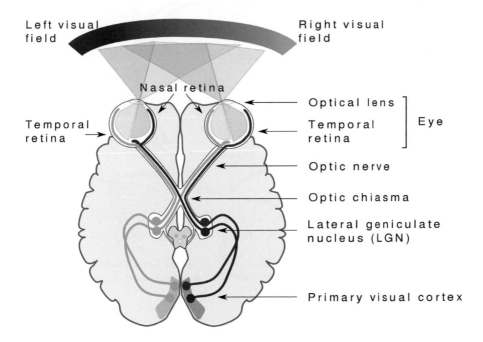

Figure 1.1 The visual pathways from eye to visual cortex. Reused from Miquel Perello Nieto (Wikimedia Commons). This figure is licensed under the Creative Commons Attribution-Share Alike 4.0 International license (https://creativecommons.org/licenses/by-sa/4.0/deed.en).

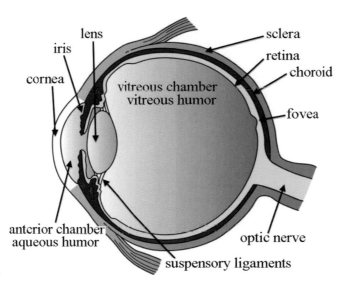

Figure 1.2 The eye structure. Reused from Holly Fischer (Wikimedia Commons). This file is licensed under the Creative Commons Attribution 3.0 Unported license. (https://creativecommons.org/licenses/by/3.0/deed.en).

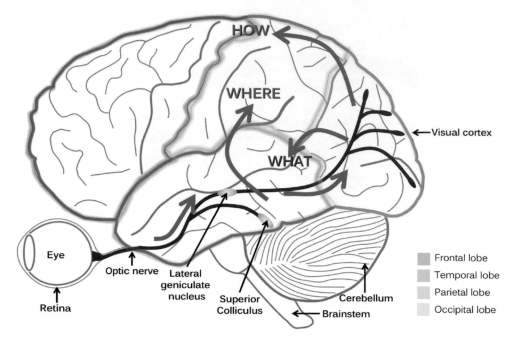

Figure 1.3 Dorsal and ventral pathways of the visual system.

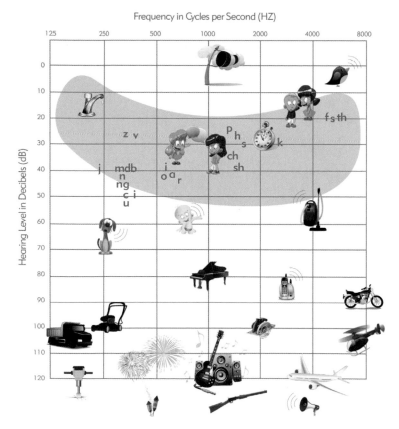

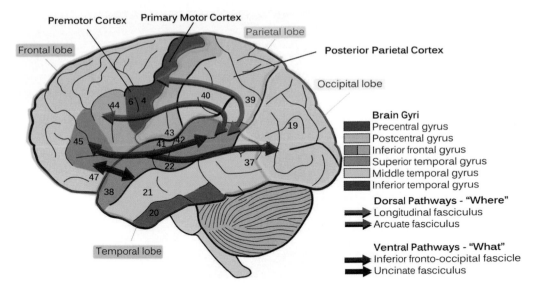

Figure 5.2 Cortical regions and white matter pathways involved in language.

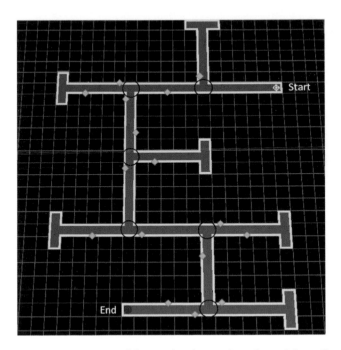

Figure 7.2 Sample maze structure used for navigation tasks, adapted from Farran et al. (2012). Landmarks are depicted as yellow diamonds. Each red circle indicates a decision point at which an error may occur.

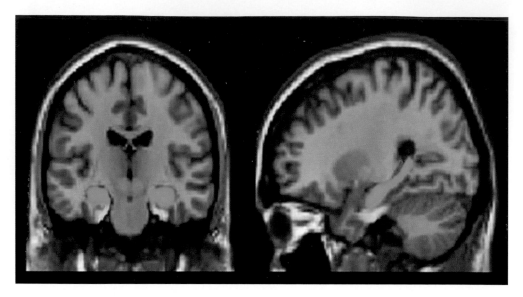

Figure 9.1 Magnetic resonance imaging scan of the brain with the hippocampus highlighted in green and the underlying rhinal cortices in yellow.

CHAPTER 4

Motor Coordination

Dido Green and Elisabeth L Hill

Presenting Concern

Jacob is an energetic 11-year-old boy who has been referred due to concerns over problems with organisation and difficulties with motor skills. He is showing increasing frustration and refusing to undertake tasks at school, particularly involving use of apparatus such as rulers and compasses, and he causes disruption in his classroom. Jacob lives at home with his twin sister, an older sister (13 years), and his parents. Jacob was born at 27 weeks gestation, the second of twins. His birthweight was 1460 grams. He was identified as having a left-sided mild hemiparesis at the age of 18 months, although computerised tomography imaging and ultrasound scanning were inconclusive. Imaging at age 11 years showed periventricular leukomalacia and intraventricular haemorrhaging at grade I in the right hemisphere with asymmetry of ventricles and white matter volume. The hemiparesis predominantly affects his ability to rotate his left forearm (supination) with slowness in fine motor skills. His twin sister has no difficulties, and she is able to perform tasks in the same way as her peers, whilst Jacob is frustrated particularly that he cannot keep up with his peers in ball games.

Jacob's motor impairments due to cerebral palsy may be classified as level I on both the Manual Ability Classification System (MACS) and the Gross Motor Function Classification System (GMFCS). The MACS ranks ability to handle objects in important daily activities (Eliasson et al. 2006), and the GMFCS documents gross motor functional capacity (Palisano et al. 2008) with higher levels reflecting greater difficulty or impairment. Young people with unilateral cerebral palsy typically fall between levels I and III on the MACS and GMFCS with skills ranging from mild restrictions to difficulties requiring mobility aids and help modifying activities. Yet Jacob's functional difficulties extended beyond those experienced by children classified as level I on both the MACS and GMFCS; to some extent reflective of problems experienced by children with developmental coordination disorder.

Jacob is keen to be involved in sports and enjoys running around with friends. He is increasingly opting out of sporting games and has difficulties following rules. His occupational therapist, involved in helping Jacob use his left hand in bimanual tasks, commented, 'How can we get him to use his left hand when he does not know what to do with his right (dominant/preferred) hand?'

This was particularly notable when attempting to use a toy bow and arrow in archery. Jacob was unable to work out how to place the end of the arrow and release the cord with his right hand, whilst holding the bow still with his left hand, and maintaining aim.

THEORY

Theoretical Perspectives of Motor Coordination

The development of motor coordination tends to fall into maturational or ecological accounts (see Sugden and Wade 2019). In this section, we discuss the most influential paradigms in order to consider Jacob's presentation and the ways in which interventions draw on theoretical perspectives.

Traditional theorists align the development of motor skills with the *maturation* of the child's neurological system. This framework defines a structured perspective in which skills develop in progressive hierarchical stages whereby graded levels of control at a neural level appear behaviourally, in a predictable and sequential fashion. More recently, alternative explanations for the acquisition of motor skills have emerged. These are termed *ecological approaches* and focus predominantly on non-linear dynamic interactions of the infant/child with the environment. For some, these two approaches are entwined. For example Gesell et al. introduced the principle of 'growth gradients', progressive stages or degrees of maturity that a child passes through towards higher levels of behaviour, with these being dependent upon the maturity of the child's nervous system but described as 'alternating stages of equilibrium and disequilibrium' (Gesell et al. 1977, p. 17). This led to more ecological approaches attesting to the individuality of each child with uniqueness or unevenness of patterns of growth, influenced by environmental and temperamental factors (Gesell et al. 1977). The ecological approaches take a dynamic perspective in which the context interacts with a person's capabilities for the development (or not) of skilled motor behaviour (Thelen and Smith 1994).

Theorists, whether maturational or ecological, have tended to study specific aspects of the movement control required to execute planned and voluntary actions. These include balance (and recovery of balance following perturbation), reach and grasp patterns, or the accuracy of judging distance, force, speed, and direction to produce the movement required. These movements are delivered from a neural basis over three main levels. Figure 4.1 illustrates a hierarchical relationship between strategy, tactics, and action execution representing the interrelationship between inter-neuronal activity in the neocortex and basal ganglia, the motor cortex and cerebellum, and the brainstem and spinal cord respectively.

Neural developmentalists tend to use descriptive models to describe stages of motor *development*, documenting the acquisition of measurable motor skills with the assumption that these reflect underlying neurological and structural changes. 'Neurological soft

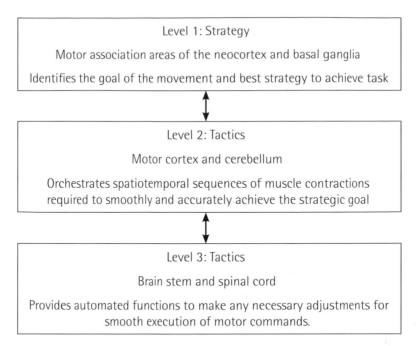

Figure 4.1 Representation of hierarchy of neural functions of motor control.

signs', such as persistence of mirror movements, primitive reflexes, etc., have commonly been considered representative of neural maturation and predictive of developmental problems of cognition, coordination, and behaviour. Whilst these indicators of 'neural' maturation continue to be used as markers for 'motor delay' or 'motor disorders' (Hadders-Algra 2010), there is limited evidence that these are important predictors of later developmental trajectories. Verification of neural maturation via brain imaging also has limitations (Weinstein et al. 2018). In most cases, it is a child's behaviour/functional difficulties observed that inform our work, and thus consideration of 'soft-signs' need to be placed in the context of other performance parameters.

Figure 4.2 considers the relationship of potential aetiological factors to neurological deficit and characteristic functional motor deficits. In a child who has sustained developmental insults or has a disorder, there is a complex interaction between brain regions. The impact of a primary insult may alter connectivity to other regions, having more diffuse effects across functional areas than seen in acquired brain injury in an adult patient (where the consequences of the injury may be more contained).

In addition to the complex dynamics influencing the behavioural outputs of motor control, scientists have investigated the organisation of the many 'degrees of freedom' (DOF) underlying any action. DOF refers to the multiple ways available to perform a movement to accomplish the same goal. The organisation of DOF and trial by trial

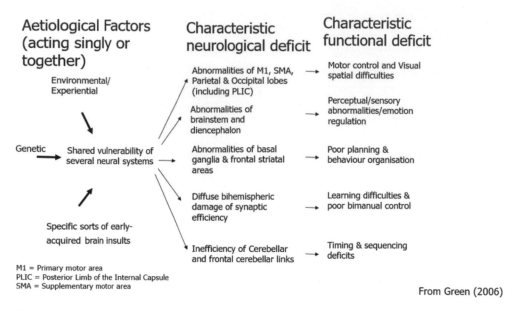

Figure 4.2 Multiple primary deficits contribution to sensory motor behaviour (from Green 2006).

adaptations, with task specific variation, are particularly important components of motor learning to ensure consistent performance (see Sternad 2009). Repetition, variability, generalisation, and transfer are critical elements of motor learning approaches in rehabilitation (Lage et al. 2015).

Applying these theories to our understanding of Jacob's motor difficulties, we can see the impact of early brain injury directly affects motor control of his left arm, with restricted range, speed, and force control of movement, particularly to forearm rotation and control of individual finger movements of the left hand. In addition, the presence of mirrored movements impedes bimanual control, which may be due to a lack of interhemispheric inhibition from cortical damage to his right hemisphere (Mayston et al. 1999) – thus when moving his left (affected) hand there are corresponding and homologous movements in the right. With so many bimanual tasks requiring divergent movements between hands, the persistence of mirrored movements will have considerable functional implications (Zielinski et al. 2017). The need for extensive practice to overcome environmental/ecological constraints on the control of movement variability and the multiple DOF will be important in intervention design for Jacob.

Focussing on 'motor milestones' and 'soft signs' (as considered in neural maturational approaches), oversimplifies the processes of motor control and motor coordination. In day-to-day life, we apparently effortlessly, make effective movements to achieve goals (e.g. dressing, tightening a screw, etc.). With practice, feedback during actions supports anticipatory motor control and planning. This process will be influenced by factors such as the use of mental imagery in action planning, the cognitive system's involvement in action selection when there are competing rewards, the influence of knowledge of end-point (goals), and the tendency to seek 'end-state comfort'. Unconscious selection of grasp patterns will differentially influence motor planning, compare for example when reaching to grasp a mug placed upside down to set it upright versus moving it from one upright position to another. Steenbergen and colleagues have further explored these issues in relation to disability (Steenbergen et al. 2004). The principle of 'end state comfort' shows reach–grasp patterns are preferentially chosen to ensure the 'end point' of action is most efficient (Solnik et al. 2013). When considering the motor planning of children with motor disorders, the timing, sequencing, and execution of their actions may differ from typically developing peers (Hill and Wing 1999), and they may treat each segment of a task as a different or new task (Rudisch et al. 2016). Thus, whilst Jacob's typical peer would learn through experience how to use the bow and arrow accurately, Jacob proceeded with incorrectly positioning the arrow and releasing the wooden bar of the bow, on each attempt only realising an error on completion of the task. Jacob's difficulties in planning and organising the 'how' of placing the arrow as well as control timing of the release of the arrow in relation to the position of the bow, can be seen as indicative of problems in anticipatory control and use of effective feedback during the task. The ability to adjust a movement or modify a plan whilst performing the action is an executive function, particularly motor planning, response inhibition, and working memory (see Chapter 11).

We have outlined various perspectives in understanding motor coordination and related impairments; assessment of these processes is a greater challenge. This is not only due to the complexity of motor control and motor coordination but due to involvement of many other processes (e.g. attention, memory) and the nature of available assessments.

ASSESSMENT AND FORMULATION

If we use the International Classification of Functioning, Disability and Health (WHO 2007) model to consider appropriate assessments for a child such as Jacob we typically start from referral information, which may be limitations to activity performance or participation expected for the child's age (e.g. riding a bicycle, using cutlery, etc.). Alternatively, our assessment may be focused on body function level and qualitative dimensions of muscle properties and motor control (e.g. spasticity, dyskinesis, or tremor). Clarifying the purpose of the assessment is an important first step in identifying what needs to be assessed and how.

Standardised assessments may be classified according to the types of tasks that are performed (e.g. fine or gross motor) or target particular activities (e.g. handwriting). But, what do these tell us about the underlying difficulties in order to assist in treatment planning? One of the fundamental problems, particularly with assessments done in the clinical setting, is determining the extent to which a measured property such as muscle strength, links to another, for example balance, and which in turn may contribute to the presenting problem – inability to hop on one leg or ride a bicycle.

Minoliti and colleagues (2020) have provided a recent review of tests of children's motor coordination highlighting nature of the task(s), psychometrics, and cultural adaptations of a number of tools. For example falling below a standardised normative value for placing pegs quickly in a pegboard may not be indicative of difficulties in doing up buttons. Table 4.1 describes commonly used assessments and observations that may support clinical reasoning and problem-solving for diagnosis and intervention planning.

For Jacob, assessment included: movement quality, frequency of use of affected hand and motor skill (Assisting Hand Assessment, Accelerometry, Jebsen-Taylor Test of Hand Function, respectively), motivation/goal identification (Children's Hope Scale, goal attainment scaling), and potential impact of mirrored movements (e.g. Woods and Teuber 1978) to guide intervention but unfortunately did not include assessment of motor planning. Assessment identified poor bimanual coordination, which was particularly affected by poor supination and executing individual finger movements of the left arm and hand and mirrored movements influencing fine motor skills, speed, and dexterity. Additional observations showed poor attention. His reluctance to engage in the assessment tasks resulted in low scores on positivity and agency (Children's Hope Scale) and reduced engagement in goal setting. Detailed observations of how Jacob benefited from repetition and practice along with experimental manipulation to explore 'anticipatory motor planning' and 'end state comfort' may give us greater insight into the 'why' of his difficulties to plan appropriate interventions.

Ecological validity is more questionable the more remote the measured skill is from the motor task (Vinçon et al. 2017). The challenge therefore is to be able to select appropriate clinical tools that can assist in meaningful understanding of the nature and extent of movement difficulties. This requires meaningful reflection on the assessments used, the context in which they have been administered, the interpretation of the findings gained from these, in conjunction with gathering information on the child's experience of daily life activities. Defining important indicators and criteria for deficits, and thus which children should then receive what treatment is problematic. At this point, many of these decisions rest with those involved directly in supporting a child in their unique context.

INTERVENTION AND MANAGEMENT

The past 30 years has shown a shift from sensory-motor and perceptual motor interventions to task-focused models. There is little evidence to recommend sensory or perceptual interventions in which components of a skill are practised such as tracing between lines or balancing on a wobble board with the aim to improve skills such as handwriting and bicycle-riding respectively. The evidence for these component-based approaches for children with coordination disorders, such as developmental coordination

Table 4.1 Standardised motor tests

Test	Purpose and age range (y or y:mo)	Skill	Additional observations
The Movement Assessment Battery for Children, Second Edition (Movement ABC-2; Henderson et al. 2007)	Motor function impairment 3–16	Fine motor Ball skills Static and Dynamic balance (strength/agility)	Differences between dominant and non-dominant sides Lack of improvement between first and second trials Repetition of error or different errors between first and second trials Quality of movement e.g. slow, tremor, force, effortful Ability to follow instructions
Bruininks/Oseretsky Test of Motor Proficiency, Second Edition (BOT-2; Bruininks and Bruininks 2005)	Motor proficiency 4–21	Fine motor precision Fine motor integration Manual dexterity Bilateral coordination Balance Running speed and agility Upper-limb coordination Strength	Same as above
McCarron Assessment of Neuromuscular Development (MAND; McCarron 1997)	Balance, fine motor, grasping, neurological, or walking disabilities Fine and gross motor 3:5–16	Fine motor: Beads in box Beads on rod Finger tapping Nut and bolt Rod slide Gross motor: Hand strength Finger/nose finger	Quantitative measurements of performance (speed, accuracy); qualitative observations

(Continued)

Table 4.1 Continued.

Test	Purpose and age range (y or y:mo)	Skill	Additional observations
		Standing long jump Heel toe walk One-foot stand	
Test of Gross Motor Development, Third Edition (GMD-3; Ulrich 2000)	Delayed gross motor skill development 3–10	Locomotor – e.g. running, galloping Ball skills – e.g. two-hand striking a stationary	Aids identification of gross motor development delay and intervention planning
Bayley Scales of Infant and Toddler Development, Fourth Edition (Bayley and Aylward 2019); Motor component	Motor skills (cognitive, language, social-emotional, and adaptive skills can be considered along with motor skills) 16 days–42 months	Fine motor Gross motor	Caregiver responses support scoring of some items Behaviour observation inventory including muscle tone
Peabody Developmental Motor Scales, Second Edition (PDMS-2; Folio and Fawell 2000)	Fine and gross motor skill 0–6	Fine motor: Grasping Visual–motor integration Gross motor: Reflexes Stationary performances Locomotion Object manipulation	Measure of developing motor skills

(Continued)

Test	Purpose and age range (y or y:mo)	Skill	Additional observations
Assisting Hand Assessment (AHA): Kids-AHA (Krumlinde-Sundholm and Eliasson 2003) Mini-AHA (Greaves et al. 2013) Ad-AHA (Adult) (Louwers et al. 2016) Related: Hand Assessment for Infants (HAI) (Krumlinde-Sundholm et al. 2017) Both-Hands Assessment (BoHA) (Elvrum et al. 2018)	Spontaneous functional use and capacity of affected hand during bimanual tasks	Semi-structured play or task based/activities documenting: frequency/initiations, reaching, grasp-release, manipulation, pacing) in tasks where two hands are typically used Same activities as AHA group with both hands scored separately and additional bimanual items	Strategy use Persistence with ineffective strategies/repetition of errors Differences in initiation of use when using items that must have two hands to achieve versus those that can be performed with one hand and supportive surfaces Amount of assistance or not provided by less affected hand Attention and behaviour
Clinical Observation of Motor and Posture Skills, Second Edition (COMPS-2) (Wilson et al. 2000)	Motor problems with a postural component Supplemental information to tests of Sensory Integration (Ayres 1972)	Six items reflecting body function skills based on Sensory Integration Theory of movement difficulties: slow movements, rapid forearm rotation, finger-nose touching, prone extension posture, asymmetric neck reflex, and supine flexion posture	No recent psychometrics to support use for children with movement difficulties; however, minor neurological impairments may be indicated if poor performance on slow movements, rapid forearm rotation, finger to nose and asymmetric neck reflex

(Continued)

Table 4.1 Continued.

Test	Purpose and age range (y or y:mo)	Skill	Additional observations
Alberta Infant Motor Scale (AIMS) (Piper and Darrah 1994)	Gross motor maturation 0–18 months	Observational assessment scale of gross motor maturation focussing on four positions: Prone Supine Sitting Standing	Performance based, observational assessment Motor development over time to identify motor development delay Differences in movement patterns
Gesture (variety of tasks available including the Gesture Imitation Test) (Bergès and Lézine 1965)	Gesture production	Motor, spatial, and temporal components of gesture production	Accuracy of gestures made under various conditions (e.g. with and without vision, from command, imitation, from picture) Quality of gesture production Nature of errors made
Woods and Teuber scale (Woods and Teuber 1978)	Mirrored movements Childhood	Finger tapping Forearm rotation Finger sequencing	Mirrored movements are affected on functional activities
Purdue Pegboard (Tiffin and Asher 1948)	Unimanual and bimanual finger and hand dexterity 5–89	Placing pegs Fine fingertip dexterity in assembly tasks	Manual dexterity and bimanual coordination incorporating cognitive speed and attentional control

disorders (Blank et al. 2019) or disorders of motor control such as cerebral palsy (Novak et al. 2013) is weak; without transfer and generalisation to daily tasks. Task focussed interventions such as neuromotor task training, virtual reality technologies (Blank et al. 2019; Farr et al. 2019), and more problem-solving approaches such as the Cognitive Orientation to daily Occupational Performance (Green 2006; Green et al. 2006; Gimeno et al. 2019) show promise for children with developmental coordination disorder as well as those with cerebral palsy.

Task-focused interventions for children with cerebral palsy, which build on motor learning theories to provide more intensive opportunities for practice with particular emphasis on repetition, variability, and transfer, have arisen out of animal models and stroke rehabilitation (Kwakkel et al. 2015). Constraint-induced movement therapy involves restraining/constraining the non-paretic arm forcing use of the affected limb in task-focused (scaffolded) training for 8 to 16 hours a day for up to 1 month. Constraint-induced movement therapy has been modified for children and the intense model adapted also for bimanual training (Novak et al. 2013; Novak et al. 2020).

Constraint-induced movement therapy might have been considered for Jacob since there is good evidence of its benefits for children with hemiparesis. However, this approach would not address Jacob's difficulties in bimanual coordination, goal selection, and error correction. The key ingredients of motor learning programmes are repetition, variability, and transfer of training, which are influenced by intensity, dosage, and self-initiated movements. With this in mind, Jacob undertook a 2-week, 6 hours per day summer day camp involving intensive magic-themed bimanual training (Green et al. 2013). Learning of magic tricks provided motivating tasks and context to ensure sufficient intensity of movement repetition whilst also requiring considerable problem-solving skills and mental imagery (to interpret the perspective of the 'audience'). Jacob showed good progress in specific skills practised through the learning of magic tricks and these generalised to daily activities. Furthermore, the opportunity to play (and work) along-side other children with unilateral cerebral palsy provided friendships that endured after the summer camp with the young people setting up their own Facebook page and giving magic shows at one another's schools. Further research into these innovative models of intervention, combining problem-solving approaches along with intensive task-oriented training in real or virtual social contexts, is needed not only to determine their effectiveness but also to understand the mechanisms by which change is occurring.

Outcome

Jacob, a young boy born preterm and suffering a brain injury, illustrates the interaction between motor control, impacted by spasticity in his left arm, and deficits in executive functions, particularly strategy generation and attention. For Jacob, assessments of motor skills involving unimanual *and* bimanual tasks helped define the extent of his motor impairment. More detailed analysis of motor planning, response inhibition, and error correction were needed to understand how to support strategy generation for skill acquisition – beyond simply providing multiple opportunities for practice and repetition. Assessment was used to understand the nature of Jacob's difficulties and potential mechanisms underpinning Jacob's motor impairments. This was important to help scaffold and shape his learning experience in a fun and meaningful manner. Jacob had the opportunity to participate in a 2-week summer day camp, following principles of motor learning and incorporating the learning of magic tricks to assist problem-solving and perspective-taking. The task-focussed evidenced-based intervention set in a group context had a long-term value for Jacob with the acquisition of new friends as well as new skills.

SUMMARY

Motor coordination is a complex dynamic skill involving multiple factors interacting with a person's capabilities, the task requirements, and environmental influences. Transactional influences between the person, task, and environment are implicit processes in learning. They reinforce learning, or negatively impact upon this, to support translation of learning to wider contexts. Unpicking these various elements during assessments and intervention is difficult, especially when trying to determine skills and capacities set against experiences and expectations. Ascertaining whether there is a significant difference in developmental trajectories involves the triangulation of information from multiple sources.

Assessments may assist diagnosis of motor capacity and performance and determine the impact on activity and participation in everyday life which also enable consideration of modifications to environmental factors to scaffold supports for learning. Other tools may provide more specific information on body functions such as spasticity or weakness. All of these have some pros and cons and the selection of assessments should be determined by the presenting concerns, particularly those of the child. Importantly, the context and ecological validity of assessments used should ensure these relate to age-appropriate everyday activities.

Intervention planning should keep in central focus the goals and needs of the child within their family and environmental contexts. Evidence for task-focussed interventions targeting skill performance and participation in meaningful tasks and situations supersedes those for component-based programmes directed to specific body functions.

Further research is needed to develop assessments which help us understand the mechanisms underpinning the motor impairments in order to design person-specific, task-focussed, evidenced-based interventions that have long term value for children in the contexts in which they need to perform and which matter to them in their daily lives.

REFERENCES

Ayres AJ (1972) *Sensory Integration and Learning Disorders*. Los Angeles, CA: Western Psychological Services.

Blank R, Barnett AL, Cairney J et al. (2019) International clinical practice recommendations on the definition, diagnosis, assessment, intervention and psycho-social aspects of Developmental Coordination Disorders. *Developmental Medicine and Child Neurology* **61**: 242–285. doi. org/10.1111/dmcn.14132.

Eliasson AC, Krumlinde-Sundholm L, Rösblad B et al. (2006) The Manual Ability Classification System (MACS) for children with cerebral palsy: Scale development and evidence of validity and reliability. *Developmental Medicine and Child Neurology* **48**: 549–554.

Farr WJ, Green D, Bremner S et al. (2019) Feasibility of a randomised controlled trial to evaluate home-based virtual reality therapy in children with cerebral palsy. *Disability Rehabilitation* **43**(1): 85–97.

Gesell A, Ilg, FL, Ames LB (1977) *The Child From Five to Ten, Revised Edition.* New York: Harper & Row.

Gimeno H, Brown RG, Lin JP, Cornelius V, Polatajko HJ (2019) Cognitive approach to rehabilitation in children with hyperkinetic movement disorders post-DBS. *Neurology* **92**: e1212–e1224.

Green D (2006) *A Qualitative and Quantitative Study of the Nature of Developmental Coordination Disorder* (Doctoral dissertation, University of Leeds).

Green D, Chambers ME, Sugden DA (2008) Does subtype of developmental coordination disorder count: Is there a differential effect on outcome following intervention? *Human Movement Science* **27**(2): 363–382.

Green D, Schertz M, Gordon A et al. (2013) A multi-site study of functional outcomes following a themed approach to hand–arm bimanual intensive therapy for children with hemiplegia. *Developmental Medicine and Child Neurology* **55**(6): 527–533.

Hadders-Algra M (2010) *Neurological Examination of the Child With Minor Neurological Dysfunction.* London: Mac Keith Press.

Hill EL, Wing AM (1999) Coordination of grip force and load force in developmental coordination disorder: A case study. *Neurocase* **5**: 537–544.

Kwakkel G, Veerbee JM, van Wegen EE, Wolf SL (2015) Constraint-induced movement therapy after stroke. *Lancet Neurology* **14**: 224–234.

Lage GM, Ugrinowitsch H, Apolinário-Souza T, Vieira MM, Albuquerque MR, Benda RN (2015) Repetition and variation in motor practice: A review of neural correlates. *Neuroscience & Biobehavioral Reviews* **57**: 132–141.

Leisman G, Braun-Benjamin O, Melillo R (2014) Cognitive-motor interactions of the basal ganglia in development. *Frontiers in Systems Neuroscience* **8**: 16.

Mayston MJ, Harrison LM, Stephens JA (1999) A neurophysiological study of mirror movements in adults and children. *Annals of Neurology* **45**: 583–594.

Minoliti R, Crepaldi M, Antonietti A (2020) Identifying developmental motor difficulties: A review of tests to assess motor coordination in children. *Journal of Functional Morphology and Kinesiology* **5**: 16.

Novak I, Mcintyre S, Morgan C et al. (2013) A systematic review of interventions for children with cerebral palsy: State of the evidence. *Developmental Medicine and Child Neurology* **55**: 885–910.

Novak I, Morgan C, Fahey M et al. (2020) State of the evidence traffic lights 2019: Systematic review of interventions for preventing and treating children with cerebral palsy. *Current Neurology and Neuroscience Reports* **20**: 1–21.

Palisano RJ, Cameron D, Rosenbaum PL, Walter SD, Russell D (2006) Stability of the gross motor function classification system. *Developmental Medicine and Child Neurology* **48**(6): 424–428.

Rudisch J, Butler J, Izadi H et al. (2016) Kinematic parameters of hand movement during a disparate bimanual movement task in children with unilateral Cerebral Palsy. *Human Movement Science* **46**: 239–250.

Solnik S, Pazin N, Coelho CJ et al. (2013) End-state comfort and joint configuration variance during reaching. *Experimental Brain Research* **225**: 431–442.

Steenbergen B, Meulenbroek RG, Rosenbaum DA (2004) Constraints on grip selection in hemiparetic cerebral palsy: Effects of lesional side, end-point accuracy, and context. *Cognitive Brain Research* **19**: 145–159.

Sternad D, editor (2009) *Progress in Motor Control*. Boston, MA: Springer US. doi: 10.1007/978-0-387-77064-2.

Sugden D, Wade MG (2019) *Movement Difficulties in Developmental Disorders: Practical Guidelines for Assessment and Management*. London: Mac Keith Press.

Thelen E, Smith LB (1994) *A Dynamic Systems Approach to the Development of Cognition and Action*. London: The MIT Press.

Vinçon S, Green D, Blank R, Jenetzky E (2017) Ecological validity of the German Bruininks-Oseretsky Test of Motor Proficiency – 2nd Edition. *Human Movement Science* **53**: 45–54.

Weinstein M, Green D, Rudisch J et al. (2018) Understanding the relationship between brain and upper limb function in children with unilateral motor impairments: A multimodal approach. *European Journal of Paediatric Neurology* **22**: 143–154. doi.org/10.1016/j.ejpn.2017.09.012.

WHO (2007) *International Classification of Functioning, Disability and Health: Children and Youth Version: ICF-CY*. Geneva: World Health Organization.

Zielinski IM, Green D, Rudisch J, Jongsma ML, Aarts PB, Steenbergen B (2017) The relation between mirror movements and non-use of the affected hand in children with unilateral cerebral palsy. *Developmental Medicine and Child Neurology* **59**: 152–159.

CHAPTER 5

Language

Anne Hoffmann, Karen Riley, and Christina Hawkins

Presenting Concern

Ryan is an 8-year-old boy enrolled in Year 3 at a mainstream primary school. A language evaluation was completed in response to concerns regarding his academic progress, attention in class, and engagement with peers. His parents note that Ryan often struggles to express his ideas clearly and sometimes seems to forget or misunderstand what they have said to him.

Ryan was born at term but sustained a perinatal stroke during his first week of life. Magnetic resonance imaging indicated an infarct in a cortical branch of the middle cerebral artery, with the lesion located in the left temporo-parietal junction. Ryan experienced seizures in the perinatal period but has remained seizure free since this time. His communication history was significant for language development delay. Whilst he babbled prior to his first birthday, he did not use his first word until 18 months and only used 20 words consistently at 24 months. There were no concerns regarding hearing or early social communication skills.

Ryan was referred to speech and language therapy during his preschool years due to his medical history and receptive and expressive language delay. He made good progress, although his language skills, both receptive and expressive, remained slightly behind his peers.

At referral, Ryan's teacher noted he had trouble with early literacy skills and was placed in an at-risk reading group. In Year 1, he continued to have difficulty keeping pace with other students in reading. He had trouble following complex directions and sometimes responded incorrectly when questions were posed to him. His vocabulary range was slightly weaker compared to peers. Currently, his teacher reports that his responses tend to be poorly organised and he struggles to understand and produce more complex narratives, both verbally and in writing. He does not seem to retain instructions or get the bigger picture from in-class reading assignments and is falling further behind the other students.

Ryan has remained in good health and his parents' primary concern is his ability to keep pace with the academic curriculum. Ryan's teachers also report a growing tendency for Ryan to isolate himself from his peers. Ryan was referred for a neuropsychological assessment in order to understand his language and academic needs in the context of his early medical history and wider cognitive development. A detailed language assessment was requested to better understand Ryan's communication profile and guide intervention approaches.

THEORY

Language Development

Communication is fundamental to interaction. In typical development, language abilities develop without direct instruction or teaching. Infants are able to perceive sound contrasts from all spoken languages, with a narrowing of contrasts specific to their native language occurring at 6 to 12 months. Comprehension of first words typically occurs around 8 to 10 months with first words spoken around 10 to 20 months and two-word utterances around 18 to 24 months. During this time, children learn how to use communication for different functions (e.g. requesting, protesting), a component of pragmatic language. Sentence complexity, vocabulary range, use of narratives, and an understanding of the social rules of language continue to develop throughout childhood and adolescence.

Classification of Language Impairments

Language difficulties may be developmental or acquired (Bishop et al. 2016). The term 'developmental language disorder' (DLD) describes a persistent language disorder without a known biomedical aetiology. A comorbid diagnosis (e.g. attention-deficit/hyperactivity disorder), however, may be present (see Figure 5.1 for pathways to language disorder diagnosis outlined by Bishop et al. 2017). Some children are likely to 'catch up' with peers during early childhood, whilst others will experience a persistent pattern of language difficulty, particularly when receptive language skills are affected. Where a persistent language impairment exists secondary to another developmental disorder or acquired brain injury, a diagnosis of 'language disorder' is given (e.g. language disorder associated with autism spectrum disorder/acquired brain injury). Children with acquired difficulties can present with variable or uneven language profiles and trajectories, depending on the underlying cause and nature of the injury, as well as the impact of other acquired or premorbid conditions. The long-term impact of language impairment on areas such as literacy, mental health, employment, and peer relationships has been recognised (Law et al. 2009; Conti-Ramsden et al. 2013), thus highlighting the importance of early identification, diagnosis, and intervention. Paediatric neuropsychologists will include speech and language evaluation in their hypotheses-driven assessments, although more detailed assessments may be carried out by speech and language therapists. The role of the neuropsychologist is likely to evaluate speech and language in relation to other areas of function and how these

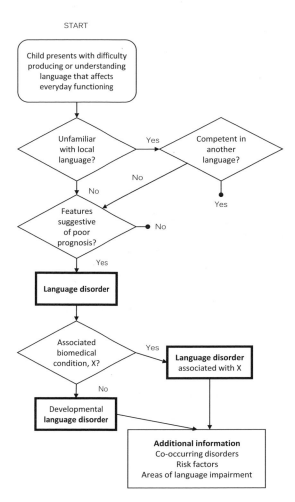

Figure 5.1 Flow chart illustrating pathways to diagnosis of language disorder. Numbers in square brackets refer to results in the Bishop et al. study and can be ignored here. Reproduced with permission from Bishop et al. (2017).

relate to brain injury or development. Bearing in mind that challenges that emerge with speech and language development may also include written language, social cognition, and attention.

Aetiology of Language Impairments

Identification of possible causes of DLD and language disorder includes exploring neurological, genetic, and environment factors. Neuroimaging studies are developing understanding of neural language networks and include exploration of ventral

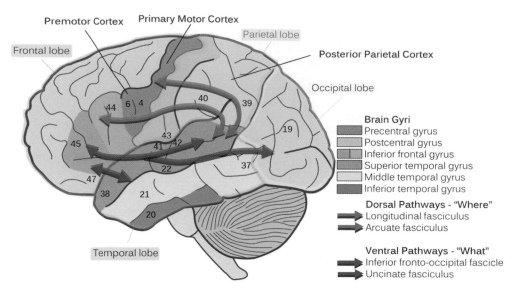

Figure 5.2 Cortical regions and white matter pathways involved in language. (A colour version of this figure can be seen in the colour plate section)

and dorsal pathways connecting the language centres of the prefrontal and temporal lobes (see Figure 5.2). The ventral pathway supports semantic skills and basic syntactic processes and may play a key role in early language development. The dorsal pathway supports phonological and syntactic processing as well as working memory. Although one dorsal stream is observable from infancy, a second longer dorsal stream is thought to mature later in childhood and could therefore be involved in more complex linguistic processing (Friederici 2012). There is growing research into underlying brain structures that might differ for individuals with DLD (De Fossé et al. 2004), with consensus that the expected left lateralisation for language functioning is reduced in this population, although cause of the impairment is a matter of debate (Bishop 2013).

In acquired language disorders, damage to the language network or associated areas can impact language development in different ways and be dependent on factors such as age, severity of injury, and/or presentation of comorbidities. For example dorsal stream damage following perinatal stroke can lead to weaker abilities in sentence repetition (Northam et al. 2018), a marker associated with language impairment in the wider population (Conti-Ramsden et al. 2003). The capacity for complete or partial inter- or intrahemispheric reorganisation of language has been well documented, particularly for children with early-acquired left hemisphere lesions (Tillema et al. 2008). Such reorganisation can lead to the sparing of language function, although due to possible 'crowding' effects, other areas of cognitive function may be negatively impacted (Kim et al. 2018).

Core Components of Language

As language encompasses multiple skills (e.g. grammar, vocabulary, interactions) and modalities (e.g. spoken, gestural, written, and augmentative/alternative) it is helpful to view it as form, content, and use.

Form

Form of language includes syntax (the rules underlying how sentences are formed), morphology (the rules underlying how words are formed), and phonology (the rules underlying how sounds can combine). Morphosyntax is the intersection of morphology and syntax and can be summarised as the grammar of language. Morphosyntax is the most frequent area of deficit for English-speaking children with DLD and a key feature of language disorders associated with another condition. Children may omit obligatory grammatical markers in spontaneous speech (e.g. past tense –ed) past the age when mistakes are expected. They may struggle with more complicated verb structures as well as using longer, more complex phrases. Children may also have impaired comprehension of different grammatical forms and complex syntax.

Content

Content is the semantic component of language, including both vocabulary knowledge and general world knowledge. Children with DLD have significantly reduced vocabularies, both receptively and expressively, that may stem from difficulty in learning new words (Jackson, Leitao, and Claessen 2016). Children with acquired language disorders can also present with lexical difficulties and patterns of severity and recovery are often dependent on the cause or nature of neurological insult. Word retrieval difficulties can be present in both developmental and acquired disorders and may relate to weaker semantic or phonological representations, disruptions to lexical access, and cognitive difficulties, such as slower information processing speed (Messer and Dockrell 2006).

Use

Use is the pragmatic component of language (i.e. social communication). Pragmatic language includes being able to match your speaking style to your audience, knowing when it is appropriate to speak, how much you should say about a subject, as well as nonverbal aspects such as body language. The foundational pragmatic skills appear early, with infants learning to pay attention to what adults are referencing (i.e. joint attention) and grow in complexity. For some children, pragmatic language difficulties may relate to a diagnosis of autism spectrum disorder or occur due to an acquired brain injury. For children with DLD, however, pragmatic language skills have been described as immature as opposed to atypical. Adolescents with DLD report having difficulty with peer relationships, despite self-reporting as being pro-social (Conti-Ramsden et al. 2013). Impairments in pragmatic language may also be affected by comorbid cognitive difficulties (e.g. processing speed) on areas such as verbal discourse or social interaction.

Relationship to Cognitive and Language Domains

The above three areas of language are each essential for successful communication, but children with language impairments frequently have weaknesses in other cognitive domains. Deficits in executive function, including inhibition, working memory, and attention control, are documented in the literature for children with DLD (Tomas and Vissers 2019). Bishop et al. (2014) demonstrate this interplay by describing a three-stream model in which (1) executive function is affected by language function; (2) language function is affected by executive function; and (3) an external factor influences both executive and language function independently. Tomas and Vissers (2019) review the impact of executive functions on language and social interaction, highlighting possible associations with auditory perception, attention control, inhibition, flexibility, and working memory. In addition, studies have reported that children with DLD can be impaired in both verbal and nonverbal domains of working memory, suggesting the association between DLD and working memory is domain-general rather than specific to auditory processes (Vugs et al. 2013). The relationship between language and literacy, including reading comprehension, is also well documented (see Chapter 14). Whilst relationships between higher-level cognition and language impairment remain an area of debate, these underlying deficits, alongside other comorbidities, such as attention-deficit/hyperactivity disorder or autism spectrum disorder, are likely to contribute to the outward manifestation of language impairment and should be taken into account in assessment and intervention planning.

ASSESSMENT AND FORMULATION

Methods of Assessment

Assessment of language presents multiple challenges, one of which is the wide spectrum of areas that may be affected. A speech-language professional must look at language skills over a variety of contexts bearing in mind that children frequently perform differently in testing situations. A comprehensive language assessment should include, at minimum: norm-referenced standardised assessment, language/communication sample, and caregiver report. Hearing evaluation and oral-mechanism examination should also be completed (see Chapters 6 and 10). Understanding the unique developmental strengths and challenges of an individual with either DLD or language disorder is imperative to determining appropriate educational placements and intervention plans. By utilising multiple assessment methods, clinicians can provide a thorough understanding of language functioning across contexts and interaction partners, which increases accuracy and precision of the diagnostic process.

COMMUNICATION HISTORY

A developmental and communication history is crucial to understanding the nature of an individual's language difficulties. Questions relating to family history, early development, and medical or developmental needs can aid the identification of possible co-occurring or contributing factors. Teacher interviews are important for understanding how language difficulties may impact academic and social functioning.

STANDARDISED ASSESSMENT

A comprehensive, norm-referenced assessment using a psychometrically sound measure provides a comparison of an individual's overall language to that of same-aged peers, which is helpful for documenting progress, understanding the child's profile, and guiding services (see Table 5.1). Whilst some children will present with an impairment across all areas of language, others may show an uneven pattern of development or a difficulty

Table 5.1 Examples of standardised language assessments/questionnaires

	Age range (y or y:mo)	Format	Key areas assessed
Clinical Evaluation of Language Fundamentals, Fifth Edition (CELF-5)	5–21	Direct assessment Picture-based Digital and nondigital formats	Receptive language Expressive language Language structure Language content Language memory Pragmatic language
Clinical Evaluation of Language Fundamentals Preschool-3 (CELF Preschool-3)	3–6:11	Direct assessment Picture based Digital and nondigital formats	Receptive language Expressive language Language structure Language content
Preschool Language Scales, Fifth Edition (PLS-5)	0–7	Direct assessment Object and picture based	Preverbal/interaction skills Auditory comprehension Expressive communication
British Picture Vocabulary Scale, Third Edition (BPVS-3)	3–16	Direct assessment Picture based	Receptive vocabulary
Expressive Vocabulary Test, Third Edition (EVT-3)	2:6–90+	Direct assessment Picture based Digital and nondigital formats	Expressive vocabulary
Children's Communication Checklist, Second Edition (CCC-2)	4–16	70-item questionnaire for school and/or parents.	Screen for language and communication problems

that affects only specific domains of language functioning. Assessments can be selected and tailored to provide a broad overview or target key areas of language function. In addition to the tests described in Table 5.1, which are those most commonly used by speech and language therapists, paediatric neuropsychologists may also draw on the receptive and language subtests included in measures of intellectual function such as the Wechsler Intelligence Scale for Children, Fifth Edition, Wechsler Preschool & Primary Scale of Intelligence, Fourth Edition, Bayley Scales of Infant and Toddler Development, Fourth Edition or other more academic focused batteries such as the Wechsler Individual Achievement Test, Fourth Edition.

QUESTIONNAIRES

Standard questionnaire instruments allow understanding of language performance across a range of contexts. Parents, teachers, and others who know the child well are valuable sources and can provide information regarding aspects of language that are difficult to assess in a clinic. This is especially useful for those individuals who perform well in a very structured environment but struggle with communication in 'real-life' scenarios. Equally, for some children, participating in standardised assessments can be a stressful experience and may have a depressing effect on performance and, by extension, scores. Questionnaires can assist in confirming or disproving opinions formed during the evaluation process.

COMMUNICATION SAMPLE

A communication sample provides information about the functionality of a child's language. For younger children and those still developing early language skills, a communication sample would include observations about any vocalisations and gestures used, as well as how the individual interacts with people and objects. Response to simple requests and reciprocity in interactions would also be noted. It may be more effective for the parent or caregiver to act as a communication partner with very young children. For children with more language skills, the language sample can take place during a joint play activity that the clinician has engineered to provide communication opportunities (e.g. providing toys that require adult assistance). School-age children and older individuals can participate in a conversation or provide a retelling of a story or movie. If permitted, it can be very helpful to audio or video record to allow for a precise observation and transcription. Transcriptions can provide information about multiple areas of language, including vocabulary, grammar, and interaction skills.

AUTHENTIC ASSESSMENT

In response to challenges associated with standardised assessments the practice of authentic assessment has emerged. This asset-oriented process to evaluating children in their natural environments has been utilised effectively, particularly in early childhood, and is particularly important for young children with significant delays. Capabilities and needs are evaluated through observation of children within familiar settings and with familiar individuals engaging in everyday activities, and includes information from a variety of sources including parents, other caregivers, teachers, and other professionals. These approaches allow children to demonstrate their knowledge, skills, dispositions, and other aspects of development by solving naturally occurring problems, interacting, and talking with individuals, and acting on and experimenting in their environments (Riley, Miller, and Sorenson 2016).

Further Assessment Considerations

Individuals with severe language impairment may perform below the lowest standard score (i.e. floor effect), which limits their usefulness in characterising level of function. Floor effects can be particularly problematic for progress monitoring as small and incremental gains may not be noted. Comparison of raw scores over time or the use of more informal assessment approaches may be more valuable in these cases. Informal assessment might involve evaluating a child's ability to follow instructions that vary in length or complexity or analysing a child's language and interaction skills during picture description tasks, conversation, or play-based activities. Consideration must also be given to the possible impact of other areas of cognitive difficulty. For example executive function difficulties may impact on areas of language processing, such as the ability to inhibit or select words or organise sentences or sequence narratives. Demands on areas such as working memory, processing speed, literacy, attention, inhibition, or planning should also be identified when selecting tasks and interpreting results. Comorbidities should be evaluated as part of an overall formulation and considered in both assessment and intervention planning.

INTERVENTION AND MANAGEMENT

Intervention Approaches

Intervention for developmental or acquired language disorders should be specific to the needs of individuals and informed by detailed assessment. It is likely that the delivery of intervention may be with a speech and language therapist but knowledge of the evidence base in addition to availability of treatment within the local community is important in meeting the needs of the child. In general, the goal(s) of interventions may include removing the underlying cause and normalise language, modifying the disorder by teaching new language behaviours or increasing the frequency of language behaviours, teaching compensatory strategies, or modifying the environment to make the child's communication more successful. Interventions for children with acquired language difficulties may focus on rebuilding areas of language following a loss of skills or regression, alongside teaching compensatory skills and supporting the child's communication environment (e.g. through training for schools or communication part-ners). For all children, the focus and design of the intervention should be established in collaboration with the child, parents/caregivers, and school to ensure targets are functional and effective.

For very young children (birth to 3 years), the focus of intervention is often on teach-ing parents how to best foster communication development. Significant research has demonstrated the benefits of parent responsivity training for children with language disorders (Roberts and Kaiser 2011).

For preschool children, nurseries and early learning centres are frequently the principal setting for interventions, which often include working on basic communication principles. For example increasing utterance length (form) and vocabulary comprehension and use (content) are common goals. Pragmatic language (use) may involve using language for a variety of functions as well as the basics of taking turns during an activity. Play should still be the primary vehicle for intervention, and most preschool classrooms are structured in a manner to make this possible.

There are multiple service delivery options for speech-language intervention with school-aged children and consideration should be given to supporting generalisation of skills from therapy sessions into real-life situations. Therapy approaches may include: one-to-one or small group sessions targeting specific areas of language function, working with the student in the classroom to provide necessary scaffolding to reach a goal, co-treating with other professionals, or providing consultation or training to other individuals on the child's team.

As children begin functioning more independently in primary school and beyond, two key areas of language need are academics and social situations. Form and content reflect the growing curricular demands, sentences within verbal teaching and task instructions are becoming longer with more complicated morphosyntax, and vocabulary becomes more specialised. This results in a greater need for interventions that are focused on curricular needs of students (Balthazar and Scott 2015). By observing the student in the classroom and involving the teacher in the process, goals relevant to daily tasks can be developed. For example if the student struggles presenting information in an organ-ised manner in class, intervention should work on developing a template for forming a cohesive response. Similarly, deficits in receptive and expressive language can be chosen based on their impact on the student's functioning during the school day.

For many children, one-to-one or group sessions can be introduced to focus on specific areas of language deficit and practise compensatory skills. Intervention packages have also been established that target functional communication and pragmatic language, with activities such as social skills groups, video modelling, and role-playing enabling students to both learn what 'should' happen in social situations and then practise them in everyday settings.

Evidence-Based Practice

Although a developing area of research, there continues to be a lack of high-quality evidence on the effectiveness of language interventions, including limited studies on the impact of frequency, duration, or intensity of therapy. A Cochrane Review, involving a meta-analysis of 25 randomised controlled trials of speech-language therapy interventions (Law et al. 2003), highlighted evidence for the effectiveness of phonological and vocabulary interventions and mixed evidence for interventions targeting expressive syntax. Little evidence was available for receptive language interventions.

The movement toward further developing evidence-based practice is of key importance in demonstrating the clinical and functional effectiveness of interventions and indicating appropriate levels of support required for each child. Within clinical practice, interventions should be informed by the integration of published research, clinical expertise (e.g. professional consensus or position statements), and service-user preferences (e.g. Patient and Public Involvement activity). Databases such as The Communication Trust's 'What Works', provided a useful tool for clinicians to review the evidence relating to specific areas of language deficit (https://www.thecommunicationtrust.org.uk/whatworks).

The need for further research is recognised and intervention studies continue to strengthen the evidence base and inform clinical practice. For example randomised control trials have demonstrated the effectiveness of 'Shape Coding' on improving aspects of grammar and sentence structure for secondary-school aged children with language impairment (Ebbels et al. 2014). This approach, designed for school-aged children, uses colours and symbols as a visual 'code' to *show* sentence structure (syntax) and link it to meaning (semantics). A recent systematic review of vocabulary interventions for adolescents with language disorder also provided tentative evidence for the effectiveness of using combined phonological and semantic approaches to target this area (Lowe et al. 2018). Evidence for narrative interventions is also documented in small scale studies that demonstrate some improvements post-intervention (e.g. Swanson et al. 2005).

Outcome

On assessment, Ryan's receptive language score was in the low average range, but specific subtests fell within the mildly impaired range, particularly those that required understanding of more complicated syntax. Classroom observation showed that Ryan found it difficult to sustain attention when his teacher gave long verbal instructions or if visual supports were not included in the lesson. Ryan reported that his difficulties impacted on his ability to follow conversations with peers. Expressively, Ryan scored well on a sentence formulation task but showed mild difficulties in sentence repetition and narrative formation. In the language sample, Ryan frequently inserted extra 'fillers' or would revise his sentence after starting it. Overall, the assessment revealed a mild receptive and expressive language disorder and Ryan qualified for speech-language services at school.

Following Ryan's assessment, his clinician met with his parents and teacher to discuss his strengths and needs and plan interventions. The team noted that Ryan had made a good recovery from his early stroke and showed nonverbal abilities in the average range on cognitive assessment. It was discussed that, whilst many children do not present with language difficulties following perinatal stroke, some children can experience ongoing language needs. In Ryan's case, his mild receptive and expressive language disorder was impacting particularly on his literacy skills and understanding in class. There was also a secondary impact on his attention in class and conversations with peers. A multilayered intervention approach was planned to include: (1) weekly group sessions focusing on understanding complex sentences and constructing narratives; (2) classroom strategies to support his understanding in class (e.g. pre-teaching vocabulary, 'chunking' verbal information, incorporated visual resources to aid processing of information) and develop his ability to use his own strategies (e.g. to seek help, ask for repetition); and (3) whole class approaches to develop Ryan's interactions with peers through supported activities focusing on shared interests and hobbies.

With these supports in place, Ryan was able to better access information and he showed improvements in his use of more complex language structures, attention in class, and interactions with peers. He was able to access support when he found lessons or situations difficult. Ryan's parents and teachers report that he is doing well and continuing to benefit from classroom strategies and targeted language interventions.

SUMMARY

Working with an individual with language disorder provides clinicians an opportunity to use knowledge across the lifespan. The presentation of language impairment shifts with age and requires clinicians to be aware of issues that may arise as language demands increase. An early goal may focus on the ability to request wants and needs, whereas later goals may shift to comprehension of information text, use of compensatory strategies, and interactions with peers. It is the responsibility of the clinician to accurately assess and treat those areas in the manner most appropriate for the specific client considering current evidence-based practice.

Further research is required into the aetiology of language disorders and effective interventions for this population. The heterogeneity of language disorders requires the clinician to provide an individualised approach to assessment and monitor interventions over time as the child's presentation changes or develops.

A key aspect of working with individuals with language impairments is collaboration across the multidisciplinary team. Parents/caregivers, teachers, neuropsychologists, speech language clinicians, and other specialists play an important part in each step of the identification, assessment, and intervention process. Involving the child in goal setting and intervention planning is important to facilitate their engagement in the intervention process. A collaborative approach helps place a child's language difficulties in the context of their cognitive skills or underlying medical condition and enhances understanding of both the functional impact of the impairment and the demands of the current communication environment. A neuropsychological evaluation can give particular insight into potential areas of weakness, such as low working memory ability, that may be associated with or impact language and academic outcomes.

REFERENCES

Balthazar C, Scott C (2015) The place of syntax in school-age language assessment and intervention. In: TA Ukraintetz, editor, *School-Age Language Intervention: Evidence-Based Practices*. Austin, TX: Pro-Ed, pp. 279–334.

Bishop D (2013) Cerebral asymmetry and language development: Cause, correlate, or consequence? *Science* 340(6138): 1230531.

Bishop D, Nation K, Patterson K (2014) When words fail us: Insights into language processing from developmental and acquired disorders. *Philosophical Transactions of the Royal Society B.* 369: 20120403.

Bishop D, Snowling MJ, Thompson PA, Greenhalgh T (2016) CATALISE: A multinational and multidisciplinary Delphi consensus study. Identifying language impairments in children. *PLOS One* 11(7): e0158753.

Bishop DV, Snowling MJ, Thompson PA, Greenhalgh T (2017) Phase 2 of CATALISE: A multinational and multidisciplinary Delphi consensus study of problems with language development: Terminology. *Journal of Child Psychology and Psychiatry* 58(10): 1068–1080.

Conti-Ramsden G, Botting N, Faragher B (2003) Psycholinguistic markers for specific language impairment (SLI). *Journal of Child Psychology and Psychiatry* 42(6): 741–748.

Conti-Ramsden G, Mok PL, Pickles A, Durkin K (2013) Adolescents with a history of specific language impairment (SLI): Strengths and difficulties in social, emotional and behavioral functioning. *Research in Developmental Disabilities* 34(11): 4161–4169.

De Fossé L, Hodge SM, Makris N et al. (2004) Language-association cortex asymmetry in autism and specific language impairment. *Annals of Neurology: Official Journal of the American Neurological Association and the Child Neurology Society* 56(6): 757–766.

Ebbels SH, Marić N, Murphy A, Turner G (2014) Improving comprehension in adolescents with severe receptive language impairments: A randomized control trial of intervention for coordinating conjunctions. *International Journal of Language and Communication Disorders* 49(1): 30–48.

Friederici AD (2012) Language development and the ontogeny of the dorsal pathway. *Frontiers in Evolutionary Neurosciences* 4: 3.

Friederici AD, Gierhan SME (2013) The language network. *Current Opinion in Neurobiology* 23(2): 250–254.

Jackson E, Leitao S, Claessen M (2016) The relationship between phonological short-term memory, receptive vocabulary, and fast mapping in children with specific language impairment. *International Journal of Language & Communication Disorders* 51(1): 61–73.

Kim J-A, Jeong J-W, Luat A, Chugani HT (2018) Metabolic correlates of cognitive function in children with unilateral Sturge–Weber syndrome: Evidence for regional functional reorganization and crowding. *Human Brain Mapping* 39(4): 1596–1606.

Law J, Rush R, Schoon I, Parsons S (2009) Modeling developmental language difficulties from school entry into adulthood: Literacy, mental health, and employment outcomes. *Journal of Speech Language and Hearing Research* 52(6): 1401–1416.

Law J, Garrett Z, Nye C (2003) Speech and language therapy interventions for children with primary speech and language delay or disorder. *Cochrane Database Syst Rev* 3: CD004110.

Lowe H, Henry L, Müller LM, Joffe VL (2018) Vocabulary intervention for adolescents with language disorder: a systematic review. *International Journal of Language & Communication Disorders* 53(2): 199–217.

Messer D, Dockrell J (2006) Children's naming and word-finding difficulties: Descriptions and explanations. *Journal of Speech, Language, and Hearing Research* **49**: 309–324.

Northam GB, Adler S, Eschmann KCJ, Chong WK, Cowan FM, Baldeweg T (2018) Developmental conduction aphasia after neonatal stroke. *Annals of Neurology* **83**(4): 664–675.

Riley K, Miller GL, Sorenson C (2016) Early childhood authentic and performance-based assessment. In: Garro A, editor, *Early Childhood Assessment in School and Clinical Psychology*, 1st edition. New York: Springer Publishing, pp. 95–117.

Roberts MY, Kaiser AP (2011) The effectiveness of parent-implemented language interventions: A meta-analysis. *American Journal of Speech-Language Pathology* **20**: 180–199.

Swanson LA, Fey ME, Mills CE, Hood LS (2005) Use of narrative-based language intervention with children who have specific language impairment. *American Journal of Speech-Language Pathology* **14**(2): 131–143.

Tomas E, Vissers C (2019) Behind the scenes of developmental language disorder: Time to call neuropsychology back on stage. *Frontiers in Human Neuroscience* **12**: 517.

Tillema JM, Byars AW, Jacola LM et al. (2008) Cortical reorganization of language functioning following perinatal left MCA stroke. *Brain and Language* **105**: 99–111.

Vugs B, Cuperus J, Hendriks M, Verhoeven L (2013) Visuospatial working memory in specific language impairment: A meta- analysis. *Research in Developmental Disabilities* **34**: 2586–2597.

CHAPTER 6

Speech

Frédérique Liégeois and Angela Morgan

Presenting Concern

Anisha is a 10-year-old girl currently attending mainstream school. She was referred to speech and language therapy and neuropsychology services primarily because of communication difficulties, but also due to suspected learning difficulties. Her speech is unclear, sounds slurred, and the volume of her voice is very quiet. In addition, she is hesitant to interact verbally with peers, relatives, and teachers. As a result, she has been withdrawing from her peer group. Anisha lives at home with her two older brothers and parents. One of her brothers has a diagnosis of attention-deficit/hyperactivity disorder. Her parents are concerned Anisha is becoming socially isolated and is not coping well within mainstream education.

At home, Anisha enjoys reading for pleasure. She also enjoys throwing a netball by herself in the yard but does not enjoy playing team sports as she does not like having to call out for the ball.

At school, Anisha struggles to make herself understood when speaking. She works well in groups but tends not to say much. She cannot complete classroom tasks on time. When given maths and English written tasks, she takes much more time than her peers and as a result fails to finish the tasks. The teachers think she may need specialist support due to learning difficulties.

Anisha's main personal concerns are frustration when communicating with peers and that teachers think she is not smart.

Developmental history shows Anisha was born at term after an uneventful pregnancy. She had an unremarkable development and reached milestones at typical ages. At the age of 5 years, however, she was involved in a road traffic accident and struck by a car as a pedestrian in a supermarket car park. She lost consciousness for 30 minutes and had a computerised tomography scan at the local hospital. The computerised tomography scan showed bilateral foci of hypointensity of the brainstem and motor cortex (implying damage to the corticobulbar tract). After 2 months she was discharged as she recovered well and did not develop seizures. Her parents noticed her speech was not clear and she struggled to hold a pen in her right hand. There are no ongoing health concerns.

THEORY

Speech Development

In the first year of life, speech development follows typical milestones from babbling to single sounds to sound clusters (see Kuhl 2004). By age 8 years, most speech sounds can be pronounced by most children, with individual variability in the acquisition and mastery of speech sounds (McLeod, Crowe, and Shahaeian 2015). There are speech sound error patterns that 10% or more of the general population produce under the age of 6 years (e.g. 'gliding' as when /w/ is substituted for /r/ as in 'wabbit' for 'rabbit'). A small percentage of children use atypical sound patterns (e.g. sound preference substitution where children replace all initial consonants with a preferred sound such as /n/). Children who use atypical sound patterns during the preschool years are at an increased risk of having persistent speech errors (Morgan et al. 2017).

Classification of Speech Disorders

Speech sound disorders affect the naturalness, quality, or precision of speech production in one or several domains, namely respiration, phonation, articulation, prosody, and resonance. Current classifications of speech sound disorders (Dodd 2014; see Fig. 6.1) are based on these speech features but not neuroscientific evidence, due to our poor understanding of their brain bases. For intervention planning, it is particularly important to discriminate language-based *phonological disorders* (errors are

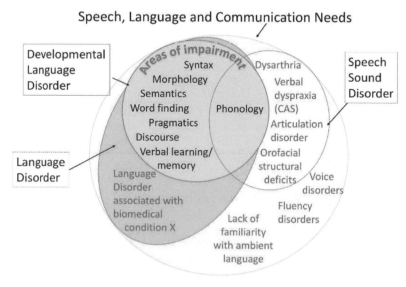

Figure 6.1 Venn diagram of speech and language disorders. Reused from Bishop et al. (2016). This figure is licensed under the Creative Commons Attribution 4.0 International (CC BY 4.0) license (https://creativecommons.org/licenses/by/4.0/).

rule-based and effect types of sounds – please see Chapter 5 for more detail) from *articulation disorders* (errors are motor-based, such as distortion of the sound /s/) (Bishop et al. 2016).

Under the category of motor speech disorders, childhood apraxia of speech (CAS or verbal dyspraxia; ASHA 2007) is hypothesised to be rooted in planning/programming difficulties, while dysarthria is typically seen as an 'execution' disorder (Liégeois et al. 2013). Dysarthria results from impairment of the central or peripheral nervous system that involves the control of neuromuscular tone and coordination. Dysarthria affects the motor production of speech sounds in isolation as well as in sequences. The strength, speed, range, steadiness, tone, or accuracy of speech sounds can be affected. By contrast, CAS is characterised by three core features (1) inconsistent speech sound errors across the same target words (e.g. upi, umba, ubella across three productions of 'umbrella'); (2) impaired coarticulatory transitions manifest in features such as groping to produce speech sounds or reducing the number of syllables in a word (e.g. disa for dinosaur); and (3) prosodic impairments (e.g. producing words with equal stress or incorrect stress; ASHA 2007). Whilst these conditions can exist in isolation, CAS and dysarthria can co-occur (Liégeois and Morgan 2012).

The Brain Basis of Speech Motor Control

Functional magnetic resonance imaging studies of overt speech have revealed a speech network that partly overlaps with other types of motor control (e.g. supplementary motor area, somatosensory cortex, premotor and motor cortices, striatum, and cerebellum). Language regions are also involved due to the necessary links between the speech and linguistic systems (inferior frontal, superior temporal, and temporoparietal cortices, see Fig. 6.2).

The integrity of white matter connections between these brain regions is crucial for accurate speech control. Of particular relevance are the corticobulbar tracts: the primary motor pathway to cranial nerves and the dorsal language stream (arcuate fasciculus, fronto-temporal, and fronto-parietal segments) (Friederici 2006). The dorsal speech network overlaps with verbal working memory, phonological loop, syntax, and 'inner speech' networks in adults (Hickok et al. 2014). This anatomical overlap highlights the need to assess co-occurring difficulties in children with developmental and acquired speech sound disorders. Speech sound disorders can be associated with developmental anomalies, lesions, or dysfunction of grey as well as white matter brain structures.

There is strong functional magnetic resonance imaging evidence that speech execution involves bilateral ventral sensorimotor cortices in adults and children (Liégeois et al. 2016). In contrast, there is converging evidence that the ventral premotor and Broca's area activations are predominantly left sided for word retrieval tasks (Weiss-Croft and Baldeweg 2015). Similarly, left activation is seen for speech initiation (supplementary motor area) and planning (anterior insula).

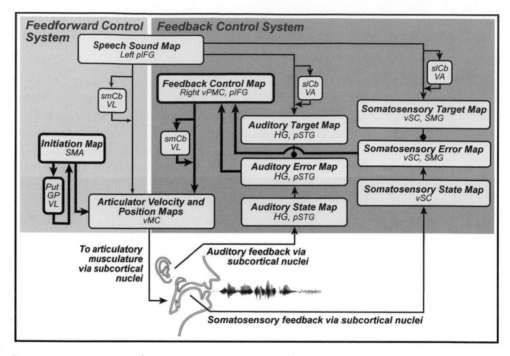

Figure 6.2 DIVA model (Tourville and Guenther 2011). Brain regions: IFG, inferior frontal gyrus; PMC, premotor cortex; MC, motor cortex; v, ventral; p, posterior; SMG, supramarginal gyrus; HG, Heschl's gyrus; SC, sensory cortex; Put, putamen; GP, globus pallidus; VL, ventralateral thalamic nucleus; SMA, supplementary motor area; slCb, superior lateral cerebellum; smCb, superior medial cerebellum.

Theoretical Models of Speech Motor Control

The architecture of theoretical models of speech overlaps with those developed for other motor control and motor learning systems. Information is sent from a 'controller' to an 'effector', which results in a 'state' change (the movement). In speech, the planned state arises from conceptual and word level systems linked to language systems (see Fig. 4 in Hickok 2012 for an adult model).

The current most informed speech model system is the Directions into Velocity of Articulators ('DIVA' model; see Tourville and Guenther 2011, Fig. 6.2).

Unlike the Hickok model, the DIVA model includes movement initiation but does not include linguistic input. In both models, an efference copy of the motor command (forward control/model) allows a prediction of the state in auditory and somatosensory modalities. Sensory systems are involved in defining the speech targets. Without this prediction, errors are made, especially in speech sequences that are not highly automated or nonsense words. The execution of the movement will result in sensory feedback, such as position of articulators, vibration of vocal chords, acoustic feedback, etc.

The predicted and actual sensory consequences are compared and this difference is used as a motor correction that is sent to the controller.

Speech motor control relies on stages of initiation, planning, programming, and execution, with crucial roles played by sensory feedback and linguistic parameters. Although a hierarchy exists, parallel processes occur, especially before the 'execution' stage. As it is highly distributed, the speech network is vulnerable to many types of developmental and neurological conditions (Liégeois and Morgan 2012).

ASSESSMENT AND FORMULATION

Children presenting with speech sound difficulties typically undergo a differential diagnostic assessment that considers developmental history, speech error types, and cognitive profile. The assessment has two objectives: (1) to identify the type and severity of communication disorder ('differential diagnosis') across speech and language, and (2) to assess whether there are co-occurring cognitive impairments outside these domains.

Developmental History via Questionnaires

An extensive developmental interview with the child's guardian allows the clinician to gather information on developmental milestones and concerns from birth. In acquired injury, the results will assess whether there were pre-existing difficulties. Of particular relevance is whether there were concerns regarding speech and language milestones and a family history of speech disorders. A structured interview (Children's Communication Checklist, Second Edition; Bishop 2003; The Vineland Adaptive Behavior Scales, Third Edition; Sparrow, Cicchetti, and Saulnier 2016) with carers will allow to rule out pre-existing social communication impairments and developmental language/speech disorder.

Tools to Provide a Differential Diagnosis of Speech Disorder

A differential diagnosis will establish at which level(s) speech processes are affected across cognitive-linguistic processes, speech planning/programming, or speech execution, and guide intervention recommendations.

Articulation can be assessed using the Goldman-Fristoe Test of Articulation, Third Edition (Goldman and Fristoe 2015), a US-normed test allowing the clinician to document the child's phonetic repertoire. When paired with the Khan-Lewis Phonological Profile, Second Edition (Lewis and Khan 2015), a clinician can also probe whether the child makes phonological errors as well.

The Diagnostic Evaluation of Articulation and Phonology (DEAP), normed in British English and Australian English (Dodd et al. 2002), allows the clinician to differentiate articulation from inconsistent phonological disorder, consistent phonological disorder, and phonological delay. There is also an oral motor screener to identify any nonspeech oral motor deficits, which may give an indication to neuromuscular involvement (dysarthria) or oral motor praxis (that frequently co-occurs with CAS).

Recording a speech in conversation or picture description (e.g. Park Play; Patel and Connaghan 2014) will allow a clinician to phonetically transcribe and identify error patterns in an ecologically valid setting. Speech intelligibility ratings can be used to provide an indication of the severity of this functional impact (e.g. Intelligibility in Context Scale; McLeod, Harrison, and McCormack 2012).

Language Assessment

Given the co-occurring speech and language disorders, a standardised assessment of language skills across different domains will allow the clinician to evaluate whether there are associated semantic and syntactic difficulties, as well as working memory. There are multiple forms of standardised language tools available that may be applied (see Chapter 5). The Clinical Evaluation of Language Fundamentals, Fifth Edition (Wiig, Semel, and Secord 2013) is one widely used standardised assessment. A receptive vocabulary test (e.g. British Picture Vocabulary Scale, Receptive One-Word Picture Vocabulary Tests, or Peabody Picture Vocabulary Test, Fourth Edition) does not require speech production and can allow the quantification of single word knowledge, even in children with limited production abilities.

Intelligence Assessment

In the case of known aetiology (neurological condition or syndrome), speech disorder is likely to co-occur with other cognitive impairments. In developmental conditions, an IQ assessment will assess whether there are global cognitive deficits and guide intervention. There are multiple examples of cognitive assessments (see Chapter 21). One appropriate tool would be an age-appropriate Wechsler scale and examination of non-verbal intelligence (Wechsler 2017).

Assessment of Other Movement Skills

Primary motor pathways for speech and hand movements are anatomically close in the corona radiata and overlap partly at the level of the posterior limb of the internal capsule. There are multiple standardised motor assessments available. To assess fine motor deficit, exemplar tests would be a pegboard task or subtest of the Movement Assessment Battery for Children, Second Edition (Movement ABC-2; Henderson, Sugden, and Barnett 2007; e.g. Beads) (see Chapter 4). In developmental conditions, speech sound disorders co-occur highly with developmental coordination disorder and developmental language disorder (Eadie et al. 2015), therefore a developmental coordination disorder questionnaire may be recommended (DCDQ, https://www.dcdq.ca/dcdq-07.html).

Assessment Results in Anisha's Case

Developmental History

Anisha had typical development up until the time of her injury. Neither teachers nor parents reported any concerns regarding pre-injury behavioural/learning difficulties, and she was performing in line with her peers.

Differential Diagnosis

The Diagnostic Evaluation of Articulation and Phonology revealed age-appropriate phonological development. During assessment, Anisha had distortions across all of her speech sounds, pointing to a potential diagnosis of dysarthria. Anisha also had oral motor deficits, such as reduced tone of the lips, tongue, and cheeks, as well as a reduced range and rate of oral motor movements. Her mother reported that her speech became less clear as she became tired. Anisha also has reduced respiratory support for speech, being able to produce only two to three words in a single breath. A conversational speech sample revealed poor intelligibility in connected speech. The Intelligibility in Context Scale (McLeod et al. 2012) confirmed that her family and friends had difficulties understanding Anisha, demonstrating an impact on everyday functioning.

Language Assessment

Anisha obtained a total language score of 87 on the CELF-5, with no discrepancy between receptive and expressive scales. Anisha's Peabody Picture Vocabulary Test, Fourth Edition score was also within the average range (standard score = 90).

Intelligence Assessment

Anisha received a low average score for Full Scale IQ on the Wechsler Intelligence Scale for Children, Fifth Edition with a specific weakness in the Processing Speed Index, with a score in the extremely low range (65).

Assessment of Other Movement Skills

Anisha obtained a score within the 5th percentile on Manual Dexterity on the Movement ABC-2, indicating clinically significant fine movement difficulties. Qualitative observation indicated that this was driven by slow movements. She obtained borderline performance on the Aiming and Catching, and Balance subtests (14th percentile).

INTERVENTION AND MANAGEMENT

High-level evidence for efficacy of speech interventions is still sparse. A few systematic reviews and observational studies, however, allow general recommendations to be made based on the differential diagnosis provided (see Assessment and Formulation section).

In the case of dysarthria, as seen for Anisha, therapy goals will focus on improving speech intelligibility and increasing communicative participation. There are no controlled randomised controlled trials in this field to date (Pennington et al. 2016). Observational studies indicate some efficacy of interventions based on the principles of motor learning (such as Prompts for Restructuring Oral Muscular Phonetic Targets or PROMPT therapy and articulation), if they are intensive and provide faded feedback, for children who acquire dysarthria before the age of 3 years (Pennington et al. 2016). Smaller-scale studies have suggested a potential role for biofeedback therapy (e.g. Pennington et al. 2016), where the child is given visual feedback on the placement of their tongue against the palate on a computer screen during the therapy sessions.

For children with a diagnosis of CAS, one recent randomised controlled trial (Murray et al. 2015) suggested some evidence of efficacy using the Nuffield Dyspraxia Programme, Third Edition (NDP-3); and the Rapid Syllable Transitions Treatment (Morgan, Murray, and Liégeois 2018). For children with phonological disorders, there is randomised controlled trial evidence suggesting that contrast therapy, also known as minimal or maximal pair therapy, is effective (Law, Garrett, and Nye 2004). For children with articulation disorders, there is evidence to suggest that traditional articulation therapy in isolation and articulation therapy with contingency management to increase home practice are effective approaches (Gunther and Hautvast 2010).

Outcome

The profile seen in Anisha is consistent with impairment at the level of the speech execution system after an acquired injury, i.e. dysarthria. In this case, there are no co-occurring learning or language difficulties, but processing speed is impaired. Adjustments at school may be required to give her more time to complete tasks. Anisha's difficulties with handwriting are likely to be linked to other fine motor difficulties.

Intensive intervention for dysarthria should be provided. There is a limited evidence base in this field; however, there are early indications that a treatment such as the Body Systems approach (Pennington et al. 2016) may improve this speech neuromuscular execution disorder. The body or speech system approach is based on motor learning theory (practice: acquisition retention transfer). The intervention aims to increase intelligibility by maintaining adequate volume, chunking speech into phrases (to ensure breath support), and slowing speech where relevant. The therapist models target words and phrases that the child repeats, while feedback is faded to encourage self-monitoring.

Post-intervention evaluation should measure intelligibility, and interviews used to quantify whether participation in communication has improved. Tests carried out before intervention should be repeated to measure intervention efficacy.

SUMMARY

Our case example demonstrates the long-term impacts of a traumatic brain injury sustained at 5 years of age in a 10-year-old female, Anisha. Here we see the critical importance of a detailed case history to identify significant life events, such as a brain injury, that may still be affecting a child many years later. Unfortunately, for many children, there are support systems in place around the time of the injury but very little monitoring to support the child later in life.

A subset of children with traumatic brain injury experience the neuromuscular execution speech disorder of dysarthria. Whilst clinicians have evidence-based methods to differentially diagnose the presence of dysarthria, there is very little research around the development or rigorous evaluation of treatments for dysarthria. We see the functional long-term impacts of dysarthria on Anisha's social life with her withdrawing from social engagement with peers and team sports. Hence dysarthria therapy should be applied to mitigate these impacts, but we do not have sufficient evidence at this time to specify which approach should be used nor can we confidently predict the benefit or outcome of this therapy. Further, dysarthria often occurs with other motor and processing deficits, so the presence of dysarthria should alert the neuropsychologist to provide a detailed cognitive assessment. In this case, the results of the neuropsychology report could help to change Anisha's teachers' perception that she is not intelligent. Anisha is an intelligent child who simply needs extra processing time due to her injury, which has affected the white matter connections in core processing regions of her brain, with resultant impacts on the communication between these brain networks.

REFERENCES

American Speech-Language-Hearing Association (ASHA) (2007) *Ad Hoc Committee on Childhood Apraxia of Speech*. Retrieved from http://www.asha.org/policy/PS2007-00277/.

Bishop DVM, Snowling MJ, Thompson PA, Greenhalgh T, CATALISE Consortium (2016) CATALISE: A Multinational and Multidisciplinary Delphi Consensus Study. Identifying Language Impairments in Children. PLOSOne. https://doi.org/10.1371/journal.pone.0158753.

Dodd B (2014) Differential diagnosis of pediatric speech sound disorder. *Current Developmental Disorders Reports* 1(3): 189–196.

Eadie P, Morgan AT, Ukoumunne OC, Ttofari Eecen K, Wake M, Reilly S (2015) Speech sound disorder at 4 years: Prevalence, comorbidities, and predictors in a community cohort of children. *Developmental Medicine & Child Neurology* 57(6): 578–584. doi: 10.1111/dmcn.12635.

Friederici AD (2006) The neural basis of language development and its impairment. *Neuron* 52(6): 941–952. doi: 10.1016/j.neuron.2006.12.002.

Gunther T, Hautvast S (2010) Addition of contingency management to increase home practice in young children with a speech sound disorder. *International Journal of Language & Communication Disorders* 45(3): 345–353.

Hickok G. (2012) Computational neuroanatomy of speech production. *Nature Reviews Neuroscience* 13(2): 135–145.

Hickok G, Rogalsky C, Chen R, Herskovits EH, Townsley S, Hillis AE (2014) Partially overlapping sensorimotor networks underlie speech praxis and verbal short-term memory: Evidence from apraxia of speech following acute stroke. *Frontiers in Human Neuroscience* 8(649). doi: 10.3389/fnhum.2014.00649.

Kuhl PK (2004) Early language acquisition: cracking the speech code. *Nature Reviews Neuroscience* 5(11): 831–843. doi: 10.1038/nrn1533.

Law J, Garrett Z, Nye C (2004) The efficacy of treatment for children with developmental speech and language delay/disorder: A meta-analysis. *Journal of Speech Language and Hearing Research* 47(4): 924–943. doi: 10.1044/1092-4388(2004/069).

Liégeois FJ, Butler J, Morgan AT, Clayden JD, Clark CA (2016) Anatomy and lateralization of the human corticobulbar tracts: An fMRI-guided tractography study. *Brain Structure and Function* 221(6): 3337–3345. doi: 10.1007/s00429-015-1104-x.

Liégeois FJ, Tournier JD, Pigdon L, Connelly A, Morgan AT (2013) Corticobulbar tract changes as predictors of dysarthria in childhood brain injury. *Neurology* 80(10): 926–932. doi: 10.1212/WNL.0b013e3182840c6d.

Liégeois FJ, Morgan AT (2012) Neural bases of childhood speech disorders: Lateralization and plasticity for speech functions during development. *Neuroscience & Biobehavioural Reviews* 36(1): 439–458. doi: 10.1016/j.neubiorev.2011.07.011.

McLeod S, Crowe K, Shahaeian A (2015) Intelligibility in context scale: Normative and validation data for English-speaking preschoolers. *Language, Speech, and Hearing Services in Schools* 46(3): 266–276. doi: 10.1044/2015_LSHSS-14-0120.

McLeod S, Harrison LJ, McCormack J (2012) The intelligibility in context scale: Validity and reliability of a subjective rating measure. *Journal of Speech, Language, and Hearing Research* 55: 648–656.

Morgan AT, Eecen KT, Pezic A et al. (2017) Who to refer for speech therapy at 4 years of age versus who to 'watch and wait'? *The Journal of Pediatrics* 185: 200–204. e201. doi: 10.1016/j.jpeds.2017.02.059.

Morgan AT, Murray E, Liégeois FJ (2018) Interventions for childhood apraxia of speech. *Cochrane Database of Systematic Reviews* 2009(3): CD006279. doi: 10.1002/14651858.CD006279.pub2.

Murray E, McCabe P, Ballard KJ (2015) A randomized controlled trial for children with childhood apraxia of speech comparing rapid syllable transition treatment and the Nuffield Dyspraxia Programme – Third Edition. *Journal of Speech, Language, and Hearing Research* 58(3): 669–686. doi: 10.1044/2015_JSLHR-S-13-0179.

Patel R, Connaghan K (2014) Park Play: A picture description task for assessing childhood motor speech disorders. *International Journal of Speech-Language Pathology* 16(4): 337–343.

Pennington L, Parker NK, Kelly H, Miller N (2016) Speech therapy for children with dysarthria acquired before three years of age. *Cochrane Database of Systematic Reviews* 2016(7): CD006937. doi: 10.1002/14651858.CD006937.pub3.

Tourville JA Guenther FH (2011) The DIVA model: A neural theory of speech acquisition and production. *Language and Cognitive Processes* 26(7): 952–981, doi: 10.1080/01690960903498424.

Weiss-Croft LJ, Baldeweg T (2015) Maturation of language networks in children: A systematic review of 22 years of functional MRI. *Neuroimage* 123: 269–281. doi: 10.1016/j.neuroimage.2015.07.046.

CHAPTER 7

Visuo-Spatial Processing

Katie A Gilligan-Lee, Elizabeth Roberts, and Emily Farran

Presenting Concern

Hamish was a fit boy until, at 12 years 2 months, he was hit by a car while he was cycling. Prior to his accident, Hamish was reported to have been of average intelligence, to have settled in well at his secondary school, to have made friends, and to have no known special educational needs. There is no family history of note, including no history of learning difficulties, non-right handedness, neurodevelopmental disorders, or visuo-spatial deficits. As a result of his accident, Hamish sustained a localised 'contrecoup' injury to his right parietal lobe due to his right hemisphere colliding with the inside of his skull because of inertia. Brain scans revealed infarction and bruising in this area. In addition, the scans showed multiple small haemorrhages throughout the brain, indicative of diffuse axonal injury (global injury to the axons of brain cells). Such damage is associated with fatigue, reduced processing speed, difficulties with attentional control, and poor memory. Hamish also acquired a left-sided hemiplegia (motor weakness). As a result, following his accident, he was fully dependent on a powered wheelchair for mobility. He was right-hand dominant prior to his accident and following the accident he retained functional control of this arm.

As a result of his brain injury, Hamish spent 3 months in an acute hospital setting, followed by 4 months of neurorehabilitation in a residential setting. On admission to the neurorehabilitation setting, Hamish was noted to be disorientated. He had particular difficulty learning his way around the site and initial screening highlighted impairment in visuo-spatial skills. A neuropsychological assessment was requested to understand the impact of Hamish's brain injury on his behaviour and to support planning post discharge, particularly with regards to supporting Hamish's transition back to the educational setting.

THEORY

Visuo-spatial processing involves making sense of what the eyes see with respect to the visual and spatial attributes of the visual array. This can involve perceiving the colour and shape of objects as well as processing the dimensions and locations of objects and their relationships with other objects in the environment. It is core to everyday living. Poor visuo-spatial abilities are associated with direct disadvantages in moment-to-moment functioning in everyday activities, for example finding one's way around, stacking a dishwasher, packing a suitcase, recognising letters and numbers. Furthermore, disruption to visuo-spatial processing in the early years can have extended negative effects on later motor, language, and cognitive outcomes (Gori et al. 2016). From an educational perspective, visuo-spatial processing has also been implicated in educational achievement including reading, mathematics, and science performance in childhood (e.g. McCandliss, Cohen, and Dehaene 2003; Hodgkiss et al. 2018; Gilligan et al. 2019). In short, there are far-reaching negative implications for both day-to day adjustment and educational success for children with deficits in visuo-spatial thinking.

The ability to diagnose and treat deficits in visuo-spatial processing depends on an understanding of the structure and development of visuo-spatial thinking in the typically developing brain. The cortical processing of visuo-spatial information can be subdivided into two pathways, the dorsal and ventral streams. Both streams originate in the occipital lobe (V1), the dorsal stream passing through V5/middle temporal visual area and terminating in the parietal lobe, and the ventral stream running through V4 to the temporal lobe (Milner and Goodale 1995; Milner and Goodale 2008). Beyond differences in their structural organisation, there is evidence that these streams are functionally distinct. The dorsal stream has traditionally been associated with motion of objects, spatial cognition, and visual motor planning (perception for action), while the ventral stream is responsible for visual memory and object recognition (form perception) (Milner and Goodale 1995; Milner and Goodale 2008; Johnston et al. 2017). This is supported by evidence from lesion studies in both primates and humans, showing that damage to parietal areas leads to deficits in perception for action, the processing of 'where' and 'how' information, while lesions in temporal areas impact form perception, or the processing of 'what' information (Kravitz et al. 2011). This distinction is useful for understanding brain–behaviour relationships; it is, however, important to recognise that these streams do not work in isolation.

In typical development, there is evidence that dorsal stream functions have relatively longer developmental trajectories than those associated with the ventral stream (Braddick, Atkinson, and Wattam-Bell 2003). Consequently, it has been proposed that dorsal functions may be more vulnerable to disruption from genetic factors (Braddick et al. 2003; Farran and Formby 2012). Traditionally, this argument has been supported by evidence that the dorsal stream is affected in several neurodevelopmental disorders, including developmental dyslexia, autism spectrum disorders, developmental coordination disorder/dyspraxia, Williams syndrome, and Fragile X syndrome (Grinter, Maybery, and Badcock 2010). However, in a recent review of dorsal and ventral processing in individuals with neurodevelopmental disorders, Johnston et al. (2017) reported that only 40% of studies found a selective deficit in motor perception (perception for action) in these groups, i.e. a dorsal stream deficit. For example in developmental coordination disorder, dorsal stream deficits are seen concurrently with ventral stream deficits (measured behaviourally using tasks proposed to measure ventral stream functions; Grinter et al. 2010). Therefore, although many atypical groups present with dorsal stream deficits, it would be simplistic to assume that they all share the same visuo-spatial profile. This also applies to individuals with acquired brain damage such as Hamish, such that it is rare for lesions to create a pure deficit; substantial variation is seen in dorsal processing deficits across disorder groups and those with acquired injuries. Furthermore, the origins of this variation likely differ between those with neurodevelopmental disorders and those who have acquired brain injuries. For the former group, specialisation of function has been within the context of an atypical brain from the infant start-state, and thus impairments can result from cascading developmental impacts of early, more subtle impairment. Equally, functions can develop via alternative neural pathways due to brain plasticity. In contrast, in the case of Hamish, and others with acquired brain disorder, disrupted processing is within the context of typical development of function prior to injury.

Although they are often presented as distinct processing streams, further evidence that the dorsal and ventral streams do not work entirely in isolation comes from work on their structural and functional interconnections. These connections lead to substantial cross-talk between the streams (Van Essen and Maunsell 1983). Moreover, both the dorsal and ventral streams are complex, multi-component systems. Each stream comprises multiple stages, any one of which may be disrupted. For example distinctions have been made in the dorsal pathway between the parieto–prefrontal pathway, a parieto–premotor pathway, and a parieto–medial temporal pathway, responsible for spatial working memory, visually guided action, and spatial navigation respectively (Kravitz et al. 2011). Owing to this complexity, damage to different parts of the dorsal (or ventral) stream in two individuals (or across two syndromes) may lead to very different profiles of cognitive task performance on a visuo-spatial task battery.

Diagnosis of compromised visuo-spatial functioning based solely on an analysis of the role of the dorsal and ventral streams is not sufficient. There are several other cortical areas known to contribute to the completion of visuo-spatial tasks. For example for spatial navigation, the parahippocampal gyrus, caudate nucleus, and hippocampus have been heavily implicated in landmark knowledge, route knowledge, and configural knowledge, respectively (Doeller, King, and Burgess 2008; Wegman and Janzen 2011). Similarly, the cortical areas responsible for domain general processes such as attention and executive functions (associated with the frontal lobe) also contribute to visuo-spatial task performance (Atkinson and Braddick 2012). Therefore, prior to diagnosing a dorsal or ventral stream deficit, it is also important to recognise both the complexity of these systems as well as the importance of other possible cognitive contributors to poor performance on visuo-spatial tasks.

Taken together, there is evidence that visuo-spatial processing can be broadly described using the dorsal-ventral stream framework, in which the dorsal and ventral streams have largely distinct structural and functional organisation. However, for clinical purposes these streams should be considered as complex, multi-component systems, such that a deficit in the dorsal (or ventral) stream may present differently in different individuals. Finally, although there is some evidence that individuals with neurodevelopmental disorders and individuals with lesions show particular dorsal stream deficits and that interventions targeting the dorsal stream may be particularly effective in these groups, intervention should be designed on an individual basis as individual variation in dorsal stream task performance may vary substantially.

ASSESSMENT AND FORMULATION

There are a range of suitable assessments that can be used to assess the processing of visuo-spatially represented information. For the ventral stream, assessments include figure copying tasks, object recognition tasks, visual search tasks, and visual memory tasks. Figure copying tasks require participants to copy an image. The image typically remains available to the participants and as such there is no memory component. Tasks of this type can be used to identify visual neglect, i.e. when participants do not attend to certain parts of the visual field. Other types of assessment for ventral processing are figure-ground tasks, such as the Children's Embedded Figures Task (CEFT; Witkin et al. 1971). In the CEFT, participants are required to identify the spatial location of one object against a distracting background, i.e. they must find a target shape in a more complicated picture (Ekstrom et al. 1976). Other ventral stream tasks, including object recognition and visual memory tasks, require participants to store or access mental images. For object recognition tasks participants must identify an object, often with limited visual cues, for example visual closure subtests of the Test of Visual Perceptual Skills, Fourth Edition (Martin 2017) and of the Developmental Test of Visual Perception, Third Edition (Hammill, Pearson, and Voress 2014). For visual memory tasks, participants must store an image in memory, and may, for example, be asked to identify whether the image is the same or different as another image, for example visual memory subtests of the Test of Visual Perceptual Skills, Fourth Edition (Martin 2017) and the equivalent subtest in the Developmental Test of Visual Perception, Third Edition (Hammill, Pearson, and Voress 2014). In combination, using a range of tasks to assess visuo-spatial processing can provide a more detailed picture of an individual's visuo-spatial abilities. For example an individual with damage to the parieto–prefrontal pathway would be expected to perform poorly on mental imagery and visual memory tasks; however, they may not have reduced performance on tasks in which there is no need to store or access an image in the mind. Conversely, an individual with an overall ventral stream deficit would be expected to perform poorly on all of these tasks.

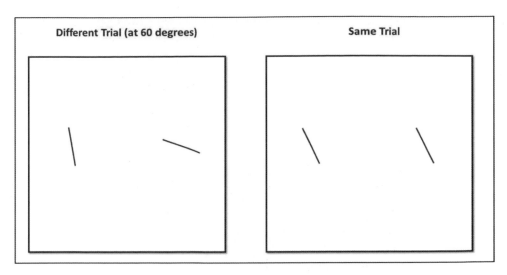

Figure 7.1 Sample items from an orientation–discrimination paradigm, adapted from Farran (2006).

For the dorsal stream, suitable measures include orientation-discrimination, mental rotation, perspective taking, navigation, and visuomotor planning tasks. For orientation-discrimination tasks, participants are required to determine whether two lines have the same, or a different orientation (see Fig. 7.1). In typical mental rotation paradigms participants must establish which images are rotated versions of a target image. Several neuroimaging studies have implicated the parietal lobe in mental rotation task performance (Hawes et al. 2019). Perspective taking tasks require participants to imagine what a scene will look like from a perspective that is different from their own. This requires an imagined movement (motion perception) to view a scene from a different perspective. In particular, damage to the posterior parietal lobe can lead to difficulties representing the locations of objects relative to the observer (Newcombe 2018). Navigation tasks also provide a wealth of information on visuo-spatial processing. In simple navigation tasks (e.g. see Fig. 7.2), participants are typically required to learn a route from a start to an end point. Performance is measured as the number of trials required for a participant to complete the route without making any errors or the cumulative number of errors made within those trials. However, as previously outlined, navigation tasks are complex and provide insight into several other brain areas beyond the dorsal stream. Newcombe (2018) claimed different navigation performance patterns can be interpreted to determine damage to different cortical areas. For example some individuals may have difficulty representing locations relative to other locations (suggestive of a retrosplenial cortex deficit) whilst others may not be able to recognise familiar landmarks (suggestive of a parahippocampus deficit). Neither of these deficits specifically relate to the dorsal stream.

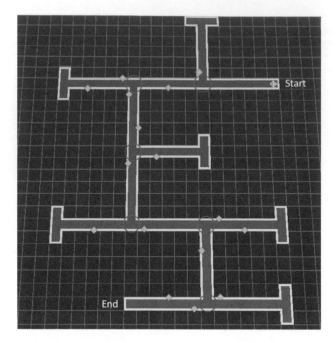

Figure 7.2 Sample maze structure used for navigation tasks, adapted from Farran et al. (2012). Landmarks are depicted as yellow diamonds. Each red circle indicates a decision point at which an error may occur. (A colour version of this figure can be seen in the colour plate section)

Case Study – Hamish

Hamish's initial screening assessment revealed significant difficulty on a task tapping visuo-spatial skills. He was unable to match the angle and orientation of lines on a line-orientation task. This led to referral for a comprehensive assessment to determine the full impact of the acquired brain injury on his visuo-spatial processing capacities. The assessment was completed whilst he was engaging in neurorehabilitation (see Table 7.1). Hamish engaged well with the assessment; he was observed to be motivated throughout the sessions and appeared to attempt all tasks to the best of his ability. The evidence from the assessment confirmed that Hamish has a significant impairment in the processing of visuo-spatial information.

As indicated by his performance on visuo-spatial measures, Hamish had difficulty learning new routes in a virtual format despite multiple learning trials, i.e. finding his way around a virtual maze. Hamish's difficulty finding his way around impacted on his ability to orientate to his surroundings, which contributed to him feeling anxious and unsettled at times. Hamish scored in the 'extremely low' range on tasks that involved line orientation and also scored in the same low range on mental rotation tasks. One explanation for these difficulties could be dorsal stream deficits, which supports visually guided behaviour. In comparison, Hamish had good object recall, which is mediated by the ventral stream. However, he also performed poorly on the CEFT, which is also proposed to recruit the ventral stream. This suggests that Hamish had ventral damage. This poor performance could, however, have been the result of the documented diffuse axonal injury influencing sustained attention, inhibition, working memory, and processing. He was also assessed as having relative strengths in his language skills (see Table 7.1), which was hypothesised as reflecting that

Table 7.1 Patient scores on the assessment battery

Assessment	Score
Visuo-Spatial Assessments	
Ventral stream tasks	
Figure Copying (Repeatable Battery for the Assessment of Neuropsychological Status, RBANS)	0.1st percentile*
Children's Embedded Figures Task	Score: 3 (Max score: 18)
Landmark recall (ability to recall common objects based on Farran et al. 2012)	100%
Dorsal stream tasks	
Line Orientation (RBANS)	<2nd percentile*
Orientation Discrimination Task (based on Farran 2006)	Overall accuracy 52% (chance performance is 50%)
Navigation (route learning). In each of 10 trials, the patient was asked to make decisions at six turning points. Therefore, chance performance is three errors per trial (based on Farran et al. 2012)	Hamish had >4 errors for every trial and failed to learn the route
Block Design (Wechsler Intelligence Scale for Children, Fifth UK Edition, WISC-V^UK)	0.1st percentile*
Other Assessments	
Matrix Reasoning measuring non-verbal reasoning (WISC-V^UK)	0.1st percentile*
Language Index (RBANS)	18th percentile*
Verbal Comprehension Index (WISC-V^UK)	17th percentile*
Fluid Reasoning Index (WISC-V^UK)	12th percentile*
Processing Speed Index (WISC-V^UK)	10th percentile*
Working Memory Index (WISC-V^UK)	10th percentile*
Vigil – subtest measuring sustained attention (Test of Everyday Attention for Children, Second Edition, TEA-Ch2)	8th percentile*
Simple Response Time – subtest measuring sustained attention (TEA-Ch2)	10th percentile*
Sustained Attention to Response Task – subtest measuring sustained attention and inhibition (TEA-Ch2)	6th percentile*

*A percentile rank gives Mark's standing relative to other same-age children. For example he achieved a percentile rank of 0.1 for his Figure Copy, which means that he performed as well as or better than the lowest 0.1% of children his age.

Hamish's left hemisphere was relatively preserved (the left hemisphere is particularly involved in language). Thus, Hamish's performance profile is likely to differ from others who have sustained, for example, a localised parietal lesion. In this way, this case study highlights the complexity of visuo-spatial processing, showing that dorsal stream deficits do not always occur in isolation and that all individuals with dorsal stream deficits do not have identical performance profiles.

Hamish had significant difficulty learning new routes within the navigation task. The navigation task has good ecological validity, as it makes use of virtual reality to attempt learning a new route. Studies have shown that route learning in a virtual environment correlates with route learning in the real world (Coutrot et al. 2019). Furthermore, Hamish's difficulty learning new routes was also observed within real life situations, as he struggled to remember his route around the rehabilitation setting, leading to him feeling disorientated and anxious.

INTERVENTION AND MANAGEMENT

Hamish's identified visuo-spatial processing difficulties were supported through his neurorehabilitation programme. An initial goal for Hamish's rehabilitation was to support him in learning his way around the site. Hamish was provided with photos of his team, a visual timetable, and a map of the site (see Fig. 7.3).

In order to support Hamish in achieving his goal, he was supported by staff to learn his route around the site using an errorless learning approach. Errorless learning is an evidence-based technique for teaching individuals following a traumatic brain injury,

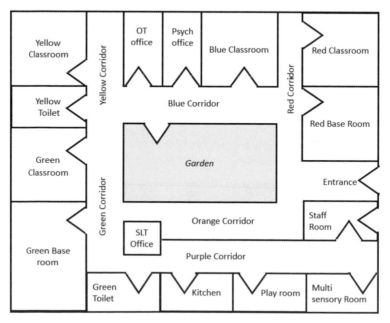

Figure 7.3 Map of the neurorehabilitation site.

Note: This map has been simplified to protect confidentiality.

particularly those with specific memory problems (e.g. Ehlhardt at al. 2008). Errorless learning involves teaching an individual in such a way that they do not make mistakes as they learn the new information. This is achieved by simplifying the task and providing adequate support and cues to ensure success. This is then repeated multiple times to ensure the new information is retained. As such, when staff were supporting Hamish to learn his way around the site they made use of compensatory cues to support this process. As highlighted, this included providing Hamish with a simple map of the site and identifying key landmarks in his environment that he could use to find his way around (e.g. the colour of the walls). Hamish was supported by a member of staff at all times when initially learning the route to prompt him to use the map and landmarks. This support was not reduced until Hamish could navigate successfully at all times. Hamish reported that becoming familiar with how to navigate around the site independently helped to reduce his anxiety, as he felt more familiar with his environment and was less worried about getting lost.

Hamish's difficulty on the block design task suggested that he had difficulty understanding how individual parts are related to the 'whole' (i.e. gestalt principles). As such, consideration was given as to whether cognitive rehabilitation should focus on visuo-spatial tasks such as completing puzzles, creating maps, and construction activities. However, there is not a strong evidence base for the cognitive rehabilitation of visuo-spatial deficits (e.g. Cicerone et al. 2000). As such, the cognitive rehabilitation programme was focussed instead on improving academic skills known to be impacted by visuo-spatial deficits, particularly mathematical skills and reading (McCandliss et al. 2003; Gilligan et al. 2019).

In addition, brain injury psychoeducation including information about severe traumatic brain injury, diffuse axonal injury, and the two visual-stream hypotheses were provided to Hamish and his parents. This information provided Hamish and his parents with a context within which they could make sense of the difficulties he was having in day-to-day life, as well as to ensure that they were able to advocate for his needs in the future (e.g. ensuring adequate support and compensations when he returned to school).

Outcome

The assessment, alongside Hamish's response to intervention, enabled a formulation of his strengths and needs to be established. This formulation was used to plan for Hamish post discharge, particularly with regards to supporting Hamish's transition back to school. Key school staff were provided with information about the brain to help them gain an understanding of Hamish's injury and the impact on his cognition, behaviour, and emotional well-being. This was achieved through psychoeducation, during which severe traumatic brain injury, diffuse axonal injury, and the two visual-stream hypothesis, were explained. This theory was then linked to the findings from Hamish's neuropsychological assessment. Based on this information, staff were supported to design personalised interventions to assist Hamish. This included having colour and object markers to support Hamish's navigation around the school site, as well as planning his lessons to ensure that his routes around school were simplified. The school also ensured that Hamish had a key member of staff allocated. This member of staff was trained in errorless learning to ensure she could apply this approach when supporting Hamish to navigate around the school environment. Hamish reported that having this support in place from the beginning of his transition back to school helped him feel less anxious about his reintegration.

Hamish's class teachers provided compensations in the classroom including careful consideration of where Hamish was seated to ensure good sight of the board; providing Hamish with additional time when copying information from the board or when completing an activity with increased visuo-spatial requirements (e.g. drawing, writing etc.); and ensuring that information on the board and worksheets was simplified to avoid overwhelming him. Hamish returned to school on a reduced timetable. This was achieved through his dropping a subject that he was not planning to take forward to GCSE level. This was useful in terms of helping him to manage his levels of fatigue and in ensuring more free lessons that could be used for one-to-one sessions focussing on academic skills known to be linked with visuo-spatial deficits, i.e. mathematics skills and reading.

SUMMARY

From a theoretical perspective, this chapter highlights how a cognitive understanding of the structure of visuo-spatial processing can be used to both understand visuo-spatial deficits and to inform intervention. Visuo-spatial processing is imperative for everyday living and independence, and deficits in this domain have significant implications for motor, language, cognitive, and educational outcomes. Within this chapter, we outlined a range of suitable assessments that can be used to measure visuo-spatial thinking across both the dorsal and ventral processing streams. Although these streams are largely structurally and functionally distinct, they are also highly complex. As such, we have emphasised that dorsal and ventral deficits may present differently in different individuals and a pure lesion that impacts upon one stream only is uncommon. Therefore, a range of assessments should be used to generate comprehensive profiles of visuo-spatial performance in those with visuo-spatial deficits. The complex, multi-component nature of visuo-spatial processing across dorsal and ventral streams, and the cross-communication between these streams, suggests that visuo-spatial interventions should be designed on an individual basis based on individual profiles of visuo-spatial strengths and weaknesses.

REFERENCES

Atkinson J, Braddick O (2012) Visual attention in the first years: Typical development and developmental disorders. *Developmental Medicine & Child Neurology* 54: 589–595. https://doi.org/10.1111/j.1469-8749.2012.04294.x.

Braddick O, Atkinson J, Wattam-Bell J (2003) Normal and anomalous development of visual motion processing: Motion coherence and dorsal-stream vulnerability. *Neuroscience and Biobehavioral Reviews* 83: 32–45. https://doi.org/10.1016/S0028-3932(03)00178-7.

Cicerone KD, Dahlberg C, Kalmar K et al. (2000) Evidence-based cognitive rehabilitation: Recommendations for clinical practice. *Archives of Physical Medicine and Rehabilitation* **81**: 1596–1615.

Coutrot A, Schmidt S, Coutrot L (2019) Virtual navigation tested on a mobile app is predictive of real-world wayfinding navigation performance. *PloS One* **14**(3). https://doi.org/ 10.1371/journal.pone.0213272.

Doeller CF, King JA, Burgess N (2008) Parallel striatal and hippocampal systems for landmarks and boundaries in spatial memory. *Proceedings of the National Academy of Sciences* **105**(15): 5915–5920. https://doi.org/10.1073/pnas.0801489105.

Ehlhardt LA, Sohlberg MM, Kennedy M et al. (2008) Evidence-based practice guidelines for instructing individuals with neurogenic memory impairments: What have we learned in the past 20 years? *Neuropsychological Rehabilitation* **18**(3): 300–342. https://doi.org/ 10.1080/09602010701733190.

Ekstrom RB, French JW, Harman HH, Dermen D (1976) *Kit of Factor-referenced Cognitive Tests*. Princeton, NJ: Educational Testing Service.

Farran EK (2006) Orientation coding: A specific deficit in Williams syndrome? *Developmental Neuropsychology* **29**(3): 397–414. https://doi.org/ 10.1207/s15326942dn2903_1.

Farran EK, Courbois Y, Van Herwegen J, Blades M (2012) How useful are landmarks when learning a route in a virtual environment? Evidence from typical development and Williams syndrome. *Journal of Experimental Child Psychology* **111**: 571–586. https://doi.org/ 10.1016/j.jecp.2011.10.009.

Farran EK, Formby SC (2012) Visual perception and visuospatial cognition. In: *Neurodevelopmental Disorders Across the Lifespan: A Neuroconstructivist Approach*. Oxford: Oxford University Press.

Gilligan KA, Hodgkiss A, Thomas MSC, Farran EK (2019) The developmental relations between spatial cognition and mathematics in primary school children. *Developmental Science* **22**: e12786. https://doi.org/10.1111/desc.12786.

Gori M, Cappagli G, Tonelli Baud-Bovy G, Finocchietti S (2016) Devices for visually impaired people: High technological devices with low user acceptance and no adaptability for children. *Neuroscience and Biobehavioural Reviews* **69**: 79–88. https://doi:10.1016/j.neubiorev.2016.06.043.

Grinter EJ, Maybery MT, Badcock DR (2010) Vision in developmental disorders: Is there a dorsal stream deficit? *Brain Research Bulletin* **82**(3–4): 147–160. https://doi.org/10.1016/j.brainresbull.2010.02.016.

Hawes Z, Sokolowski HM, Ononye CB, Ansari D (2019) Neural underpinnings of numerical and spatial cognition: An fMRI meta-analysis of brain regions associated with symbolic number, arithmetic, and mental rotation. *Neuroscience and Biobehavioural Reviews* **103**: 316–336. https://doi.org/10.1016/j.neubiorev.2019.05.007.

Hodgkiss A, Gilligan KA, Tolmie AK, Thomas MSC, Farran EK (2018) Spatial cognition and science achievement: The contribution of intrinsic and extrinsic spatial skills from 7 to 11 years. *British Journal of Educational Psychology* **88**: 675–697. https://doi.org/10.1111/bjep.12211.

Johnston R, Pitchford NJ, Roach NW, Ledgeway T (2017) New insights into the role of motion and form vision in neurodevelopmental disorders. *Neuroscience & Biobehavioral Reviews* **83**: 32–45. https://doi.org/10.1016/j.neubiorev.2017.09.031.

Kravitz DJ, Saleem KS, Baker CI, Mishkin M (2011) A new neural framework for visuospatial processing. *Nature Reviews Neuroscience* **12**: 217–230. https://doi.org/10.1038/nrn3008.

McCandliss BD, Cohen L, Dehaene S (2003) The visual word form area: Expertise for reading in the fusiform gyrus. *Trends Cogn Sci* **7**(7): 293–299. https://doi.org/10.1016/S1364-6613(03)00134-7.

Milner AD, Goodale MA (1995) *The Visual Brain in Action*. Oxford: Oxford University Press.

Milner AD, Goodale MA (2008) Two visual systems re-viewed. *Neuropsychologia* **46**: 774–785. https://doi.org/10.1016/j.neuropsychologia.2007.10.005.

Newcombe NS (2018) Three kinds of spatial cognition. In: Wixted J, Thompson-Schill SL, editors, *Stevens' Handbook of Experimental Psychology and Cognitive Neuroscience*, 4th edition. New York: John Wiley & Sons, pp. 521–552.

Van Essen DC, Maunsell JHR (1983) Hierarchical organisation and functional streams in the visual cortex. *Trends in Neurosciences* **6**(9): 370–375. https://doi.org/10.1016/0166-2236 (83)90167-4.

Wegman J, Janzen G (2011) Neural encoding of objects relevant for navigation and resting state correlations with navigational ability. *Journal of Cognitive Neuroscience*, **23**(12): 3841–3854. https://doi.org/10.1162/jocn_a_00081.

CHAPTER 8

Attention

Megan N Scott and Tom Manly

Presenting Concern

Caleb is a 13-year-old black boy, referred for evaluation due to concerns about attention, depressed mood, social functioning, and academic progress. He lives with his mother with whom he has a strong relationship.

Caleb was born extremely preterm at 28 weeks with the extremely low birthweight of 822 grams. He suffered a grade 3 intraventricular haemorrhage at birth. His lungs were underdeveloped, and he was mechanically ventilated for 1 month after birth for mild bronchopulmonary dysplasia. He was discharged from the neonatal intensive care unit at 2.5 months of chronological age. There is a family history of congenital heart defect and attention-deficit/hyperactivity disorder (ADHD).

Caleb received early intervention services including speech, occupational, physical, and developmental therapy, and, with extensive input, met his major developmental milestones on time (without correction for gestational age). He participated in speech therapy, occupational therapy, and physical therapy until he was 3 years old, at which point he aged out of early intervention and entered the public-school system.

Throughout elementary school, Caleb received special education services through an Individualised Education Program including speech therapy, additional time to complete tests, and support for executive functioning. Although he attained A and B grades at school, according to his mother these were achieved only through extensive support for poor attention, poor organisation, and difficulty remembering and turning in assignments. Caleb's problems included daydreaming during class, making careless mistakes, forgetting to turn in assignments or bring work home, and losing materials. He had a tendency to leave his seat and wander around the classroom.

His mother decided to home-school Caleb, beginning at age 13 years, due to concerns that he was not getting services recommended in his special education plan, was falling behind, and was refusing to go to school due to bullying. He was taking online courses and working with a tutor. Caleb's academic strength was reading, whilst he struggled with maths and organising his writing. Initiating and completing homework was frequently a challenge, as was remaining seated and on-task. His mother indicated that home-schooling was helpful in allowing him flexibility with task completion.

Throughout his childhood, Caleb faced challenges in his peer relationships where his behaviour could be perceived by others as disruptive or malicious. According to his mother, this was largely due to difficulty stopping himself from acting impulsively in social situations, difficulty reading cues that peers did not want him to join, and some reactive behaviour when he was overtly rejected by peers. Caleb continues to struggle with social interactions and does not have many friends. Caleb has been seeing a social worker for outpatient psychotherapy for the past year to address his mood. He reported depressed mood, low self-esteem, social withdrawal, decreased motivation to participate in social and extracurricular activities, and negative beliefs about his ability.

THEORY

In this chapter, we focus on the features primarily affecting Caleb's learning: daydreaming, problems initiating and detecting errors in his work, difficulty staying on task, and disorganisation. These can be interpreted as reflecting problems in attention and are consistent with symptoms of ADHD.

Defining Attention

Our senses constantly receive information from numerous events on which we could focus. In our interior worlds there are many things that we could remember, think about, or imagine, and bodily sensations of which we could become particularly aware. At any moment, only one (or very few) of these will dominate subjective awareness and, as one thing dominates, our ability to be aware of all of the others, in that moment, declines. It seems that we have a very limited capacity for a certain kind of processing. We call that capacity our 'attention'. This idea of a competition between stimuli for our limited capacity for attention is useful (e.g. 'I wasn't paying attention!' or 'That really caught my attention!'). Some stimuli have features to which our senses are particularly responsive, such as being bright or loud, suddenly appearing or moving quickly. Some have great biological significance (e.g. potentially threatening stimuli) or learned associations (e.g. hearing our name at a party). These things tend to 'grab' our attention, regardless of our wishes. Other competitors in the battle will be things on which we need to focus to complete our goals (e.g. what the teacher is saying). The idea is that, if these things are not naturally very good at capturing our attention, we must invest effort ('pay') to keep them in focus if we are to achieve our aims and/or avoid negative consequences. The job of our neural system is to negotiate this battle for attention in the most adaptive way – being sufficiently goal-directed to get things done whilst allowing important information (e.g. indicating opportunity or threat) to impinge where necessary.

Different Types of Attention

There are several features that would be useful in determining the outcome of this battle for attention. For example reducing the influence of information that may distract from the current task, that is for the system to be appropriately *selective*. Ideally, it could *sustain* this level of selectivity for as long as is required to get a task done. The ability to wilfully *switch* attention from one thing to another would be essential. At times, we may want to *divide* our attention between two important streams of information. Experimental psychologists developed tasks that emphasised these different characteristics and called them 'selective attention', 'sustained attention', 'attention switching', and 'divided attention' tasks. This does not, in itself, mean that the tasks are measuring distinct attention systems. It could be that they are measuring different capacity limits of the same system. Nevertheless, as discussed below, these apparent distinctions between different types of attention are often made in the experimental and clinical literature and can be useful in thinking about the types of tasks with which a child may most struggle in everyday life.

The Cognitive Neuroscience of Attention

It is not within the scope of this chapter to summarise the vast neuroscientific literature on attention. Rather we will provide one, well-worked through example from the visual system that highlights the degree to which attentional selection and limited attention capacity are built into our processing (Desimone and Duncan 1995). This account discusses how the brain's early visual processing areas are dealing with huge amounts of information (e.g. colours, shapes, and edges) in parallel; that is that the amount of processing given to one feature does not vary according to how much is being given to another. However, as this visual information travels forwards in the brain's ventral stream from the occipital towards the temporal lobes, these separate features (colour, shape, etc.) are bound together to create representations of objects. Now, rather than being parallel, the amount of processing given to one object begins to vary enormously depending on the amount given to another. In effect, objects now compete for representation and only a very limited set will pass further forwards at any given time. The system has become highly selective.

The features that will determine the outcome of this competition are the inherent and learned salience of the objects/events, and their relevance of our current goals. Within this view, the frontal cortex is important in the development and maintenance of goals (e.g. 'look for your pen'). These frontal representations then influence other brain areas such that things that look like your pen are enhanced and nonpenlike things suppressed. An important implication is that 'it' is not in the frontal lobes (or temporal, parietal, or occipital) but emerges from interactions *between* regions. An interesting question is why a system computationally capable of processing all the visual information within your visual fields, all of the time, in parallel should discard much of this information to get down to a very narrow subset at any given moment. One potential reason is that we can generally only do one thing at a time and cutting out things that are currently irrelevant is important in the smooth production of coherent action.

Distinct Attentional Networks

As discussed, psychologists developed different tasks that would emphasise different aspects of attention. Not surprisingly, researchers using early neuroimaging techniques were keen to see whether there were different patterns of neural activation associated with different tasks. A review of this area proved very influential (Posner and Petersen 1990; Petersen and Posner 2012). Petersen and Posner (2012) proposed an anatomical basis for distinct attention networks. The anterior cingulate was particularly active during fast target-detection tasks and in situations where you need to inhibit a relatively automatic response – hence an important component within a 'selective attention' network. In contrast, damage to the right prefrontal cortex caused problems with long and tedious monitoring tasks – hence part of a 'vigilance' or 'sustained attention' network. Damage to the parietal cortex caused problems in moving attention around space – hence part of a 'spatial attention' network.

More recently, Gallo and Posner (2016), moving the emphasis from regions to brain networks, reviewed the research with a particular emphasis on those networks in which abnormal function had been associated with ADHD. Within this view a frontoparietal circuit was particularly involved in remaining alert and orienting to salient events. The dorsal frontostriatal circuit was involved in inhibitory control, response selection, and aspects of executive function. Finally, the mesocorticolimbic circuit was involved in motivation and reward processing.

It is important to emphasise that these task-based distinctions are relative; a particular network is significantly more active during one type of task than another. It does not mean that other brain areas and networks are not also involved or that damage/atypical development in these regions would not have an effect on performance.

The inclusion of ideas of reward and motivation in the discussion is useful at this point. A presumption sometimes in the experimental literature is that research participants are all equally motivated to pay attention to the often abstract tasks/stimuli used and that performance differences arise from the relative efficiency of attention processes (rather than the ability to self-motivate). An interesting question when it comes to interventions for poor attention (e.g. in the classroom) is whether one can enhance 'attention' by increasing the motivational and reinforcing qualities of the material (see below).

Disorders of Attention

Given the number of regions involved and the connections needed to support attention, it is not surprising that a very wide range of childhood problems have been linked with attention impairments (e.g. preterm birth, Fragile X syndrome, Williams syndrome, Turner syndrome, autism spectrum disorder, epilepsy, leukaemia, acquired brain injury, dyslexia, conduct disorder, anxiety, depression). Difficulties with attention can be secondary to another disorder. For example inattention can occur secondary to anxiety as a result of distraction by ruminative thoughts. At the same time, anxiety can arise from one's own perceived difficulties in paying attention and from negative feedback from others. Similarly, problems in attention will tend to co-occur with problems in learning, including challenges with reading (see Chapter 14 for more detail) and maths.

Whilst attention difficulties are common across many developmental conditions there is one to which attention is considered so central that it has it in its title. ADHD first made its appearance in the Diagnostic and Statistical Manual (DSM) of the American Psychiatric Association in 1980 (taking over from the 'hyperkinetic' [moving around excessively] terminology of the 1960s). Although there have been various revisions since, it is important to note that the ADHD diagnosis was, and is, entirely based on reports of behaviour and whether a problem (e.g. difficulty waiting one's turn) is considered excessive in a given context. This is not, in itself, a bad thing; such reports may (1) capture things missed by cognitive testing under highly focused one-to-one conditions and (2) be of greater relevance to real-world outcomes (Is a cognitive test better at determining whether a child will tend to run around the school than direct observation of that child in school?). Perhaps inevitably, such an approach leads to quite wide variations in diagnosis rates. There is also a lack of specificity in that two children can both meet diagnostic criteria for ADHD despite having few symptoms in common, whilst symptom-overlap between children with ADHD and those with other diagnoses, such as dyslexia, can be considerable.

ASSESSMENT AND FORMULATION

In assessing attention, multiple methods should be applied. These will include: obtaining a detailed history, gathering information from multiple informants (e.g. parents and teachers), understanding the child's perspective, quantitative self- and informant-report rating scales, behavioural observations, and performance-based cognitive assessments (American Academy of Pediatrics 2000).

As with other areas, a detailed history will include the family context, birth, and subsequent developmental and medical history, school experiences, peer and sibling relationships, and access to adequate opportunities to learn. Clinicians need to strike a delicate balance of having useful constructs in mind (e.g. selective attention, impulsivity) and being 'too ready' to see these in the presentation (e.g. problems in 'sustaining attention whilst reading' may be more attributable to the TV blaring away in the background). Important areas to probe will include when the problems emerged, when and in what situations they are most likely to occur, times when problems are less likely to happen, and the negative and potentially positive consequences of the difficulties (e.g. possible increased parental attention, avoidance of difficult situations). It is always useful to gauge for whom these difficulties are a problem – the child? Parents? School? Additionally, what are the expectations concerning assessment, potential interventions, and outcomes if a formal diagnosis is given. In addition, clinicians should be aware that the presentations may differ across different populations. For example research has described differences in the ADHD symptom presentation (e.g. more inattentive symptoms and related internalising symptoms, lower rates of co-occurring disruptive behaviours) and differences in identification of ADHD in females compared to males (Hinshaw et al. 2021). Diagnosis may be important for parents, siblings, schools, and peers, and for children in reducing self-blame or perception of the self as 'stupid' or 'lazy'. A formal diagnosis may also be critical in gaining resources to better support schools and families. It is important to also consider and minimise the potentially negative consequences of diagnosis including stigma, self-fulfilling negative expectations, and over reliance on medication rather than working with children to help develop their skills and resilience, or changing the context/ environment to allow a child to better cope. Inattention will often co-occur with other symptoms and thought needs to be given to the most appropriate diagnosis.

Rating Scales

DSM-IV-TR and DSM-5 diagnosis of ADHD and its variants requires particular problems to be reported across at least two contexts (generally school and home). The use of multiple-informant rating scales for children, parents, and teachers is useful in gaining information on attention problems across environments. Clinically, the completion of both broad and narrow band assessments is helpful when considering a differential diagnosis of ADHD along with other diagnoses that may impact attention and behaviour. These diagnoses can include disruptive behaviours, anxiety or depression, language impairment, etc. Broad-band measures (e.g. Behavior Assessment System for Children, Third Edition or Child Behavior Checklist) include subscales that assess some symptoms of ADHD and common co-occurring difficulties. In contrast, there are narrow measures that specifically assess symptoms and behaviours related to DSM criteria for ADHD.

Many of these narrow-band instruments have strong internal psychometric properties and reasonable normative samples (Collett, Ohan, and Myers 2003). A recent meta-analysis indicated that several commonly used ADHD scales (e.g. Conners Rating Scale-Revised; Conners et al. 1998; Child Behavior Checklist – Attention Problem Scale; Achenbach and Rescorla 2001) had only moderate sensitivity and specificity in diagnosing ADHD (Chang, Wang, and Tsai 2016). Parent and teacher ratings of ADHD symptoms may also only modestly intercorrelate (Rescorla et al. 2013). Where this reflects actual variation in symptom presentation across contexts, it is, of course, clinically useful information about observations of behaviour across settings but may also reflect differences in informant bias, awareness of typical development, and comprehension (De Los Reyes 2013).

Neuropsychological Assessments of Attention

ADHD diagnosis is based on reports of particular behavioural characteristics. There has been limited research assessing the added value of neuropsychological assessment in diagnosing and treating ADHD. It is, however, well documented that there are significant group differences between children and adolescents with and without ADHD on neuropsychological assessments, and that performance on tests may be useful for identifying children with ADHD who are at risk for academic underachievement and predicting response to treatment with methylphenidate (Molitor and Landberg 2017). Thus, neuropsychological assessments are useful in clinical assessments of attention in understanding the underlying deficits associated with an individual's symptom presentation and to guide treatment recommendations.

There are several discrete neuropsychological tests that assess individual subdomains of attention. Given the conceptual overlap with the tests discussed in Chapter 11 on executive functioning, this section will focus on measures that are less likely to tap into the executive function domain. There are, however, many executive measures that have proved sensitive to ADHD.

Individual Assessments of Attention

The most commonly used objective assessments of attention, specifically *sustained attention*, are continuous performance tests (CPTs). In CPTs a child is asked to monitor a lengthy stream of stimuli and respond to the presentation of targets, whilst withholding responses to nontargets. There is a balance between the likely sensitivity and specificity of the tasks as well as their reliability and overall task duration. Increasing the number of targets (i.e. observations of whether or not they are detected) will tend to increase reliability but could diminish demands on sustained attention through presenting frequent goal-relevant events, or make the task impractically lengthy. Having a high ratio of targets to nontargets will reduce children's expectation of non-targets and make 'inhibitory' errors more likely; having a low ratio will tend to increase error propensity on targets with, in both cases, the same trade-off between number of observations and overall task duration. Two widely used measures reflect different approaches. Conners' Continuous Performance Test, Third Edition (Conners 2014) has a target:non-target ratio of 4:1, whilst the Gordon Diagnostic System Vigilance Task (Gordon 1986) uses 1:9. The Test of Variables of Attention (Leark et al. 2016) uses a hybrid design, switching between a majority of nontargets in the first half of and a majority of targets in the second. Various metrics can be derived from the tasks including target/nontarget response accuracy, reaction time, and variability in reaction time. Numerous studies show relative impairment in children with ADHD on CPTs, and both reaction time and variability in reaction time have reported high correlations with ADHD symptoms (time-on-task decrements tend to be more variable [e.g. Epstein et al. 2003; Huang-Pollock et al. 2012]). The literature remains somewhat inconsistent regarding the most sensitive form of CPT for ADHD, which, in part, may reflect the heterogeneity of the condition or psychometric (e.g. reliability/validity) aspects of the CPT task itself.

Visual search and cancellation tests are often administered to assess selective or focused attention. There are a host of embedded tasks in broader neurocognitive batteries or individual tests of attention (examples include: Trails A, Condition 1 on the Trail Making test on the Delis–Kaplan Executive Function System, Cancellation on the Wechsler tests). Examples of attentional switching tasks include Trails B, Response Set on the Developmental Neuropsychological Assessment, Second Edition, verbal fluency switching tasks. Finally, divided attention tasks include Letter-Number Sequencing, Trails B, Color Word Interference from the Delis–Kaplan Executive Function System, or aspects of the Stroop Color-Word Test.

Broader Neuropsychological Assessments of Attention

The Test of Everyday Attention for Children (TEA-Ch; Manly et al. 1998; TEA-Ch2; Manly et al. 2016) takes a rather different approach by presenting a battery of tasks designed to emphasise different aspects of attention. One of its measures of sustained attention, for example, asks children to keep a silent count of tones presented separated by long and unpredictable silent intervals. The rationale is that a lapse at any stage during the string will show up in an erroneous total. By looking *across* three very different TEA-Ch measures of, for example, sustained attention (auditory CPT and frequent go/infrequent no-go tasks in TEA-Ch; computerised simple reaction time and frequent go/infrequent no-go tasks in TEA-Ch2), the argument is that a clinician can better get at the underlying construct somewhat independently of the particular task used to capture it. Whilst the TEA-Ch was not developed as a diagnostic tool for ADHD, not surprisingly, significant impairments in performance have been reported in this group, particularly on the sustained attention measures (e.g. Heaton et al. 2001).

INTERVENTION AND MANAGEMENT

In considering interventions for attention problems, it is useful to think about the individual, the context (e.g. classroom), and functional goals that inattention may act to undermine. For example a child's attention may be better in the morning, after a good night's sleep, during an enjoyable task, or after a break. Attention may well be worse if a child is hungry, unwell, in conflict with others, or anxious. Tasks might be easier without background distraction or in small groups. Extra time may be needed to achieve the same academic goals (one of the benefits of becoming a proficient reader or having maths knowledge is that it reduces the attentional demands as tasks become more automatic). Useful 'attention' interventions can therefore include working on barriers to good sleep, thinking about meals, scheduling breaks into tasks, finding ways to maximise enjoyment in tasks, and improving mood and self-image. The underlying tendencies may persist, but functional goals may be more easily achieved.

In this respect, given his history, Caleb's academic performance (high range performance in reading and writing, average range in maths) is encouraging. It suggests that the cognitive 'scaffolding' provided by his mother in the home-schooling environment has paid off. Part of an intervention would be to reflect this back and encourage continued experimentation on getting the best from him. In addition, that he was able to achieve these levels in standardised tests *without* extra time or support, suggests that this repeated positive experience of structure may have helped develop his own strategies, skills, and persistence.

Mood problems can exacerbate poor attention and vice versa. Accordingly, continued outpatient psychotherapy is an important aspect of Caleb's attention intervention.

Whilst there is some positive evidence for the sole use of psychosocial interventions for ADHD, combined psychosocial and pharmacological approaches have received stronger support (Chan, Fogler, and Hammerness 2016). The American Academy of Pediatrics and the American Academy of Child and Adolescent Psychiatry both support the use of stimulant medication as the first-line treatment for ADHD in school-aged children (Pliszka and AACAP Work Group on Quality Issues 2007; Wolraich, Brown, and Brown 2011).

Caleb's treatment primarily focused on cognitive behavioural therapy to address his depressive symptoms. Following evaluation, a trial of stimulant medication was found beneficial with minimal side effects. In addition, behaviour therapy, contingency management, and/or direct skill training may provide further support. The bulk of the research on psychosocial approaches to ADHD has focused on parent-training/parent interventions, and whether these can reduce ADHD symptoms and co-occurring behavioural challenges. Evidence on efficacy is particularly strong in early childhood (Mulqueen et al. 2015). Moreover, there is evidence that intensive, manualised treatment summer programs specific for children with ADHD can be effective (Evans, Owens, and Bunford 2014). For readers based in the UK, the guidance given in the National Institute for Clinical Excellence on ADHD may be beneficial (https://www.nice.org.uk/guidance/ng87). In addition, please see Chapter 13 (on disruptive behaviour) for details on parenting interventions for children with ADHD.

Finally, Caleb was experiencing social difficulties and overt peer rejection, which is not uncommon in individuals with ADHD. Therefore a six-session intervention focused in building social skills and response inhibition was carried out with the paediatric neuropsychologist (Garcia-Winner 2007; also see Chapter 12).

Outcome

In a neuropsychological evaluation, Caleb showed relative strengths in working memory and relative weakness in visuospatial tasks, resulting in an overall average Full Scale IQ of 98 on the Wechsler Intelligence Scale for Children, Fifth UK Edition. The strength of his working memory performance may seem surprising given his everyday difficulties. Such apparent anomalies highlight how a test's context (e.g. an examiner gaining a child's attention before reading relative short strings of numbers) can help some children maintain concentration and perform well, at least for a period. Identifying variability across tests, and the conditions that can produce good performance, are important in interpreting results and in thinking about maximising function in everyday tasks.

Other areas of notable strength included average to high-range verbal learning and memory when information was presented with repetition.

Caleb's difficulties with visuospatial skills and graphomotor coordination were consistent with his history of extremely preterm birth and he met diagnostic criteria for ADHD based on parent and self-report ratings, which occurs at a higher rate in children with a history of extremely preterm birth (Johnson and Marlow 2011). He achieved low average to borderline-level performance across assessments of selective, sustained, and divided attention on the TEA-Ch2. Caleb required frequent redirection and prompting to attend to task demands and was easily distracted by environmental stimuli and his own thought, often tangentially initiating conversation, or commenting on things unrelated to the task at hand. His problems with sustained attention and inhibitory control are impacting his social functioning as he is easily distracted in the social environment, has difficulty inhibiting himself from engaging in unrelated conversation, and has difficulty with behavioural inhibition and regulation (e.g. maintaining personal boundaries, keeping his hands to himself, interrupting others), which is leading to peer rejection. This has led Caleb to feel down and socially isolated. In addition, he is aware of some of his cognitive difficulties leading to decreased self-esteem, withdrawal from activities, and low mood.

SUMMARY

The cognitive domain of attention is complex and encompasses a number of subdomains that impact our ability to perform a range of cognitive tasks both in the assessment setting and in daily life. Given the complexity of these subdomains, a number of neural circuits and networks have been implicated in various aspects of attention though there is still a great deal to learn. Disorders of attention are behaviourally based diagnoses and thus there are no specific tests that can definitively identify the presence or absence of ADHD. Thorough interviewing, information from multiple sources regarding functioning across environments (e.g. school, home, and the social setting), as well as behavioural observations are crucial in making an appropriate diagnosis. It is also critical to understand that attention difficulties can be the primary issue, co-occurring with another presentation, or secondary to another diagnosis (e.g. anxiety or learning difficulties). Thus, a thorough diagnostic evaluation is imperative to provide an appropriate conceptualisation and recommendations. Whilst neuropsychological evaluation data is not sufficient for making a diagnosis of an attentional disorder, it does provide helpful information to understand an individual's presentation and guide treatment planning. This may be particularly useful in patient populations with complex medical and neurodevelopmental histories that increase the risk for ADHD or attention difficulties as well as other neurocognitive difficulties (e.g. extremely preterm birth, certain genetic disorders, epilepsy, etc.) as was the case for Caleb.

Given the heterogeneity of this population and the fact that there is still a great deal that is unknown about the genetic contribution and neurobiology of the disorder, future research focused on understanding causal mechanisms will be beneficial. In addition, continued research exploring the efficacy of psychosocial and behavioural intervention across the lifespan will be beneficial including a clear focus on the impact of commonly provided academic accommodations on outcomes.

REFERENCES

American Academy of Pediatrics (2000) Clinical practice guideline: diagnosis and evaluation of the child with attention-deficit/hyperactivity disorder. *Pediatrics* **105**(5): 1158–1170.

Chan E, Fogler JM, Hammerness PG (2016) Treatment of attention-deficit/hyperactivity disorder in adolescents: A systematic review. *JAMA* **315**(18): 1997–2008.

Chang L, Wang M, Tsai P (2016) Diagnostic accuracy of rating scales for attention-deficit/hyperactivity disorder: A meta-analysis. *Pediatrics* **137**(5): 1–13.

Collett BR, Ohan JL, Myers KM (2003) Ten-year review of rating scales. V: Scales assessing attention-deficit/hyperactivity disorder. *Journal of American Academy of Child & Adolescent Psychiatry* **42**(2): 1015–1037.

Conners CK, Sitarenios G, Parker JD, Epstein JN (1998) The revised Conners' Parent Rating Scale (CPRS-R): Factor structure, reliability, and criterion validity. *Journal of Abnormal Child Psychology* **26**(4): 257–268.

De Los Reyes A (2013) Strategic objectives for improving understanding of informant discrepancies in developmental psychopathology research. *Development and Psychopathology* **25**(3): 669–682.

Desimone R, Duncan J (1995) Neural mechanisms of selective visual attention. *Annual Review of Neuroscience* **18**: 193–222.

Epstein JN, Erkanli A, Conners CK, Klaric J, Costello JE, Angold A (2003) Relations between Continuous Performance Test performance measures and ADHD behaviors. *Journal of Abnormal Child Psychology* **31**(5): 543–554.

Evans SW, Owens JS, Bunford N (2014) Evidence-based psychosocial treatments for children and adolescents with attention-deficit/hyperactivity disorder. *Journal of Clinical Child & Adolescent Psychology* **43**(4): 527–551.

Gallo EF, Posner J (2016) Moving towards causality in attention-deficit hyperactivity disorder: Overview of neural and genetic mechanisms. *The Lancet. Psychiatry* **3**(6): 555–567. https://doi.org/10.1016/S2215-0366(16)00096-1.

Garcia-Winner M (2007) *Thinking About You, Thinking About Me*, 2nd edition. Santa Clara, CA: Think Social Pub.

Gordon M (1986) *Instruction Manual for the Gordon Diagnostic System*. DeWitt, NY: Checkmate Plus.

Heaton SC, Reader SK, Preston AS et al. (2001) The test of everyday attention for children (TEA-Ch): Patterns of performance in children with ADHD and clinical controls. *Child Neuropsychology* **7**(4): 251–264.

Hinshaw SP, Nguyen PT, O'Grady SM, Rosenthal EA (2021) Annual research review: Attention-deficit/hyperactivity disorder in girls and women: Underrepresentation, longitudinal processes, and key directions. *Journal of Child Psychology and Psychiatry*. https://pubmed.ncbi.nlm.nih.gov/34231220/.

Huang-Pollock CL, Karalunas SL, Tam H, Moore AN (2012) Evaluating vigilance deficits in ADHD: A meta-analysis of CPT performance. *Journal of Abnormal Psychology* **121**(2): 360–371.

Johnson S, Marlow N (2011) Preterm birth and childhood psychiatric disorders. *Pediatric Research* **69**: 11–18.

Manly T, Robertson IH, Anderson VA, Nimmo-Smith I (1998) *TEA-Ch – The Test of Everyday Attention for Children*. London: Pearson Assessment.

Molitor SJ, Langberg JM (2017) Using task performance to inform treatment planning for youth with ADHD: A systematic review. *Clinical Psychology Review* **58**: 157–173.

Mulqueen JM, Bartley CA, Bloch MH (2015) Meta-analysis: Parental interventions for preschool ADHD. *Journal of Attention Disorders* **19**(2): 118–124.

Petersen SE, Posner MI (2012) The attention system of the human brain: 20 years after. *Annual Review of Neuroscience* **35**: 73–89.

Pliszka S, AACAP Work Group on Quality Issues (2007) Practice parameter for the assessment and treatment of children and adolescents with attention-deficit/hyperactivity disorder. *Journal of the American Academy of Child & Adolescent Psychiatry* **46**(7): 894–921.

Posner M, Petersen S (1990) The attention system of the human brain. *Annual Reviews of Neurology* **13**: 25–42.

Rescorla LA, Ginzburg S, Achenbach TM (2013) Cross-informant agreement between parent-reported and adolescent self-reported problems in 25 societies. *Journal of Clinical Child and Adolescent Psychology* **42**(2): 262–273.

Wolraich M, Brown L, Brown RT (2011) Subcommittee on quality improvement and management. ADHD clinical practice guideline for the diagnosis, evaluation and treatment of attention-deficit/hyperactivity disorder in children and adolescents. *Pediatrics* **128**: 1007–1022.

CHAPTER 9

Memory

Rachael Elward, Patricia Martin-Sanfilippo,
and Faraneh Vargha-Khadem

Presenting Concern

Mark is a right-handed, 10-year-old boy with a history of pharmacoresistant epilepsy. He was referred for neuropsychological assessment as part of the evaluation to check his suitability for epilepsy surgery to relieve his seizures. Mark was born via normal delivery, and his early milestones were met on time. His first seizure was at age 3 years and he was formally diagnosed with epilepsy at the age of 4 years. Mark experienced stereotyped seizures characterised by a strange feeling in his stomach accompanied by lip smacking, inability to talk, and making mumbling noises. He then became unresponsive, his legs began to shake, he fell, and lost consciousness. The whole episode lasted less than 1 minute, and he would then sleep for up to 2 hours. The seizures occurred every 2 weeks in clusters. The seizures occurred every 2 weeks in clusters and were not associated with motor weakness on the right side. Mark was prescribed sodium valproate. Five antiseizure medications had been tried, some in combination, to control his seizures.

Mark attended a mainstream primary school. His parents and teachers expressed concerns about his behaviour and cognition, such as word retrieval, language, concentration, and memory. His seizures affected his sleep, schoolwork, and quality of life. He was given support for his seizures at school but not for his educational and cognitive needs.

Mark was admitted to the hospital for 4 days to carry out video telemetry and presurgical evaluations. Magnetic resonance imaging (MRI) revealed left hippocampal sclerosis. Seizure semiology and ictal video electroencephalogram were consistent with left temporal onset, but with rapid spread to the contralateral right temporal lobe. However, there was no indication of an independent seizure focus on the right side. His ophthalmology assessment was unremarkable. Neuropsychiatric evaluation indicated that Mark exhibited verbal and physical aggression at home and at school. He also suffered from anxiety. He had been referred to his local child and adolescent mental health services for intervention.

Based on all of the information gathered, we formulated hypotheses to guide Mark's neuropsychological assessment (see Table 9.1) and administered neuropsychological protocols developed for a local epilepsy surgery programme. The protocols are sensitive to developmental changes in cognitive and behavioural status as a function of increasing age and experience. The protocol assesses several cognitive domains reflecting the connectivity and interactions between neural networks underlying intelligence, memory, perception, and executive function.

Table 9.1 Symptom to function mapping

Semiology/presenting features	Neuropsychological hypotheses and protocols
Seizure onset at age 3 years; confirmed diagnosis of epilepsy at age 4 years	Early onset of epilepsy could lead to interhemispheric reorganisation of verbal functions
Seizure onset preceded by a strange feeling in the stomach; lip smacking	Epigastric symptoms and lip smacking suggest temporal lobe involvement
Inability to talk, speech arrest	Seizures disrupt the language production network – Broca's area
	Functional magnetic resonance imaging (fMRI) of language lateralisation required
Slurred speech and mumbling noises	Motor speech evaluation; differential diagnosis of dysarthria versus dyspraxia
Word retrieval problems	Seizures disrupt access to stored semantics
Concerns for behaviour	Evaluate aspects of behaviour affected; identify seizure burden; assess quality of life
Concentration problems	Evaluate attention and orientation
Epilepsy impacted overnight sleep	Sleep disturbance interferes with memory consolidation
MRI revealed left hippocampal sclerosis	Is hippocampal sclerosis unilateral or bilateral? If bilateral, memory function is disproportionately reduced relative to IQ. If unilateral, material specific deficit verbal memory deficit is more likely
	Is there concordance between MRI lesion and fMRI results?
Seizure semiology and ictal video electroencephalogram were consistent with left temporal onset but with rapid spread to the contralateral right temporal lobe	Seizure spread could affect function of the right temporal lobe

THEORY

Learning and memory are the processes through which all knowledge about the world is encoded, consolidated, stored, and subsequently retrieved. Memory is fundamental to our social existence, day-to-day functioning, and educational success. Unfortunately, memory function is particularly vulnerable to different types of brain disease or injury. Mnemonic impairments, either selectively or more generally, have been documented in a range of neurodevelopmental disorders including genetic conditions, severe acute infection, perinatal brain insults, acquired ischaemic stroke, and epilepsy (Vargha-Khadem et al. 1997; Gadian et al. 2000; Cormack et al. 2012; Alloway and Gathercole 2015; Elward and Vargha-Khadem 2018). From this diverse range of disorders affecting brain function, a broad spectrum of memory impairments can emerge depending on the aetiology and the pattern of underlying neuropathology. Although mnemonic function as a whole is associated with a distributed network of brain regions, the medial temporal lobes are particularly important for memory (Squire 2004; Wixted and Squire 2011). Furthermore, the neuropsychological literature shows that different structures within the medial temporal lobe are associated with different aspects of memory processing (see Bauer and Dugan 2020 for an overview). Neuropsychological assessment of memory using standardised scales will often identify the integrity of different components of learning and memory in relation to their underlying neural substrates.

Attention and Working Memory

In order to complete any complex cognitive task (e.g. mental arithmetic), one must focus attention on the task and also keep in mind relevant information (e.g. the numbers and the operations). Working memory refers to this kind of attention-directed, online memory for small amounts of information that are currently relevant to an immediate goal (Baddeley 2010). Information (including phonological and visuospatial material) may be maintained in an active state for a short time in the service of a goal. However, when attention turns to another task, the information can pass out of working memory and be forgotten, or it may be maintained in an intermediate, or in long-term memory for more permanent storage. Because working memory is specific to immediate goals, deficits in this domain are more closely associated with executive control of attention and self-monitoring functions, than with memory problems specifically (Diamond 2013). However, children with working memory difficulties may have difficulty encoding information into long-term memory and this may affect their learning. For example if you have difficulty repeating a phone number in working memory, then it is unlikely that the sequence of numbers will be correctly learned and stored in long-term memory. Therefore, the status of working memory and executive function should be investigated alongside that of long-term memory so that any deficits can be appropriately characterised.

Long-Term Memory

Long-term memory refers to the retention or storage of information over an extended period of time. Long-term cognitive memory is traditionally divided into two main categories: episodic memory and semantic memory (Squire 2004).

Episodic Memory

Episodic memory refers to the storehouse of past events of our lives and our personal autobiography. It enables us to bring back to mind events from our past so that we can re-experience these events in our mind. Events can be either incidentally or intentionally encoded into the episodic memory system as we experience the world. Some of these memories fade and are forgotten, so that we would not be able to recall them vividly with the passage of time, but special events (such as a wedding day or a heated argument) can be remembered with high fidelity for decades. The integrity of the hippocampal circuit is critical for episodic memory. The hippocampus has a protracted course of development. Its functions begin to emerge in early childhood, but with increasing age, experience, and independence, they reach maturity later in childhood/adolescence (Schacter and Moscovitch 1984).

Semantic Memory

Semantic memory refers to general world knowledge that we have accumulated. It consists of facts, ideas, meaning, words, and concepts (e.g. Paris is the capital city of France). In contrast to episodic memory, the defining feature of semantic memory is explicit knowledge devoid of context. Young children develop a huge amount of semantic knowledge in their early years as they learn language and come to understand the world around them. Semantic memory is thought to occur over multiple exposures to new material and requires consolidation of new information into existing conceptual structures. Semantic learning develops early whilst the hippocampus is still immature. Therefore, it does not depend on the integrity of the hippocampus in early life but on efficient processing of cortical regions, particularly the temporal neocortex.

In later childhood, the extent to which semantic memory can proceed as normal following damage to the medial temporal lobe is under some debate. In extreme cases, where children have suffered selective, hippocampal damage bilaterally during the perinatal period (e.g. due to asphyxia, circulatory problems, etc.), a developmental form of an amnesic syndrome can emerge later during childhood. Remarkably, despite their amnesic syndrome, such patients develop age-appropriate semantic memory and language skills throughout childhood and adolescence (Vargha-Khadem et al. 1997; Elward and Vargha-Khadem 2018). These notable cases suggest that semantic and episodic memory may have different neural substrates, further indicating that semantic learning can proceed, possibly via compensatory mechanisms, despite extensive damage to the hippocampal circuit. However, typically developing children rely on the hippocampus to support semantic learning. Children with any form of hippocampal-dependent memory problems will be at a disadvantage in education. In high school, children are expected to learn information over a relatively short amount of time, such as navigating around school buildings. Typically developing children are likely to use both the episodic and semantic memory systems to support their learning experiences in these circumstances, whilst those with episodic memory deficits will struggle to keep up with their peers.

Recall

Recall is the process through which we explicitly retrieve episodic and semantic memories from memory. Recall is usually self-generated in that the person has to reactivate a stored memory at will. The integrity of the hippocampal circuitry is critical for both episodic memory and recall (Tulving 2002). The physical trajectory of hippocampal development coincides with the onset of earliest explicit childhood memories. Before this age, children may not remember their personal past, and can experience difficulty with accurate recall of events in time and space (Bauer 2008). Similarly, older children with hippocampal damage may experience the same difficulties with recall (e.g. remembering instructions, forgetting their belongings).

Recognition

Recognition is a simpler memory process than recall because it does not solely rely on self-generation of information, or require bringing back to mind past events or facts. Instead, it is triggered by an external cue that evokes a stored memory. Recognition requires the identification of items that have been encountered before and stored in memory (e.g. identifying a familiar person in a series of photographs) (for review of recognition in relation to recall, see Yonelinas 2002). Within the first few days of life, infants demonstrate recognition memory by responding to familiar faces long before they are able to form and retrieve episodic memories (Fagan 1972). Recognition memory is associated with the function of cortical areas within the medial temporal lobe subjacent to the hippocampus (viz. the rhinal cortices, see Fig. 9.1) as well as the overlying temporal neocortex. When the hippocampus is selectively and severely damaged by disease or injury early in life, these neighbouring cortical regions may compensate remarkably well for some mnemonic processes, such as recognition memory.

Verbal and Nonverbal Memory Processing

The processes of recognition and recall encompass both verbal and visual information. However, depending on the status of hemispheric specialisation and lateralisation of function, the left hippocampus and the medial temporal lobe regions may be preferentially

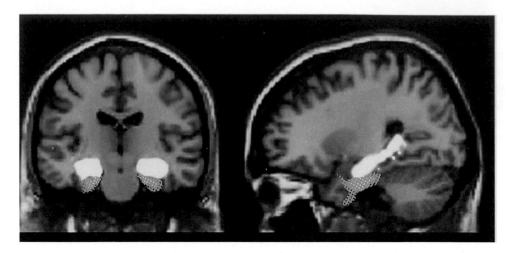

Figure 9.1 Magnetic resonance imaging scan of the brain with the hippocampus highlighted in white and the underlying rhinal cortices in cross-hatch. (A colour version of this figure can be seen in the colour plate section)

recruited for recall/recognition of verbal information, and their homologue on the right may be recruited for the processing of visual-spatial memoranda. In paediatric temporal lobe epilepsy, however, regardless of hemispheric side of involvement, verbal memory function, particularly verbal recall, is frequently compromised. This may be partly related to the fact that hemispheric specialisation and lateralisation of function, especially for speech and language, are evolving processes that do not become crystallised until early adolescence (Vargha-Khadem et al. 1992; Vargha-Khadem et al. 2011). Consequently, depending on the age at insult, lateralisation of function, and the hemisphere involved (Cormack et al. 2007; Cormack et al. 2012), the pattern of language and memory representation may be overwritten by compensatory mechanisms operating in the immature brain (Cacucci and Vargha-Khadem 2019; see Gonzalez and Wrennall 2020 for a review). In general, verbal memory and language difficulties impact educational attainment, and so these may be particularly important in the assessment of paediatric populations.

ASSESSMENT AND FORMULATION

In order to identify memory impairments in children, it is important to rule out deficits in other cognitive domains (see chapters in this volume that give further detail on language, attentional, intellectual disability, mental health difficulties, executive functions, hearing and vision, and motivation or effort). Hypotheses may be tested to determine which skills underlie an impairment (e.g. language tests are administered when a child obtains low scores on measures of verbal memory to rule out a language disorder).

Evaluation of learning and memory in children was initially based on adult memory batteries with little or no consideration of developmental factors. This practice was based on the assumption that the same memory domains found in adults were present in children and developed to the same extent. It has since been demonstrated, however, that different aspects of memory develop at different rates, and the development of the memory system as a whole depends on the maturation of other brain systems with which they are associated (Saklofske et al. 2013). Memory capacity increases alongside the development of more efficient information processing and recall strategies. This illustrates, for example, how memory is associated with processing speed and executive functions (Anderson, Northam, and Wrenall 2019).

Several well-validated memory tests for children are now available (see Table 9.2). Memory assessments typically include different modalities for presenting the stimuli

Table 9.2 Examples of standardised memory tests and subtests for each memory domain

Memory domain	Behavioural deficit[a]	Standardised tests – subtests
Working memory	Following instructions Vocabulary Speech Literacy Second languages Academic subjects with high verbal load	Children's Test of Nonword Repetition (CN REP) Wechsler Intelligence Scale for Children, Fifth Edition (WISC-V): Digits Forwards; Letter-Number Sequences Clinical Evaluation of Language Fundamentals, Fifth Edition (CELF-5): Repeating Sentences
	Mental manipulation Planning Revision Maths	WISC-V: Digits Backwards Working Memory Test Battery for Children (WMTB-C): Corsi Block Span Backwards; Listening Span; Counting Recall: Self-Ordered Pointing Task
	Nonverbal ability Social communication skills Academic subjects (art, science, geography, maths)	WMTB-C: Corsi Block Span Forward WISC-V: Picture Span Children's Memory Scale (CMS): Dot Location Rey Complex Figure Test: Immediate Recall
Long-term memory: Semantic	Factual knowledge Meaning of words Concepts	Pyramids and Palm Trees WISC-V: Information; Vocabulary; Similarities British Picture Vocabulary Test, Third Edition (BPVS-III) Expressive and Receptive One-Word Picture Vocabulary Tests, Fourth Edition (EOWPVT-4 and ROWPVT-4)

(*Continued*)

Table 9.2 Continued

Memory domain	Behavioural deficit[a]	Standardised tests – subtests
Long–term memory: Episodic	Recall of own experiences	Rivermead Behavioural Memory Test for Children (RBMT-C)
	Orientation in time and space	CMS: Delayed Recall
	Remembering to do things in the future	Rey Complex Figure Test: Delayed Recall
	Identifying source of memory	Children's Auditory Verbal Learning Test, Second Edition (CAVLT-2)
	Autobiographical and prospective memory	California Verbal Learning Test – Children's Version (CVLT-C)
	Social interaction	Child and Adolescent Memory Profile
	Independent living skills	A Developmental Neuropsychological Assessment, Second Edition (NEPSY-2)
	Organisation	Test of Memory and Learning, Second Edition (TOMAL-2)

[a]The behavioural deficits are presented only as some examples of the areas that may be affected as a consequence of the specific type of memory impairment. Deficits in other cognitive domains (e.g. language, attention) can also be associated with difficulties in these areas.

(e.g. auditory, visual), different types of recall intervals (e.g. immediate, delayed), types of material (verbal, nonverbal, spatial), exploration of different stages of processing (encoding, consolidation, storage, and retrieval), vulnerability to interference, and retrieval access (free recall, cued recall, recognition).

The neuropsychological formulation is a crucial aspect of the assessment. Formulation integrates information from all sources into an evidence-based interpretation. Radiological data may be included in a clinical formulation (see Table 9.1). These techniques are routinely used in specialist centres and multidisciplinary settings to identify the location, type, and extent of lesions causing seizures.

The formulation should also consider the possible side effects of medication(s). In the case of epilepsy, the preoperative neuropsychological formulation includes the potential risks and benefits of surgery for long-term outcome in relation to seizure control, quality of life, and subsequent cognitive development. After careful consideration of all the available information, the neuropsychologist can determine whether the child has a selective memory impairment, which parts of the memory system are affected, and if other cognitive systems are compromised. The assessment findings are integrated with the child's developmental, cognitive, psychosocial, medical, and family history. Following formulation, the clinical neuropsychologist provides input to the multidisciplinary team, and highlights risks to memory using evidence from the neuropsychological profile of the child.

Results of Neuropsychological Assessment

Mark's behavioural, socioemotional, and cognitive functioning was assessed with a series of questionnaires (Table 9.3) and neuropsychological tests (Table 9.4). Mark was found to have significant verbal memory problems, sufficient to interfere with everyday life. This pattern is not uncommon in young people with left temporal lobe epilepsy. Mark's memory difficulties are consistent with the history of early onset epilepsy and left hippocampal sclerosis. Performance on a measure of reading comprehension was impaired relative to other cognitive domains. This deficit is more than likely related to the impact of verbal memory problems on higher-level aspects of verbal processing during reading. Parental questionnaires found no evidence of comorbidity with attention-deficit/hyperactivity disorder, autistic spectrum disorder, or high risk of mental health disorders, although heightened levels of anxiety and aggressive outbursts were most likely related to the seizure burden.

Functional MRI using the covert verb generation task was also conducted to assess language lateralisation. During the verb generation task Mark showed bilateral inferior frontal activation with a predominance on the left. This suggests Mark is left lateralised for language processing.

Table 9.3 Parental and self-report questionnaires

Domain of function	Questionnaire	Results
Adaptive behaviour	Adaptive Behaviour Assessment System, Third Edition	General Adaptive=Low Average Conceptual=Low Average Social=Low Average Practical=Low Average
Social communication skills	Social Communication Questionnaire	Below the clinical cut-off for autism spectrum disorders
Quality of life	Paediatric Quality of Life Inventory	Parental ratings and self-ratings indicated no concerns about quality of life in the domains of physical health Ratings of emotional, social, and school functioning were all below average
Impact of epilepsy	Impact of Paediatric Epilepsy Scale	High impact on self and family life
Memory	Everyday Memory Questionnaire, Revised	Difficulty remembering memory scenarios in everyday life Episodic memory problems reported by carers
Attention	Conners, Third Edition – Parent	Mild concerns about attention
Executive functions	Behaviour Rating Inventory of Executive Function, Second Edition	Significant concerns about working memory, behavioural, and emotional regulation

Table 9.4 Neuropsychological test results

Domain	Measures	Results
Intelligence	Wechsler Intelligence Scale for Children, Fifth Edition	Verbal Comprehension=Low Average
		Visual Spatial=Average
		Fluid Reasoning=Average
		Working Memory=Low Average
		Processing Speed=Low Average
		Full Scale IQ=Low Average
Memory	Children's Memory Scale	Verbal Immediate=Low Average
		Verbal Delayed=Low
		Poor performance particularly on the Word Pairs Subtest
		Visual Immediate=Low Average
		Visual Delayed=Low Average
		Delayed Recognition=Low
	Child and Adolescent Memory Profile	Verbal Memory=Low
		Visual Memory=Low Average
		Immediate Memory=Low Average
		Delayed Memory=Low
	Rey Complex Figure Test and Recognition Trial	Copy=Average
		Immediate Recall=Low Average
		Delayed Recall=Low
		Recognition=Low
Language	Clinical Evaluation of Language Fundamentals	Core Language=Low Average
		Receptive Language=Low Average
		ExpressiveLlanguage=Low Average
	Expressive One-Word Picture Vocabulary Tests	Low Average (word retrieval problems)
Motor	Grooved Pegboard Test	Average
Visuo-motor	Beery-Buktenica Developmental Test of Visual-Motor Integration, Sixth Edition	Average
Attention	Conners' Continuous Performance Test, Third Edition	Average performance in all domains
Executive functions	Behavioural Assessment of the Dysexecutive Syndrome in Children	Low Average
	Delis-Kaplan Executive Function System	Low Average
Academic attainments	Wechsler Individual Achievement Test, Third Edition	Word Reading=Low Average
		Spelling=Low Average
		Reading Comprehension=Low
		Numeracy=Low Average

The findings in Table 9.3 and 9.4 were discussed at the multidisciplinary team meeting. There was clear concordance between the clinical history, seizure semiology, MRI and fMRI findings, and the neuropsychological results. The risks for heightened verbal memory deficits post-surgery were highlighted, but in view of the seizure burden, and its impact on quality of life, it was recommended to the family that a lesion-focused left anterior temporal lobectomy would be advisable. The chances of seizure freedom and ultimate weaning from antiseizure medication were considered good. The potential risks were that Mark would develop a right upper quadrant visual field defect and further memory impairment, affecting more verbal memory than nonverbal visuospatial memory.

Outcome

At age 12 years, Mark underwent a left temporal lobectomy and hippocampectomy involving the removal of the epileptogenic tissue. The operation was successful in arresting the seizures, and the patient and his family were pleased with the outcome of surgery. Relief from seizures enabled Mark to participate more fully in education and make friends. His sleep was no longer disrupted at night and he enjoyed playing football. His behaviour improved considerably, and he was less anxious following surgical intervention.

Mark's verbal memory problems escalated, however, coinciding with the start of secondary school, which required increased independent studies and production of homework. Mark reported that he had difficulty remembering lessons (in particular, French and history). He had to write everything down but frequently forgot his homework at school.

At 1 year follow-up, Mark's postoperative neuropsychological assessment revealed a pattern of strengths and weaknesses consistent with hippocampal pathology (Cormack et al. 2012). The cognitive impairment was selective to memory and was now significantly impaired (performance in the extremely low range). The difficulties included delayed recall and learning of verbal information (stories and paired associates) and word retrieval problems. Mark's abilities in all other aspects of cognition were consistent with his previous assessment and not a concern. It is likely that at least some aspects of Mark's verbal memory deficits were exacerbated by the pressures of secondary school.

INTERVENTION AND MANAGEMENT

The following strategies for memory support were implemented for Mark's specific case; however, they are applicable for any child with memory impairments stemming from other aetiologies such as a traumatic brain injury or neurodevelopmental conditions.

Mark was provided with psychoeducation about his memory difficulties to encourage productive learning strategies that were tailored to his individual needs. A revision plan was agreed. The use of visual aids such as mind maps and flowcharts was recommended. These techniques made information more memorable given Mark's stronger visual memory abilities. Mark was taught how to use a flashcards app to design his own flashcards to help with his learning. He was also trained to use several strategies adapted from Wilson (2009), including: elaboration (linking the new information to his prior knowledge on templates that he was given before his lessons), PQRST (Preview, Question, Read, State, Test), and spaced retrieval (better to revise material on several occasions spaced apart than to revise frequently or in one block). The importance of 'test after study' to help with consolidation was emphasised.

A clinician provided the teaching team at school with guidance about the type of information Mark found difficult, highlighting his strengths as well as his memory difficulties. A plan to set goals and interventions was agreed between the clinician, Mark, his parents, and the school. Mark was given permission to record his lessons on his mobile phone so that he could listen to them later. One of Mark's teachers agreed to work with him after school to support his revision, help him with his homework, and encourage Mark to organise his work using the school calendar. His teacher supported Mark's semantic learning by providing quizzes based on multiple-choice tests. He was able to use recognition memory to solve these. He was exempted from studying French and used the time to study for core subjects. He was offered training sessions at school to use different types of assistive technology (e.g. smartphone, Talking Tin, dictation software, etc.). He was also trained to use cloze procedures, essay scaffolds, and writing frames (to prompt, remind, and guide Mark in written tasks and tests). Mark's parents encouraged him to use reminders, calendars, and memory aids to foster his growing independence and develop lifelong strategies to compensate for his memory difficulties. Advice was given that strategies needed to be first modelled with Mark until he was familiar with them.

Interventions to Scaffold Memory and Learning

As discussed above, mnemonic problems in children can occur because of disruption of a range of memory-related processes. At present, there are no 'cures' for these organically based memory problems. Instead, intervention takes the form of encouraging children to use strategies that optimise learning. This can be done by finding optimal methods of learning and remembering and to support memory (for more information see Kapur 2017). In addition, children may not have full insight into their memory difficulties so realistic expectations will have to be set for them to promote their sense of self-esteem and achievement.

Children with memory problems are at a disadvantage in education. Where appropriate, modifications to the curriculum should be made to enable these children to get the most out of education. Technological aids, such as smartphones, may be used to support learning and improve day-to-day functioning. Such technologies need to be tailored to the developmental age of the child, their intellectual ability, and be compatible with their motor and language abilities. As children are increasingly adept at using technology, they may find creative solutions for memory problems and limit the impact on their quality of life.

SUMMARY

Memory is a broad term that includes several cognitive processes and recruits multiple brain networks. In order to thoroughly evaluate memory abilities, a clinician will need to assess: recall, recognition, semantic memory, episodic memory, and working memory. Neuropsychological test scores must be interpreted in the context of wider cognitive, emotional, motor, and perceptual difficulties, as well as evidence of brain pathology or aetiology. It will also be important to investigate variation in a child's own learning profile (i.e. relative strengths and difficulties in abilities). Psychoeducation about memory and how it impacts the individual when it is impaired will enable schools, carers, and children to develop compensatory strategies that are most compatible with their strengths.

REFERENCES

Alloway TP, Gathercole SE, editors (2015) *Working Memory and Neurodevelopmental Conditions*. Hove, UK: Psychology Press.

Anderson V, Northam E, Wrenall J (2019) *Developmental Neuropsychology: A Clinical Approach*, 2nd edition. London: Routledge.

Baddeley A (2010) Working memory. *Current Biology* **20**(4): R136–R140. https:doi.org/10.1016/j.cub.2009.12.014.

Bauer PJ (2008) Infantile amnesia. In: Haith MM, Benson JB, editors, *Encyclopedia of Infant and Early Childhood Development*. San Diego, CA: Academic Press, pp. 51–61.

Bauer PJ, Dugan JA (2020) Memory development. In: Rubenstein J, Rakic P, Chen B, Kwan KY, editors, *Neural Circuit and Cognitive Development*, 2nd edition. London: Academic Press, pp. 395–412.

Cacucci F, Vargha-Khadem F (2019) Contributions of nonhuman primate research to understanding the consequences of human brain injury during development. *Proceedings of the National Academy of Sciences* **116**(52): 26204–26209. doi: 10.1073/pnas.1912952116.

Cormack F, Vargha-Khadem F, Wood SJ, Cross JH, Baldeweg T (2012) Memory in paediatric temporal lobe epilepsy: Effects of lesion type and side. *Epilepsy Research* **98**: 255–259.

Cormack F, Cross JH, Harkness W et al. (2007) The development of intellectual abilities in pediatric temporal lobe epilepsy. *Epilepsia* **48**(1): 201–204. doi: 10.1111/j.1528-1167.2006.00904.x.

Diamond A (2013) Executive functions. *Annual Review of Psychology* **64**: 135–168. https://doi.org/10.1146/annurev-psych-113011-143750.

Elward RL, Vargha-Khadem F (2018) Semantic memory in developmental amnesia. *Neuroscience Letters* **680**: 23–30. doi: 10.1016/j.neulet.2018.04.040.

Fagan JF III (1972) Infants' recognition memory for faces. *Journal of Experimental Child Psychology* **14**: 453–476.

Gadian DG, Aicardi J, Watkins KE, Porter DA, Mishkin M, Vargha-Khadem F (2000) Developmental amnesia associated with early hypoxic–ischaemic injury. *Brain* **123**(3): 499–507. https://doi.org/10.1093/brain/123.3.499.

Gonzalez L, Wrennall JA (2020) A neuropsychological model for the pre-surgical evaluation of children with focal-onset epilepsy: An integrated approach. *Seizure* **77**: 29–39.

Kapur N (2017) *Cambridge Memory Manual: A Manual For Improving Everyday Memory Skills.* Available at: https://www.cambridgememorymanual.com/.

Schacter D, Moscovitch M (1984) Infants, amnesics, and dissociable memory systems. In: Moscovitch M, editor, *Infant Memory: Its Relation to Normal and Pathological Memory in Humans and Other Animals.* New York: Plenum, pp. 173–216. doi: 10.1007/978-1-4615-9364-5_8.

Saklofske DH, Reynolds CR, Schwean V, Adams W (2013) Memory assessment. In Saklofske DH, Reynolds CR, Schwean VL, editors, *The Oxford Handbook of Child Psychological Assessment.* New York: Oxford University Press, pp. 494–525.

Squire LR (2004) Memory systems of the brain: A brief history and current perspective. *Neurobiology of Learning and Memory* 82: 171–177.

Tulving E (2002) Episodic memory: From mind to brain. *Annual Review of Psychology* 53: 1–25.

Vargha-Khadem F, Gadian DG, Watkins KE, Connelly A, Van Paesschen W, Mishkin M (1997) Differential effects of early hippocampal pathology on episodic and semantic memory. *Science* 277: 376–380.

Vargha-Khadem F, Isaacs E, van der Werf S, Robb S, Wilson J (1992) Development of intelligence and memory in children with hemiplegic cerebral palsy. The deleterious consequences of early seizures. *Brain* 115(1): 315–329.

Vargha-Khadem F, Isaacs E, Watkins K, Mishkin M (2011) Ontogenetic specialization of hemispheric function. In: Ganesan V, Kirkham F, editors, *Stroke and Cerebrovascular Disease in Childhood.* London: Mac Keith Press.

Wilson B (2009) *Memory Rehabilitation: Integrating Theory and Practice.* New York: The Guilford Press.

Wixted JT, Squire LR (2011) The medial temporal lobe and the attributes of memory. *Trends in Cognitive Sciences* 15(5): 210–217. https://doi.org/10.1016/j.tics.2011.03.005.

Yonelinas AP (2002) The nature of recollection and familiarity: A review of 30 years of research. *Journal of Memory and Language* 46(3): 441–517. https://doi.org/10.1006/jmla.2002.286.

CHAPTER 10

Auditory Processing

Teresa Bailey

Presenting Concern

Jaime, aged 10 years, was referred for neuropsychological assessment to rule out an attention disorder due to difficulty following multi-step directions, daydreaming, and drifting off-topic in class discussions. Coaches reported confusion about following directions during participation in team sports. In addition, although there was no reported problem in learning to read and write, reading speed was somewhat below expectations, and his spelling was not consistent, even within the same essay. Parents reported that Jaime did not always know what the homework assignment was and was reluctant to ask questions in class or to engage with classmates for clarification. As a result, homework took excessive time to complete, and grades suffered because the assignment had been misunderstood. Written assignments and tests lost points for 'careless' spelling errors.

Early history included a normal-term pregnancy and delivery, with several days receiving phototherapy for jaundice. Developmental milestones were all on time. Although there were no serious behavioural problems, Jaime had more difficulty staying focused and following directions in noisy environments compared to peers. There were no problems developing social relationships. Parents and teachers reported that Jaime preferred individual conversations and small groups rather than large groups at school or on sports pitches. Recently, Jaime indicated a preference for individual sports and has refused to participate in some group physical education activities.

School observation showed that Jaime appeared to be attentive and well-integrated socially in the classroom. Decibel meter readings ranged from very quiet (40dB–C), to moderate when the ventilation system was running (60dB–C), to levels that interfered with listening during transition times when instructions were being given (75dB–C). When the class broke into discussion groups, class noise level rose to and remained around 70dB–C, for the duration of the work period. Jaime appeared to attend but did not participate much in the discussion. When it was time to write about the discussion, Jaime asked the teacher to repeat the instructions.

THEORY

Auditory processing is a complex neurophysiological phenomenon that refers to what the central auditory nervous system (CANS) does with the auditory signal after it leaves the mechanical hearing processes of the outer, middle, and inner ear, and is then transmitted to the brain by the auditory nerve. From there, the signals are relayed through a series of both ipsilateral and contralateral subcortical and cerebellar regions, and are eventually processed and interpreted as sound by bilateral concentric cortical auditory processing areas. These processing areas are arranged to process and coordinate incoming signals according to frequency (pitch), intensity (loudness), duration, and differences of timing of the signal's arrival between the two ears. Additional specialised areas process whether a signal is speech or nonspeech. Higher cortical areas interpret meaning and, in feedback loops with the frontal lobes and the cerebellum, determine saliency and formulate behavioural responses to the processed signals. The seven auditory processes include sound localisation, lateralisation, discrimination (e.g. gap detection, testable example of sound discrimination), pattern recognition, temporal (timing) aspects pattern recognition, performance in the presence of competing signals (e.g. dichotic listening), and performance when presented with degraded signals (e.g. speech in noise). Thus, auditory processing is not a single event, but a unifying concept that encompasses multiple processes that take place both sequentially and simultaneously, in constantly shifting listening conditions, including during sleep (Bailey 2010). Compared to what is known about visual processing, however, the roles of each relay station and their complex networks are relatively poorly understood. Recently, Kraus (2021) published a work on laboratory research and applied intervention and outcome studies on the relationship of auditory processing to core paediatric neuropsychological concerns such as language and literacy development, early identification of difficulties, effects of noise on listening, as well as prevention and remediation strategies. Kraus's work could serve as a foundation text for neuropsychology's integration of auditory processing into evaluation and case conceptualisation.

No controversy exists that these processes take place in the brain. Disagreement focuses on the extent to which it is possible to assign the term 'disorder' to disruptions and/ or decrements in processing. This is the case regarding developmental, and to a lesser extent, acquired, disorders that can be assessed and documented in persons who have difficulty with various aspects of listening, usually in the presence of a normal audiogram for hearing perception. Peripheral hearing decrements and impairments, however, result in degraded incoming signals. This directly affects the quality of the subsequent central neural signals.

Central auditory disruptions or decrements in functioning can be caused by lesions, developmental delay, physiological problems, and diseases. These are referred to, individually and collectively, as (central) auditory processing disorder(s) or (C)APD(s). It is recognised in the current International Classification of Diseases and Related Health Problems, 10th Revision as H93.25 (World Health Organization 2016). APD is the subject of national professional health organisations' position statements and treatment guidelines (e.g. American Academy of Audiology, British Society of Audiology). A barrier to cross-disciplinary consultation regarding APDs is that although APDs may occur as a standalone diagnosis, they are often comorbid with other developmental disorders with overlapping symptoms, including, but not limited to, attention deficit disorders, autism spectrum disorder, language disorders, learning disorders, cognitive deficits such as borderline or lower intellectual functioning, and non-pathological 'tuning out' due to disinterest.

APDs are estimated to affect approximately 10% of the general population. Estimates range from 1% for a standalone APD to up to 30% to 70% comorbidity with various developmental and learning disorders (Brewer et al. 2016). Given the high prevalence of comorbidities in people with developmental and learning disorders, APDs should be considered a potential comorbidity as a matter of course in neuropsychological evaluations.

APDs are a heterogeneous group of conditions that manifest differently depending on where the problem(s) is/are within the central auditory system. They range from uncommon but identifiable lesions, to transient difficulties associated with decreased input into the central system (such as chronic otitis media with effusion), to common population difficulties such as difficulty understanding speech in noisy or sound-reflective environments (which itself has a developmental trajectory stretching into adolescence), including everyday classroom settings and restaurants (Bailey 2010).

Aetiology varies widely depending on the specific disorder. Studies of speech perception in noise have found heritability in the range of $h^2 = 0.32$ to 0.74 (Brewer et al. 2016). The statistic h^2 ranges in value from 0 to 1. Recent research has identified a new possible aetiology site in the density of dendrites at the cochlear-auditory-nerve junction. Dysfunctional signal transmission may occur even when both the cochlear function and the auditory nerve impulse conductivity are intact, but reduced dendritic density at this particular junction results in impaired transmission of signals at the very start of the central processes (Petitpre et al. 2018). Some of the known aetiologies of specific dysfunctions are: prenatal and perinatal exposure to nicotine (Baumann and Koch 2017), neonatal jaundice (Shapiro and Nakamura 2001), otitis media with and without effusion, and Chiari malformations (Bailey 2010). Commonly co-occurring developmental disorders include attention deficit disorder, dyslexia, speech and language disorders (Bailey 2013), and autism and autism-related genetic syndromes (Otto-Meyer et al. 2018).

ASSESSMENT AND FORMULATION

There is no pathognomonic sign that indicates an APD. It has been observed that whether a child or adolescent is diagnosed with an APD or an attention disorder may depend on whether the initial referral is to an audiologist or a psychologist or another health professional such as a speech and language therapist. Some of the interdisciplinary questioning about the existence of APDs comes from the overlap of symptoms among various developmental disorders, and whether there is anything that is specific to the CANS. It was noted that many of the symptoms associated with attention-deficit hyperactivity disorder, primarily inattentive type, were related to the failure to respond adequately to auditory sensory input, especially the ability to follow directions and being able to follow conversations (Bailey 2013).

This raises questions about hearing, attention, understanding language, working memory, and executive function to carry out multi-step instructions. While no one currently questions these functions, the idea that someone who is paying attention, who can hear, has at least minimally adequate language and can reasonably function in most areas of life, might have difficulty because of an auditory processing deficit, tends to be discounted in neuropsychology because we have so many other explanations and tests that are purported to measure discrete functions in the other domains, such as attention and memory. Most neuropsychological tests, however, measure more than one construct at a time. The auditory processing functions, while originally a neuropsychological construct to describe aspects of children with communication disorders (Myckelburst 1954), have become a subspecialty of audiologists. This is not only because of the specialised equipment used to deliver the test stimuli but also because neuropsychology as a field did not sustain interest in this area of sensory processing compared to its ongoing involvement in central visual processing as distinct from visual acuity. The American Academy of Audiology Clinical Practice Guidelines listed 13 behavioural markers that should raise diagnostic suspicion of a possible APD.

Table 10.1 Thirteen common behavioural symptoms that may indicate the presence of an auditory processing disorder

1. Difficulty understanding speech in the presence of competing background noise or in reverberant acoustic environments
2. Problems with the ability to localise the source of a sound signal
3. Difficulty hearing on the phone
4. Inconsistent or inappropriate responses to requests for information
5. Difficulty following rapid speech
6. Frequent requests for repetition and/or rephrasing of information
7. Difficulty following directions
8. Difficulty or inability to detect the subtle changes in prosody that underlie humour and sarcasm
9. Difficulty learning a foreign language or novel speech materials, especially technical language
10. Difficulty maintaining attention
11. Tendency to be easily distracted
12. Poor singing, musical ability, and/or appreciation of music
13. Academic difficulties, including reading, spelling, and/or learning problems

Reproduced with permission from the American Academy of Audiology (2010).

Several definitions of APD currently exist and are under revision within the fields of audiology and interdisciplinary groups such as speech-language and hearing associations. One concern in the evaluation of APD is the lack of up-to-date age-related norms for most of the behavioural methods for assessing auditory processing. Many of the older audiology behavioural tests are based on site-of-lesion studies in adults that were 'renormed' often using percentage correct or cut scores when applied to paediatric populations. This raises the same psychometric issues as other classical neuropsychological tests that followed the same test development and interpretation process. Except for the SCAN-C-3 and SCAN-A-3 (tests for auditory processing disorders) that were normed for American English, most currently available behavioural tests do not have age-related scaled scores that follow a normal curve. For tests that are based on raw scores with known age averages, these are not necessarily easily available to neuropsychologists, nor is information about the population on which they were normed. This does not render them useless, but it is an area where better standardisation is needed. An additional concern is that some of the research being done by audiologists lacks some of the psychometric rigor in sample norming, research design, and data interpretation that is a baseline assumption in neuropsychological test development and research.

Multiple diagnostic tests measure different aspects of APD. Good or poor performance on one CANS function does not predict performance on other CANS functions. As a result, each function must be measured independently. There are questions about the overlap of symptoms among diagnoses and the non-specificity of many neuropsychological measures, especially for attention, memory, and executive function, all of which can be components of APD. Although there is discussion in the literature about the overlap in symptoms and how to distinguish among them, few researchers have done the experiments to demonstrate the extent to which attention affects auditory processing testing any more than it affects other neuropsychological measures and diagnoses. Neurophysiological measures such as P300 and mismatch negativity, which bypass focused attention, have been available for many years, but have not yet achieved common clinical usage (Bailey 2013; Hall 2015). Kraus (2021) presents a strong case for measuring the frequency following response.

Another consideration in diagnosis arises with the accent-specificity of language-based auditory stimuli. Research has shown that performance on language-based stimuli, such as those found in the SCAN batteries, is affected by the patient's primary language and accent. This is because the listener may not be proficient in the accent used in the recorded test stimuli. Dawes and Bishop (2007) proposed correction formulae of the SCAN-C when used in a British English-speaking population. Due to these limitations, some suggest that only nonlanguage stimuli be used in diagnostic procedures. Although this makes sense on the surface, and there are auditory functions, such as gap detection and pitch discrimination, that can be assessed reliably without a linguistic stimulus, it has also been demonstrated that there are CANS functions that are specialised for language perception and can only be tested with language-based stimuli (Zatorre and

Gandour 2008). This places responsibility on both neuropsychologists and audiologists to ensure that both language and nonlanguage aspects of auditory processing are assessed in the diagnostic process and that language-based test stimuli have been normed and validated for native speakers of different languages and dialects (Illadou et al. 2017). Test developers need to develop language-based auditory processing tests in major languages and dialects, and have these as easily accessed modules within the test. Some nonlanguage stimuli, such as gap detection, are already included as part of the SCAN batteries. Other nonlanguage tests that are within the purview of neuropsychology are pitch patterning and pitch duration, which have historically been part of older batteries in neuropsychological assessment.

Becoming aware of the auditory demands of other neuropsychological tests can sensitise the practitioner to the extent that auditory processing is already subsumed into tests. For example the auditory attention version of the Test of Variables of Attention relies on accurate pitch discrimination and working memory for pitches. The Integrated Variables of Attention-Plus uses sensory modality switching and tracks whether there is a preference and/or response timing advantage for auditory or visual processing. Tests of language and auditory working memory aspects of repetition, span, and following directions tasks, have significant auditory processing demands. Another consideration is that testing conditions are not always ideal, and background noise can affect scores in individuals with APD.

Recent research in cross-disciplinary early identification of deficits includes identifying preschool children with difficulty perceiving speech in noise, as a biomarker for identifying children who are at risk for language-based learning disorders such as dyslexia. This was undertaken with the aim of starting intervention sooner than is currently practised, in order to prevent academic failures. While this work has not yet found its way into common clinical practice, it is an area that holds promise for paediatric neuropsychologists working with primary care clinics and in-school consultation (White-Schwoch et al. 2015; Kraus 2021).

Another aspect of diagnosis is professional training and scope of practice. Some auditory processing test batteries such as the SCAN are designed to be used both as a screening (when administered without professional grade audiological equipment) and as a diagnostic battery (when using audiological equipment to control presentation levels and sound quality). Using sound-cancelling headphones does not solve the equipment or background noise problem, as the sound-cancelling process is dependent on the headphones generating sound waves that are out of phase with a subset of Hertz ranges, which need to be present for accurate assessment of hearing and listening. With professional audiometric equipment and a sound isolation booth, where the exact control of the delivery of the stimuli can be assured, diagnosis is more reliable. Training and scope of practice may restrict availability of professional audiology equipment. Most audiometers and professional grade headphones that are available to non-audiologists state that their use is for screening purposes only. This does not mean that neuropsychologists should avoid doing screenings. Rather, neuropsychologists must be aware of the limitations of the equipment they are using, and the interdisciplinary need to integrate neuropsychological auditory processing data with additional audiometric data that is the professional scope of the audiologist.

Finally, there are electrophysiological measures, especially evoked potentials, which have been developed to assess central auditory functions while bypassing the need for directed attention, or the ability to respond either verbally or motorically. Evoked potentials are used routinely in developed countries to screen newborns and very young children for hearing problems, as well as to assess the integrity of central processes (Hall 2015). Auditory attention is already assessed by some using an electrophysiological oddball paradigm. Depending on how the data is gathered, information about the central auditory processing waves may also be included.

Case Study – Jaime

Jaime, a native speaker of American English, was administered the SCAN-3-C. Scores were within normal limits for all subtests except Auditory Figure-Ground (speech-in-noise), and Filtered Words (low-pass filtered presentation of single words, that partially deleted high frequencies). Normal performance on dichotic tests that required more cognitive effort, such as Competing Words and Competing Sentences, argued against a primary attention disorder. On the Integrated Variables of Attention-Plus, error and timing variability scores were within normal limits for visual targets, with below expectations scores for auditory target omissions, and indications of fatigue for auditory targets only as the test progressed. Reading and rapid automatic naming tests showed scatter from average to low average. Writing tests showed good idea development and logical presentation of ideas. Error analysis showed few spelling errors for simple words learned in the first years of school. Errors were seen on easily confused sounds such as /d/ and /t/, diphthongs, and consonant clusters such as /sh/ versus /sch/, and irregular spelling such as /ow/ versus /ough/, and /f/ versus /ph/. Behavioural observations included Jaime misunderstanding multi-step directions and asking for some directions to be repeated or clarified before starting a task. There was no resistance to doing any task, and no off-task behaviour across several hours of testing. Jaime worked steadily with no obvious cognitive or motor fatigue. When asked about being distracted and off-task at school and in noisy community environments, Jaime reported difficulty understanding what was being said in these environments, even when directions were repeated. Screening was carried out for co-occurring conditions such as reading disorder, which is beyond the scope of this chapter to describe.

Differential diagnosis of an APD requires an understanding that in children and adolescents, APDs are not usually found as a stand-alone diagnosis (Brewer et al. 2016). Comorbidity with one or more attention, working memory, language, learning, and executive functioning disorders is to be expected, as is often the situation with other paediatric developmental disorders. Behavioural symptoms overlap among these disorders, making the diagnosis of a contributing auditory processing problem unlikely unless there is already a high index of suspicion and an understanding of auditory processing, as well as the willingness to entertain the possibility of yet another contributor to the already complex problems that typically present to paediatric neuropsychologists.

One of the most important differential diagnosis questions is to distinguish between attention and auditory processing problems. Tillery, Katz, and Keller (2000) found that stimulant medication does not improve auditory processing in children diagnosed with a stand-alone APD or co-morbid attention-deficit/hyperactivity disorder. Listening in noise tests (Figure-Ground subtest in the SCAN battery) can be extremely important in differential diagnosis. Some patients only exhibit attention difficulties in the presence of noise or in highly reflective listening conditions such as gymnasia, restaurants, classrooms, and home environments without sound-absorbing materials such as upholstered furniture, carpeting, and curtains.

Other common co-occurring conditions such as language and learning disorders, as well as aspects of working memory, often have significant listening components. Only thorough evaluation of the auditory processing aspects alongside the other possible comorbidities will yield data that allow the neuropsychologist to understand the contribution of the CANS to cognitive and/or behavioural difficulties that likely were the primary reason for the neuropsychological referral. If any neuropsychological tests indicate there is a possible or probable auditory processing component, the neuropsychologist should do enough screening to document the need for referral for further audiological evaluation. If no audiologist is available, the neuropsychologist may have to employ a screening battery and describe both the child's performance and the test presentation's functional limitations.

INTERVENTION AND MANAGEMENT

There is no commonly agreed-upon treatment for APDs that cures or fully remediates the identified problem. Although newer paradigms are emerging for auditory training for various aspects of APDs (Dacewicz et al. 2018), and there is increasing evidence that participation in musical activities boosts skills for reading and listening in noise (Kraus et al. 2014; Kraus 2021), most of the focus is on accommodations, many of which are already familiar to neuropsychologists. These include preferential seating, assignment to classrooms with few distractions, quiet settings, presenting information in more than one sensory modality, speaking clearly at a moderate or slowed pace, and use of local FM other personal amplification systems (Smart, Purdy, and Kelly 2018). Accommodations that are not generally helpful are audio recording conversations or classes, because having to repeat and search through recordings can extend homework time beyond practical limits. As stated above, noise-cancelling headphones can block some of the sound frequencies that need to be heard, the headphones are not designed for continuous use day after day, and research is lacking on the effects of long-term use of these devices by children or adolescents.

Participation for at least 2 years in formal music instruction, whether in school or privately, has been shown to be protective across the lifespan for supporting the ability to perceive speech in noise (Kraus et al. 2014). The contribution of music instruction is presumed to result from the repetitive experience of listening to one's own contribution to a complex auditory scene while simultaneously adjusting one's contribution to a constantly shifting whole.

Given the lack of standard interventions with a strong evidence base, there are no reliable outcome studies involving large populations. There are several interventions in clinical use, which have smaller studies associated with them. Song et al. (2012) reviewed auditory training models that aim to improve listening in noise and the physiological underpinnings of the training phenomena. Fast ForWord, which addresses auditory rapid temporal processing problems, has not shown efficacy in a meta-analytic review (Strong et al. 2011). Commercially available auditory training interventions such as Berard Auditory Integration Training and the Tomatis Method have no research with sufficient power to recommend them as evidence-based interventions at this time.

Outcome

After neuropsychological evaluation, including the SCAN battery and behavioural observations, indicated a possible APD, Jaime was referred to an audiologist for comprehensive auditory processing evaluation. Findings were normal for peripheral processes, except mild hypersensitivity for some higher frequencies (hyperacusis). Perception of speech in quiet was excellent, but perception of speech in noise was notably diminished. Further testing of low-pass filtered speech confirmed screening findings of difficulty understanding speech with high, fast onset consonant sounds. Jaime was able to sing and match low and high pitch sequences, but had difficulty naming them as low or high relative to one another. Jaime's school implemented use of a classroom FM transmitter to focus listening. Jaime's parents elected to enrol him in an auditory training program that aimed at improving speech in noise perception. After training, Jaime reported it was becoming easier to understand the teacher, and that conversing in a restaurant or on the playground was not as stressful as it had been. Behaviourally, Jaime was more focused and better able to follow directions at school and at home without the FM system. Spelling improved parallel to better speech perception. Follow-up audiological evaluation a year later showed mild regression toward difficulty perceiving speech in noise. Brief booster training restored listening in noise to normal limits. Jaime began individual and music ensemble lessons to support listening with more focus when multiple sound sources were present.

SUMMARY

Auditory processing is a complex, mostly subcortical, process that begins at the junction between the mechanical ear processes and the auditory nerve's connection to the brain. Auditory processing is what the brain does with the auditory signal on its journey to higher cortical interpretation of language and environmental sounds. The study of auditory processing is rooted in neuropsychology in the 1950s and was largely abandoned until the 2000s. As a result, most research today takes place in auditory neuroscience laboratories rather than neuropsychology departments. Only a few, such as Kraus' 'Brainvolts' laboratory at Northwestern University, focus on applied paediatric research.

Auditory processing needs to be recognised as a distinct process from hearing, attention, and language, although it is related to all three. Obstacles include construct overlap, difficult to interpret behavioural testing in younger children, relative lack of objective tests in clinical practice, and the need for standardised language-based stimuli in each child's language. Once there is wider recognition of the developmental trajectory of auditory processing and the ways in which it contributes to academic and interpersonal skills, evaluation techniques can be better developed to track the seven separable auditory processing functions. The manifestations are subtle, yet crucial, components to assess.

Collaboration with hearing and language specialists is essential to integrate auditory processing contributions to linguistic skills and perception. We must also differentiate auditory processing's contribution to attention, so that, especially in sub-optimal responders to attention medications, we do not overlook the opportunity to improve a child's developmental trajectory.

REFERENCES

American Academy of Audiology (2010) *Clinical Practice Guidelines*. Available at: https://audiology-web.s3.amazonaws.com/migrated/CAPD%20Guidelines%208-2010.pdf_539952af956c79.73897613.pdf (Accessed 20 January 2019).

Bailey T (2010) Auditory pathways and processes: Implications for neuropsychological assessment and diagnosis of children and adolescents. *Child Neuropsychology* 16(6): 521–548. doi: 10.1080/09297041003783310.

Bailey T (2013) Beyond DSM: The role of auditory processing in attention in its disorders. *Applied Neuropsychology: Child* 1(2): 112–120. doi: 10.1080/21622965.2012.703890.

Baumann VJ, Koch U (2017) Perinatal nicotine exposure impairs the maturation of glutamatergic inputs in the auditory brainstem. *The Journal of Physiology* 595(11): 3573–3590. doi: 10.1113./JP274059.

Brewer CC, Zalewski CK, Kelley AK et al. (2016) Heritability of non-speech auditory processing skills. *European Journal of Human Genetics* 24(8): 1137–1144. doi: 10.1038/3jhg2015.277.

Dacewicz A, Szymaszek A, Nowak K, Szelag E (2018) Training-induced changes in rapid auditory processing in children with specific language impairment: Electrophysiological indicators. *Frontiers in Human Neuroscience* 12(3): 10. doi: 10.3389/fnhum.2018.00310.

Dawes P, Bishop DV (2007) The SCAN-C in testing a sample of British children. *International Journal of Audiology* 46(12): 780–786.

Hall JW III (2015) *eHandbook of Auditory Evoked Responses: Principles, Procedures, Protocols* [no publisher or place of publication listed]. Kindle Edition. ASIN: B1045G2FFM.

Illadou VV, Ptok M, Grech H et al. (2017) A European perspective on auditory processing disorder: current knowledge and future research focus. *Frontiers in Neurology* **8**: 622. doi: 10.3389/fneur.2017.00622.

Kraus N (2021) *Of Sound Mind: How Our Brain Constructs a Meaningful Sonic World*. Cambridge, MA: The MIT Press.

Kraus N, Slater J, Thompson EC et al. (2014) Auditory learning through active engagement with sound: Biological impact of community music lessons in at-risk children. *Frontiers in Neuroscience* **8**: 351. doi: 10.3389fnins.2014.00351.

Myckelburst H (1954) *Auditory Disorders in Children*. New York: Grune and Stratton.

Otto-Meyer S, Krisman J, White-Schwoch T, Kraus N (2018) Children with autism spectrum disorders have unstable neural responses to sound. *Experimental Brain Research* **236**(3): 733–743. doi: 10.1007s00221-0017-5164-4.

Petitpre C, Wu H, Sharma A et al. (2018) Neuronal heterogeneity and stereotyped heterogeneity in the auditory afferent system. *Nature Communications* **9**: 3691. doi: 10.1038/s41467-018-06033-3.

Shapiro SM, Nakamura H (2001) Bilirubin and the auditory system. *Journal of Perinatology* **21**: S52–S55.

Smart JL, Purdy SC, Kelly AS (2018) Impact of personal frequency modulation systems on classroom behavioral and cortical auditory evoked potential measures of auditory processing and classroom listening in school-aged children with auditory processing disorder. *Journal of the American Academy of Audiology* **29**(7): 568–586. doi: 10.3766/jaa.16074.

Song JH, Skoe E, Banai K, Kraus N (2012) Training to improve hearing speech in noise: Biological mechanisms. *Cerebral Cortex* **22**(5): 1180–1190. doi: 10.1093/cercor/bhr196.

Strong GK, Torgeson CJ, Torgeson D, Hulme C (2011) A systematic meta-analytic review of evidence for the effectiveness of the Fast ForWord language intervention program. *Journal of Child Psychology and Psychiatry* **52**(3): 224–235. doi: 10.1111/j.1469-7610.2010.02329.x.

Tillery J, Katz J, Keller WD (2000) Effects of methylphenidate (Ritalin) on auditory performance in children with attention and auditory processing disorders. *Journal of Speech, Language, and Hearing Research* **43**: 293–301.

White-Schwoch T, Carr KW, Thompson EC et al. (2015) Auditory processing in noise: A preschool biomarker for literacy. *PLOS Biology* **13**(7): e1002196. doi.org/10.1371/journal.pbio1002196.

World Health Organization (2016) *International Classification of Diseases and Related Health Problems 10th Revision*. Available at: https://icd.who.int/browse10/2016/en (Accessed 20 January 2019).

Zatorre RJ, Gandour JT (2008) Neural specializations for speech and pitch: Moving beyond the dichotomies. *Philosophical Transactions of the Royal Society B Biological Sciences* **363**(1493): 1087–1104.

CHAPTER 11

Executive Function

Deborah Budding and Laura Flores Shaw

Presenting Concern

Tommy was referred for evaluation due to concerns about self-regulation and school refusal. He was described as a bright, athletic, and creative 9-year-old white child. Tommy lived with his 4-year-old sister, mother, and father and attended a Montessori school. He had been diagnosed with autism spectrum disorder and attention-deficit/hyperactivity disorder.

Tommy enjoys sports, LEGO®, watching videos, and telling stories. His parents and Montessori teachers reported that he dislikes academic work and adaptive, skill-related tasks such as cleaning his room. He tells them, 'I don't like it when people tell me what to do.' Additionally, he was described as emotionally reactive, with periodic tantrums. His family was unable to determine the trigger for these outbursts; however, there appeared to be a link between days Tommy complains about school and later tantrums at home. Attempts to find either reward or consequence-related solutions at home were unsuccessful. Whilst he did not typically demonstrate significant dysregulation at school, both family and teachers perceived him as wilful.

Regarding developmental history, there were no issues with Tommy's gestation or birth. Developmental milestones developed unevenly. He did not crawl but walked early. He had some difficulty with dexterity and motor planning. His speech was mildly delayed, and he received intervention focusing on articulation and word-finding. Tommy had difficulty with his sleep schedule. As an infant, he needed to be rocked or driven in a car to sleep. At the time of referral, he had difficulty settling to sleep, but generally slept through the night. He was described as a picky eater with strong aversions to tastes and textures. Toilet training was attained at 4 years of age for both bladder and bowel. Whilst he enjoyed imaginative play, his play style tended to be structured, and he often lined up his toys.

School observations showed that Tommy preferred working alone, though he did have friends. However, he rarely initiated interaction with them. When his friends initiated interaction, which was fairly rare, his response was friendly, but he frequently continued working alone, even though the Montessori elementary program he attended was designed for group work. Additionally, sometimes Tommy misunderstood his classmates' behaviours, interpreting them as bullying when they were not. Conversely, he was sometimes controlling with the other children, which they misunderstood as bullying.

Academically, he enjoyed and was very competent at reading. However, he used reading as escape behaviour for unwanted tasks. He disliked and tended to avoid writing tasks and had difficulty making sight words automatic. Tommy had difficulty manipulating a pencil and was inconsistent in his spelling and grammar. His math calculation skills were age- and grade-appropriate, but his ability to retrieve math facts was inconsistent, which was considered to be due to a lack of effort.

THEORY

Neuropsychological evaluations typically feature a strong emphasis on assessing executive function. Traditionally, executive function is defined as a heavily cognitively mediated set of skills, emphasising top-down, conscious control, and intentional goal-directed behaviour (Miyake et al. 2000). Executive functions are typically broken down into three main subdomains: working memory, inhibition, and cognitive flexibility (Diamond 2013). Each of these areas can also be further subdivided. For instance, working memory features both maintenance (holding things in mind) and updating components (Eriksson et al. 2015). From these perspectives, frontal systems are primarily considered paramount with 'lower' systems sub-serving those higher-level systems (Parvizi 2009).

Executive function skills continue to develop throughout childhood and adolescence into young adulthood (Diamond 2000). Children and students who are seen as having self-regulatory challenges are encouraged to better develop their 'thinking' skills and their ability to engage formal sequential reasoning strategies in the face of unfamiliar or frustrating circumstances (Roebers et al. 2012). Accordingly, clinical assessments tend to focus on measuring these aforementioned subdomains (Miyake et al. 2000). The various subcomponents of attention (initial registration, sustained attention, etc.), which are presumed to intersect with working memory, are also emphasised and are largely viewed from the perspective of conscious control (Posner, Rothbart, and Tang 2013).

Whilst not incorrect, this traditional view of executive function is incomplete and lacks both ecological and ethological validity. It emphasises deliberate, intentional behaviour but leaves out important components of adaptive functions that are not consciously controlled (Koziol and Budding 2009). This traditional view is also inconsistent with current understanding of both structural and functional neuroanatomy (Cisek and Kalaska 2010) and supports an outdated model of cognition based on serial processing – the see–think–act view of cognition – rather than current action-oriented models more aligned with current neural data (Engel, Friston, and Kragic 2016). Current neuroscientific thinking regarding human cognitive and adaptive function emphasises interacting networks existing across brain regions that have evolved together over millennia (Cisek 2019). Further, clinical practitioners solely considering and measuring intentional skills can only suggest interventions addressing those skills, which can result in incomplete and ineffective treatment planning. For example emotional regulation is also an essential aspect of executive function and has been found to involve multiple cortical and subcortical networks (Morawetz et al. 2020).

A more inclusive and comprehensive view of executive function could be defined as 'those functions an organism employs to act independently in its own best interest as a whole, at any point in time, for the purpose of survival' (Koziol, Budding, and Chidekel 2012, p. 506, paraphrased from Miller 2008, p. 7). This conceptualisation of executive function involves, as Pezzulo and Cisek (2016) describe, 'parallel processes of competition and selection among potential action opportunities ("affordances") expressed at multiple levels of abstraction' (p. 414). This means that rather than serving as a serial processor, 'the brain is a feedback control system whose primary goal is not to understand the world, but to guide interaction' with it (p. 414).

Ultimately, human adaptive function involves a combination of behavioural content and process not only involving the 'what' and 'where' of information guiding behaviour, but also the 'when' and 'how' mediated by cortical and subcortical circuitry (Koziol and Budding 2009). This more holistic view of executive function recognises that actions are selected via both conscious, intentional control, *and* automatically, with the latter actions comprising the majority of movements (Torres 2011). It also recognises that affordances – 'environmental opportunities for organism-salient action and intervention' (Clark 2016, p. 133) – help us to organise ourselves as we implicitly and explicitly learn to predict outcomes of our actions. Such predictions can either lead to effective or ineffective adaptability. The affordance landscape can comprise human relationships, the physical environment, and the larger cultural context, with the latter often minimised as an important contributor to developmental expectations (Ramstead, Veissière, and Kirmayer 2016). Thus, treatment planning should include subconscious learning systems (adaption and reinforcement), not merely those involved in thinking (see Table 11.1). Myriad systems contribute to action selection (Roemmich and Bastian 2018), self-regulation (Van Overwalle et al. 2020), and, ultimately, effective environmental adaptability (Pezzulo and Cisek 2016).

Within this more holistic view of executive function wherein all actions and learning systems are considered for treatment planning, it is also necessary to understand the reafference principle. This long-standing principle refers to a person's ability to differentiate sensory information as coming from the external versus internal environment (Von Holst and Mittelstaedt 1950). Essentially, self-generated movements themselves produce reafferent signals that can feed back into one's sensory system and are used to help the organism predict outcomes of an action. Noisy reafferent signals can disrupt an individual's ability to learn from the environment in specific circumstances as well as their ability to generalise learning (Brincker and Torres 2017). This disruption is thought to contribute to the implicit learning differences autistic individuals frequently demonstrate (Foti et al. 2015). Predictive action control negatively impacted by signals with unclear origins can contribute to someone developing and maintaining compensatory yet maladaptive behaviours that allow a subjective sense of predictive control

Table 11.1 A holistic view of adaptive behaviour/executive function

Executive functions and behaviour	
Bottom–up ↑	**Top–down ↓**
Automatic	Deliberate
• Arousal	• Working memory
• Vulnerability to fight/flight	• Deliberate inhibition
• Processing speed	• Cognitive flexibility
Quick consistent responses to familiar circumstances requiring little energy	Flexible problem-solving requiring energy
Without conscious thought	With conscious, intentional thought
Predictable environmental aspects	Unpredictable environmental aspects
Procedural/implicit learning	Declarative learning
Behavioural process ('when' and 'how' responses to affordances)	Behavioural content ('what' and 'where' responses to affordances)
Aligning treatment approach	
Bottom–up ↑	**Top–down ↓**
Procedural memories/habits	Declarative memories
• Relational approaches to self-regulation	• Psychodynamic therapies
• Environmental front-loading	• Cognitive and behavioural therapies
• Sensorimotor-based interventions	▪ Cognitive behavioural therapy
▪ Occupational therapy	▪ Dialectical behaviour therapy
▪ Neurologic music therapy	• Mindfulness and metacognitive training
• Pharmacological interventions	
Neuromodulation techniques	

Note: These area divisions are not rigid.

whilst failing to accurately consider and adapt to the environment (Torres, Yanovich, and Metaxas 2013). Populations diagnosed with autism (Brincker and Torres 2017), attention-deficit/hyperactivity disorder (Torres and Denisova 2016), and schizophrenia (Nguyen et al. 2016) have all been found to generate movements with noisy reafferent signals, commonly accompanied by deficits in executive functions, illustrating an underlying sensorimotor component to these disorders that should be included for effective treatment.

ASSESSMENT AND FORMULATION

Children like Tommy are generally seen for a full neuropsychological evaluation comprising multiple standardised tests, emphasising qualitative as well as quantitative aspects of performance in relation to both task-related and non-task-related sensorimotor behaviour

(Koziol and Budding 2009). Measures may include the Wisconsin Card Sorting Test (Heaton 2004), Tower of London (Culbertson and Zillmer 1999), Developmental Neuropsychological Assessment, Second Edition (NEPSY-II; Korkman, Kirk, and Kemp 2007), and the California Verbal Learning Test – Children's Version (CVLT-C; Delis et al. 1994). Other frequently used measures include rating scales such as the Behavior Rating Inventory of Executive Function, Second Edition (Gioia et al. 2015), normed batteries such as the Delis–Kaplan Executive Function System (Delis et al. 2001) and the Behavioural Assessment of the Dysexecutive Syndrome in Children (Emslie et al. 2003). The Tasks of Executive Control (Isquith, Roth, and Gioia 2010) is a computerised set of tasks also often used to systematically assess the relationship between a child or teen's ability to manage increasing working memory and inhibitory function demands in the context of game-like presentation. Most of these tasks are considered measures of executive function in the traditional sense; the CVLT-C is considered a learning and memory test but features a number of embedded executive function demands that provide useful information about explicit and implicit learning skills.

Administered measures of intellectual function placed Tommy in the overall high average range, albeit with a scattered subtest profile. Typically, most measures of executive function assume IQ falling grossly within the average range. This can, of course, be problematic in relation to individuals with intellectual function falling significantly outside this range in either direction (Duggan and Garcia-Barrera 2015). Among 'classic' tests of executive function, Tommy was administered a computerised version of the Wisconsin Card Sorting Test, which required him to sort cards into a variety of simple categories such as colour or shape with immediate feedback regarding whether his choice was correct but not why. Tommy was able to use this somewhat vague but constant feedback effectively, but only after needing extensive time to adjust – he needed 28 attempts to complete the first category, which is below average for his age and shows weak performance. Tommy also struggled when asked to independently sort cards featuring pictures of animals into groupings of his own choosing (NEPSY-II Animal Sorting). He was required to sort eight cards into two groups of four using shared elements (e.g. four little animals and four big animals). He appeared to find the material overwhelming and had trouble directing his attention and problem-solving, ultimately creating only a few out of more than 10 possible groupings.

Tommy also had difficulty with aspects of sequential reasoning and was inefficient in solving problems on the Tower of London task. He often needed additional moves and problem-solving time. Tommy additionally performed variably in relation to a set of inhibition-type tasks requiring him to engage in rapid naming while at times also withholding automatic responses, thus requiring him to alternate between automatic and deliberate processing. He tended to perform better under circumstances requiring him to be more deliberate as opposed to automatic in his naming style (NEPSY-II Inhibition).

Tommy's performance on a verbal learning and memory task was notable (CVLT-C). This task required him to listen to and repeat two lists of 15 words presented in shopping list form. One list was read a total of five times, while a second was read once. No explicit preparation is given in relation to how many words or how many lists will be presented. The lists feature underlying categories that, if discovered, can be used to more efficiently chunk the words by categories, but the existence of these categories is not explained. Upon first presentation of the first list, Tommy appeared to be overwhelmed and was able to recall only three of the 15 words, which is below average. His performance improved with each presentation, but Tommy did not take advantage of the available chunking strategy, leading to inefficient learning. Despite being familiar with the shopping list format, when the second list was presented, he did not respond as if the task was familiar but instead again only recalled three words. His later independent recall for the first list was within normal limits upon both short and long delay, as was his ability to recognise relevant material. His performance on this task illustrates his need for explicit structure during aspects of learning. The implicit aspects of this task are thus extremely helpful for clarifying an individual's self-regulatory and self-organising skills – central features of executive function.

Overall, Tommy's assessment results demonstrated a need for some degree of scaffolding and preparation via general 'front-loading' of the gist of what will happen when presented with novel material, as well as time to adjust in such circumstances. Given his trouble adjusting to novelty, his vulnerability to rapidly enter a fight/flight state made sense. At the same time, he benefits from flexibility and being allowed a sense of agency and control.

INTERVENTION AND MANAGEMENT

Interventions for Tommy and his family included a combination of bottom-up sensorimotor and top-down cognitively mediated interventions. Medication support was provided by a psychiatrist and was aimed at stabilising his arousal and impulsivity. Sensorimotor interventions included play-based occupational therapy with a sensory/arousal focus (Rodger and Ziviani 1999; Lillas et al. 2018; Nestor and Moser 2018). There are numerous occupational therapy approaches that have been found to assist sensorimotor and adaptive function, particularly those featuring an emphasis on aspects of sensory integration; some clinicians and researchers view sensory integration as a separate area of disorder/diagnosis, whilst others view this as an important piece of most neurodevelopmental disorders but not as a standalone diagnosis. Nevertheless, most agree that sensory integration represents an important aspect of functional adaptation (Christensen et al. 2020).

Tommy also engaged in neurologic music therapy (Thaut 2005), an intervention using rhythm in a nonmusical setting to aid with arousal and behavioural fluency. Neurologic music therapy has long been used with adults in rehabilitation settings, particularly in relation to fall prevention with poststroke and patients with Parkinson disease (Thaut,

McIntosh, and Hoemberg 2015). This intervention is also increasingly used with children both in relation to brain injury and cerebral palsy (Peng et al. 2011; Wang et al. 2013) as well as with children diagnosed with neurodevelopmental disorders (Koshimori and Thaut 2019).

A variety of other physiological interventions have also become available, including neurofeedback and other neuromodulatory approaches such as transcutaneous vagus nerve stimulation and cranial electrotherapy stimulation but were not used in this case. Research supporting these interventions is variable, particularly in regard to neurofeed-back, where there are a variety of different protocols available that presumably address different behaviours and neural circuitry, with limited consensus regarding efficacy, particularly as various protocols have been used in relation to disorders ranging from epilepsy to anxiety to attention-deficit/hyperactivity disorder (Kadosh and Staunton 2019; Arns et al. 2020). Research support for transcutaneous vagus nerve stimulation is also variable and has focused primarily on use in epilepsy and anxiety-related disorders, with much research focusing upon efficacy of transcutaneous vagus nerve stimulation in comparison to invasive implanted internal vagus nerve stimulation devices (Hamer and Bauer 2019).

Several deliberate cognitively oriented approaches were also employed, including mind-fulness meditation, metacognitive strategies via a combination of individual cognitive behavioural therapy and more systems-oriented dialectical behaviour therapy for Tommy and his family. The treatment team together created a plan that included addressing conceptual skills, inhibition (both consciously and unconsciously driven), shifting, overall arousal (how readily someone flips into fight/flight modes), and explicitly managing expectations. For example when someone does not know how or when to use chunking as a learning strategy, they are more likely to become overwhelmed. However, when someone else provides the structure without warning or explanation, the added information can be experienced as overwhelming instead of supportive. Use of frequent repetition or feedback removes aspects of novelty for better or worse. In some circumstances, novelty is beneficial, whilst in others it is experienced as det-rimental. Often, removing the overall structural novelty can make it easier to manage novel content within a familiar framework. It needs to be remembered that academic and social environments encompass both procedures and content. Thus, it is impor-tant to learn how to navigate both and students will vary in their abilities to manage this navigation.

In Tommy's case, helping him to learn what circumstances need more versus less scaf-folding helped him to feel more empowered within his environment. Thus, his parents were taught explicit strategies to help manage this as well as to be able to assist him in determining his need for direct assistance versus seeking space to sort things out himself. Education around executive function and how it applies to everyday life can be useful for children, their families, and educators and this proved to be the case for Tommy.

Practical, applied, and accessible information was available from the self-guided literature (e.g. Dawson and Guare 2018; Cannon et al. 2021).

School

Depending upon the educational environment, the environment itself can be therapeutic. Although this will not be available universally, our case presents one example: a Montessori environment which emphasises community involvement and problem-solving. Montessori environments in particular are designed to simulate life in society, which includes opportunities to manage and self-direct within the affordance landscape (Zimmerman 2006). In this way, offering fewer choices is one strategy to help students navigate their affordances, as choices can sometimes become overwhelming. Montessori schools also tend to be highly implicit in their expectations. Thus, for some students the environment needs to be adapted to provide more explicit direction. A conventional environment, on the other hand, which tends to be inherently more structured, might offer more scaffolding by (1) providing more time to adjust to changes in the academic and social focus, and (2) pre-teaching or front-loading the gist of upcoming material to help offset some of the novelty.

As noted above, parents, teachers, and peers also serve as affordances – opportunities for action. All can help organise and navigate the environment. In Montessori, classrooms consist of children of multiple ages, which allows older children to help orient younger children to the environment in a supportive manner. In conventional school structures, teachers can provide opportunities for high-performing students to support and assist other students as well. Parents benefit from understanding their own arousal levels and adaptive styles, as well of their own executive function strengths and weaknesses. Often, children are viewed in a relative vacuum, without sufficient consideration of how differing parental neurological and adaptive styles impact family communication and function. Clinical attention to similarities and differences in adaptive styles among family members allows for more effective co-regulation and scaffolding. The role that these variables play within the larger affordance landscape, which include ethnic, cultural, socioeconomic status, and religious context, also needs to be considered, particularly in areas where there are intersecting differences between children, parents, and treatment/education providers.

Outcome

Once Tommy's parents understood his need for circumstances that in some way match his expectations and to receive unambiguous directions given his trouble managing unexpected novelty, they shifted the way they treated him. They began to provide more consistent and explicit affordances – opportunities for action – for him to navigate, resulting in fewer misunderstandings and associated meltdowns. For example they began outlining plans for the day each morning and on days where they could anticipate disruption, they gave him advance notice. His treatment team began to explicitly address how distressing unexpected things were to him, which helped him to feel better understood. His Montessori teachers also began making classroom expectations explicit, such as not disturbing another child's work left on a floor mat. In both environments, adults began providing explicit links about overlapping circumstances that appeared unrelated to Tommy, helping him to generalise.

As he became more capable of maintaining a more consistent arousal state, Tommy began to show greater ability to use top-down, deliberate problem-solving strategies. He increasingly recognised growing distress and sought physiological means of calming, such as going outside to work in the garden, before escalating. Additionally, now that teachers were better able to recognise when Tommy was showing physiological signs of increasing distress, they scaffolded and redirected him using a nonshaming approach.

Front-loading the school day's activities and expectations and assisting with social interactions dramatically diminished Tommy's school refusals. Additionally, opportunities to repair social peer relationships were provided as they arose. For example his teacher facilitated a 'peace' conversation with a child Tommy assumed was bullying. The teacher helped navigate each child's misinterpretations of the other's intentions. This is critical as it should be considered that theory of mind deficits attributed only to autistic individuals may be more effectively viewed as mismatched expectations of the environment and affordances between autistic and neurotypical individuals (Heasman and Gillespie 2018; see also Chapter 12). Hostile attribution bias – the tendency to interpret the behaviour of others, across situations, as threatening, aggressive, or both – is an issue that impacts communication among adults as well as children and is often largely implicitly driven (Bondü and Richter 2016; Hiemstra, De Castro, and Thomaes 2019).

In the context of these supports coupled with outside services, such as those mentioned above, Tommy's function improved significantly and continues to progress.

SUMMARY

Previously accepted corticocentric views of executive function are no longer sufficient for understanding or supporting neurodevelopmentally based challenges, nor do they align with current understanding of both structural and functional neuroanatomy and evolutionary frameworks of adaptive function (Cisek and Kalaska 2010; Pezzulo and Cisek 2016). Instead, a vertically oriented and large-scale brain network informed perspective that considers deliberate, intentional behaviours *as well as* automatically selected behaviours can allow for more comprehensive and effective treatment planning (Koziol and Budding 2009). Key messages herein include:

• Treatment should include a combination of 'bottom-up' sensorimotor and 'top-down' cognitively mediated interventions to address the sensorimotor foundations underlying many neurological differences and disorders.

• The entirety of our environments serve as affordances (teachers, peers, and parents as well as built environments) and opportunities for action (Clark 2016). Parents and teachers, in particular, can provide important scaffolding and co-regulation at home and school.

- Given this, it is important that involved adults understand their own arousal systems, executive function strengths and weaknesses, and potential biases as they interact with children's arousal systems and various sensitivities to novelty and familiarity.
- Significant questions remain regarding individual differences in sensorimotor sensitivities and abilities to manage novel versus familiar circumstances as well as abilities to tolerate verbal and nonverbal interventions.

REFERENCES

Arns M, Clark CR, Trullinger M, deBeus R, Mack M, Aniftos M (2020) Neurofeedback and attention-deficit/hyperactivity-disorder (ADHD) in children: Rating the evidence and proposed guidelines. *Applied Psychophysiology and Biofeedback* **45**(2): 39–48. https://doi.org/10.1007/s10484-020-09455-2.

Bondü R, Richter P (2016) Interrelations of justice, rejection, provocation, and moral disgust sensitivity and their links with the hostile attribution bias, trait anger, and aggression. *Frontiers in Psychology* **7**(795). https://doi.org/10.3389/fpsyg.2016.00795.

Brincker M, Torres EB (2017) Why study movement variability in autism? In: Torres EB, Whyatt CP, editors, *Autism: The Movement Sensing Approach*. Boca Rotan, FL: CRC Press, pp. 1–39.

Cannon L, Kenworthy L, Alexander L, Adler Werner M, Gutermuth Anthony L (2021) U*nstuck and On Target!: An Executive Function Curriculum to Improve Flexibility, Planning, and Organization*, 2nd edition. Baltimore: Brookes Publishing Co.

Christensen JS, Wild H, Kenzie ES, Wakeland W, Budding D, Lillas C (2020) Diverse autonomic nervous system stress response patterns in childhood sensory modulation. *Frontiers in Integrative Neuroscience* **14**(6). https://doi.org/10.3389/fnint.2020.00006.

Cisek P (2019) Resynthesizing behavior through phylogenetic refinement. *Attention, Perception, & Psychophysics* **81**(7): 2265–2287. https://doi.org/10.3758/s13414 019-01760-1.

Cisek P, Kalaska JF (2010) Neural mechanisms for interacting with a world full of action choices. *Annual Review of Neuroscience* **33**(1): 269–298. https://doi.org/10.1146/annurev.neuro.051508.135409.

Clark A (2016) *Surfing Uncertainty: Prediction, Action, and the Embodied Mind*. New York, NY: Oxford University Press.

Dawson P, Guare R (2018) *Executive Skills in Children and Adolescents: A Practical Guide to Assessment and Intervention*, 3rd edition. New York, NY: Guilford Press.

Diamond A (2000) Close interrelation of motor development and cognitive development and of the cerebellum and prefrontal cortex. *Child Development* **71**: 44–56. https://doi.org/10.1111/1467-8624.00117.

Diamond A (2013) Executive functions. *Annual Review of Psychology* **64**: 135–168. https://doi.org/10.1146/annurev-psych-113011-143750.

Duggan EC, Garcia-Barrera MA (2015) Executive functioning and intelligence. In: Goldstein S, Princiotta D, Naglieri J, editors, *Handbook of Intelligence*. New York, NY: Springer. pp. 435–458.

Engel AK, Friston KJ, Kragic D (2016) *The Pragmatic Turn: Toward Action-Oriented Views in Cognitive Science*. Cambridge, MA: MIT Press.

Eriksson J, Vogel EK, Lansner A, Bergström F, Nyberg L (2015) Neurocognitive architecture of working memory. *Neuron* **88**(1): 33–46. https://doi.org/10.1016/j.neuron.2015.09.020.

Foti F, De Crescenzo F, Vivanti G, Menghini D, Vicari S (2015) Implicit learning in individuals with autism spectrum disorders: A meta-analysis. *Psychological Medicine* **45**(5): 897–910. https://doi.org/10.1017/S0033291714001950.

Hamer HM, Bauer S (2019) Lessons learned from transcutaneous vagus nerve stimulation (tVNS). *Epilepsy Research* **153**: 83–84. https://doi.org/10.1016/j.eplepsyres.2019.02.015.

Heasman B, Gillespie A (2018) Neurodivergent intersubjectivity: Distinctive features of how autistic people create shared understanding. *Autism* **23**(4): 910–921. https://doi.org/10.1177/1362361318785172.

Hiemstra W, De Castro BO, Thomaes S (2019) Reducing aggressive children's hostile attributions: A cognitive bias modification procedure. *Cognitive Therapy and Research* **43**(2): 387–398. https://doi.org/10.1007/s10608-018-9958-x.

Kadosh KC, Staunton G (2019) A systematic review of the psychological factors that influence neurofeedback learning outcomes. *NeuroImage* **185**: 545–555. https://doi.org/10.1016/j.neuroimage.2018.10.021.

Koshimori Y, Thaut MH (2019) New perspectives on music in rehabilitation of executive and attention functions. *Frontiers in Neuroscience* **13**: 1245–1245. https://doi.org/10.3389/fnins.2019.01245.

Koziol LF, Budding DE (2009) *Subcortical Structures and Cognition: Implications for Neuropsychological Assessment*. New York, NY: Springer.

Koziol LF, Budding DE, Chidekel D (2012) From movement to thought: Executive function, embodied cognition, and the cerebellum. *The Cerebellum* **11**(2): 505–525. https://doi.org/10.1007/s12311-011-0321-y.

Lillas C, TenPas H, Crowley C, Spitzer SL (2018) Improving regulation skills for increased participation for individuals with ASD. In: Watling R, Spitzer SL, editors, *Autism Across the Lifespan: A Comprehensive Occupational Therapy Approach*, 4th edition, pp. 319–338.

Miller R (2008) *A Theory of the Basal Ganglia and Their Disorders*. Boca Raton: CRC.

Miyake A, Friedman NP, Emerson MJ, Witzki AH, Howerter A, Wager TD (2000) The unity and diversity of executive functions and their contributions to complex 'frontal lobe' tasks: A latent variable analysis. *Cognitive Psychology* **41**(1): 49–100. https://doi.org/10.1006/cogp.1999.0734.

Morawetz C, Riedel MC, Salo T et al. (2020) Multiple large-scale neural networks underlying emotion regulation. *Neuroscience & Biobehavioral Reviews* **116**: 382–395. https://doi.org/10.1016/j.neubiorev.2020.07.001.

Nestor O, Moser CS (2018) The importance of play. *Journal of Occupational Therapy, Schools, & Early Intervention* **11**(3): 247–262. https://doi.org/10.1080/19411243.2018.1472861.

Nguyen J, Majmudar U, Papathomas TV, Silverstein SM, Torres EB (2016) Schizophrenia: The micro-movements perspective. *Neuropsychologia* **85**: 310–326. https://dx.doi.org/10.1016/j.neuropsychologia.2016.03.003.

Parvizi J (2009) Corticocentric myopia: Old bias in new cognitive sciences. *Trends in Cognitive Sciences* **13**(8): 354–359. https://dx.doi.org/10.1016/j.tics.2009.04.008.

Peng Y-C, Lu T-W, Wang T-H et al. (2011) Immediate effects of therapeutic music on loaded sit-to-stand movement in children with spastic diplegia. *Gait & Posture* **33**(2): 274–278. https://doi.org/10.1016/j.gaitpost.2010.11.020.

Pezzulo G, Cisek P (2016) Navigating the affordance landscape: Feedback control as a process model of behavior and cognition. *Trends in Cognitive Sciences* **20**(6): 414–424. https://doi.org/10.1016/j.tics.2016.03.013.

Posner MI, Rothbart MK, Tang Y (2013) Developing self-regulation in early childhood. *Trends in Neuroscience and Education* **2**(3–4): 107–110. https://dx.doi.org/10.1016/j.tine.2013.09.001.

Ramstead MJD, Veissière SPL, Kirmayer LJ (2016) Cultural affordances: Scaffolding local worlds through shared intentionality and regimes of attention. *Frontiers in Psychology* **7**(1090). https://doi.org/10.3389/fpsyg.2016.01090.

Roebers CM, Cimeli P, Röthlisberger M, Neuenschwander R (2012) Executive functioning, metacognition, and self-perceived competence in elementary school children: An explorative study on their interrelations and their role for school achievement. *Metacognition and Learning* **7**(3): 151–173. https://doi.org/10.1007/s11409-012-9089-9.

Roemmich RT, Bastian AJ (2018) Closing the loop: From motor neuroscience to neurorehabilitation. *Annual Review of Neuroscience* **41**(1): 415–429. https://doi.org/10.1146/annurev-neuro-080317-062245.

Rodger S, Ziviani J (1999) Play-based occupational therapy. *International Journal of Disability, Development and Education* **46**(3): 337–365. https://doi.org/10.1080/103491299100542.

Thaut MH (2005) *Rhythm, Music, and the Brain*. New York, NY: Routledge.

Thaut MH, McIntosh GC, Hoemberg V (2015) Neurobiological foundations of neurologic music therapy: Rhythmic entrainment and the motor system. *Frontiers in Psychology* **5**:1185. https://doi.org/10.3389/fpsyg.2014.01185.

Torres EB (2011) Two classes of movements in motor control. *Experimental Brain Research* **215**(3–4): 269–283. https://doi.org/10.1007/s00221-011-2892-8.

Torres EB, Denisova K (2016) Motor noise is rich signal in autism research and pharmacological treatments. *Scientific Reports* **6**: 37422. https://doi.org/10.1038/srep37422.

Torres EB, Yanovich P, Metaxas DN (2013). Give spontaneity and self-discovery a chance in ASD: Spontaneous peripheral limb variability as a proxy to evoke centrally driven intentional acts. *Frontiers in Integrative Neuroscience* **7**: 46. https://doi.org/10.3389/fnint.2013.00046.

Van Overwalle F, Manto M, Cattaneo Z et al. (2020). Consensus paper: Cerebellum and social cognition. *The Cerebellum* **19**: 833–868. https://doi.org/10.1007/s12311-020-01155-1.

Von Holst E, Mittelstaedt H (1950) The principle of reafference: Interactions between the central nervous system and the peripheral organs. In: Dodwell PC, editor, *Perceptual Processing: Stimulus Equivalence and Pattern Recognition*. New York, NY: Appleton-Century-Crofts, pp. 41–72.

Wang T-H, Peng Y-C, Chen Y-L et al. (2013) A home-based program using patterned sensory enhancement improves resistance exercise effects for children with cerebral palsy: A randomized controlled trial. *Neurorehabilitation and Neural Repair* **27**(8): 684–694. doi: 10.1177/1545968313491001.

Zimmerman BJ (2006) Enhancing students' academic responsibility and achievement. In: Sternberg RJ, Subotnik RF, editors, *Optimizing Student Success in School With the Other Three Rs: Reasoning, Resilience, and Responsibility*. Scottsdale, AZ: Information Age Publishing, Inc, pp. 179–199.

CHAPTER 12

Social Functioning

Miriam Bindman, Sarah Cole, and Rhonda Booth

Presenting Concern

Seamus, 10 years old, presents for assessment at a specialist social communication assessment clinic. Seamus has had longstanding difficulties with friendships, following instruction and direction in the classroom, group work, and team sports. He complains that other children are mean to him, but his teachers say he is not bullied. In the playground, Seamus likes to pretend to be a 'wild animal' and will run around roaring at other children; he often plays by himself as the other 10-year-olds no longer play this type of game. Seamus is friendly and enjoys meeting new people. He will usually start a conversation by asking the person's date of birth – he then tells them what day of the week they were born. Seamus enjoys amazing people with this skill and will then ask them about other key dates. This pattern becomes repetitive and Seamus does not seem to know what else he could talk about or how to pay attention to whether or not the other person is interested. He has told his parents he feels different to the other children.

Seamus gets on well with his current class teacher, but last year he was frequently in trouble. He complained that the teacher was 'always shouting'. The relationship between school and parents deteriorated. Seamus's parents felt that he was being treated as naughty, whilst they felt that his behaviour was due to him feeling anxious and uncertain. While Seamus's teachers feel that he is bright, he is performing approximately 3 years behind his chronological age in reading and writing, and 2 years behind for maths. This surprises them given Seamus can calculate and remember dates so well.

At home, Seamus enjoys playing with his younger brother but tends to dominate the game. The brothers easily annoy each other and argue, and Seamus can lash out physically when angry. Seamus spends a great deal of time watching videos and looking at books on wild animals. He also enjoys making detailed drawings of animals. Seamus has occasional 'meltdowns' at home, although these are less frequent than last year. They seem to occur mostly during term time after school. It is not always obvious what has triggered the events, but sometimes Seamus will report days or even weeks later, what had upset him at school.

THEORY

The set of processes required to interpret social information and behave in socially expected ways in a social environment are complex and wide-ranging (Happé and Frith 2014). Many of the building blocks of social cognition are considered innate; for example newborns prefer to look at faces that engage them in mutual gaze, establishing an important communicative link (Farroni et al. 2002). As the young child seeks out social interaction, an understanding of their own and other people's minds gradually builds over time. In the latter years of childhood and adolescence social experiences become richer and more complicated. Understanding the subtleties of social behaviour, such as deception, white lies, and nonliteral speech, all contribute to the development of the 'social mind' (Blakemore 2018).

Given the complexities and importance of our social world, a large proportion of the human brain is dedicated to understanding other people and for social interaction (Kennedy and Adolphs 2012). With the increase of functional imaging studies conducted with children, researchers are discovering distinct developmental trajectories of brain networks implicated in different aspects of social behaviour (e.g. Gunther Moor et al. 2010; Richardso et al. 2018). The development of the 'social brain' is considered a complex interplay between 'fundamentally different and dissociable functional brain processes that evolve and adapt to the social demands of a given environment and a specific phase of development' (Nelson, Jarcho, and Guyer 2016, p. 119).

As a multifaceted process, difficulties with social functioning can result from a number of different underlying cognitive causes and manifest as an even greater number of different behavioural presentations (Happé and Frith 2014). Given the reliance on several brain regions for successful social interaction, it is not surprising that these skills are often compromised in a child with an acquired or neurodevelopmental disorder. In this chapter we focus on those manifestations involving social interaction and communication difficulties akin to behaviours typically seen within the autism spectrum.

While the description of Seamus's difficulties may not appear to be specifically social, atypical development of social cognition could be a significant underlying factor. In particular, difficulty with developing theory of mind, which has been found in children with social difficulties (Baron-Cohen, Leslie, and Frith 1985). Theory of mind refers to the ability to understand another's thoughts, beliefs, and other internal states, with the skills of joint attention, imitation, and emotion recognition as precursors to its development (Fletcher-Watson et al. 2014). In addition, difficulties with social perception (reading nonverbal cues and drawing inferences), social problem-solving (thinking flexibly to generate alternative strategies), and social execution (knowing what to say and do) all make 'reading' and responding dynamically to social situations challenging. As alluded to above, the ability to function socially relies on executive functioning and 'bigger picture thinking' (central coherence) as well as social cognition (Happé and Frith 2006).

ASSESSMENT AND FORMULATION

Assessment

As difficulties with social communication and interaction are core to the diagnosis of autism spectrum disorder (ASD) in the main classificatory systems for psychiatric and neurodevelopmental conditions (Diagnostic and Statistical Manual of Mental Disorders, Fifth Edition [DSM-5] and International Classification of Diseases, 11th Revision), many of the tools and frameworks for assessment of social functioning in children have been developed for this population. We propose that many of these tools used to assess for current social functioning in children with ASD may also be relevant in children with other causes of social difficulties.

As we have seen, social functioning is impacted by many factors, some intrinsic to the child, and others related to the fit between their information processing style and the social environment. For example an intense interest in a specific topic may not have a negative impact on social functioning at a specific point in development if a peer is available who shares this interest, and the interest is valued within the social context. The impact of weakness in mentalising on social reciprocity can be mitigated when support is available from trusted adults (and in some cases helpful peers or siblings), for example by explicitly explaining or suggesting conversation strategies or rules of play.

Contexts in which the child's profile is not well understood or supported often lead to iterative difficulties and amplified problems over time. Therefore, whilst the available tools generally focus on describing the child's individual differences, social functioning is by definition determined also by social context. This should be factored into the clinical formulation to move beyond a 'deficit' model.

Assessment of social functioning requires a clinician to include a wide range of intrinsic and extrinsic assessment information about the child in their formulation. A broad overview of assessment is offered by Ashton (2018).

Seamus was assessed by the multidisciplinary clinical team comprising developmental paediatrician, clinical psychologist, and speech and language therapist. Standardised questionnaires were completed by parents and teachers prior to clinic-based assessment (Child Communication Checklist, Second Edition, Bishop 2003; Conners-3 ADHD questionnaire, Conners 2008; Social Responsiveness Scale, Second Edition, Constantino and Gruber 2012) to gather information about language and pragmatic language use, social responsiveness, restricted and repetitive behaviours, attention, behaviour, and strengths. The Development and Well-Being Assessment (Goodman et al. 2000) was completed online by parents and Seamus to screen for neurodevelopmental and mental health difficulties and focus the assessment.

In clinic, the Developmental, Dimensional and Diagnostic Interview and Autism Diagnostic Observation Schedule, Second Edition (ADOS-2®) were completed, and

Table 12.1 Standardised measures of social communication and interaction

Measure type	Name	Authors	Method and age group
Parent interview	The Developmental, Dimensional and Diagnostic Interview (3Di)	Skuse et al. (2004)	Computer-based interview Age: 3+ years (but can be modified for children aged 2+ years)
	Autism Diagnostic Interview-Revised (ADI-R)	Le Couteur, Lord, and Rutter (2003)	Paper-based; standardised, semi-structured, investigator-based interview Age: 2+ years
	Diagnostic Interview for Social and Communication Disorders 11th Edition (DISCO-11)	Wing (2006)	Semi-structured investigator-based interview Age: 1+ years
Standardised observation	Autism Diagnostic Observation Schedule, Second Edition (ADOS-2®)	Lord et al. (2012)	Semi-structured observation using standardised kit of materials and specific 'presses' to elicit social, communication/interaction behaviours, restricted and repetitive behaviours. Organised by language level into 5 modules, covering all ages
	Childhood Autism Rating Scale, Second Edition (CARS-2)	Schopler et al. (2010)	Combination of interview and direct observation of the child during an unstructured activity completed by the clinician Age: 2+ years
Questionnaires	Child Communication Checklist, Second Edition (CCC-2)	Bishop (2003)	70-item questionnaire Screens for communication problems Age: 4 to 16 years Parent and teacher forms
	Social Responsiveness Scale, Second Edition (SRS-2)	Constantino and Gruber (2012)	65-item questionnaire Screens for presence and severity of social impairment and DSM-5 classification of autism spectrum disorder Age: 2 years 6 months to adult (pre-school, school age, adult forms available) Rated by parents or other caregivers/teachers Self-report (adult) also available

(Continued)

Measure type	Name	Authors	Method and age group
	Social Communication Questionnaire (SCQ)	Rutter, Bailey, and Lord (2003)	40-item questionnaire rated yes/no. Completed by parent/caregiver Current and lifetime forms available Age: 4+ years
	Autism Spectrum Screening Questionnaire (ASSQ)	Ehlers, Gillberg, and Wing (1999)	Screener for the broader phenotype of autistic traits completed by parents/teachers Age: 7 to 16 years
	Gilliam Autism Rating Scale, Third Edition (GARS-3)	Gilliam (2013)	Parent or teacher questionnaire Age: 3 to 22 years
	Theory of Mind Inventory, Second Edition (TOMI-2)	Hutchins and Prelock (2016)	Measure of multiple theory of mind abilities using questionnaires/interviews Age: 2+ years
	Modified Checklist for Autism in Toddlers, Revised with Follow-Up (M-CHAT-R/F)	Robins, Fein, and Barton (2009)	20-item questionnaire rated yes/no. Completed by parent/carer Age: 16 to 30 months
Cognitive measures	Social Perception Domain of the Developmental Neuropsychological Assessment, Second Edition (NEPSY-II)	Korkman, Kirk, and Kemp (2007)	Affect Recognition: assesses the ability to recognise six basic emotions in photographs of children's faces Theory of Mind: assesses the capacity to understand others perspectives, intentions, and beliefs from pictured scenarios Age: 3 to 16 years
	Awareness of Social Inference Test, Third Edition (TASIT)	McDonald, Flanagan, and Rollins (2017)	Assesses understanding of social exchanges as shown in videos of naturalistic everyday conversations between two actors Age: 13+ years
	Reading the Mind in the Eyes Test, Children's Version	Baron-Cohen et al. (2001)	Child is shown 28 photographs of the eye region and is asked to select which of four words best describes what the person is thinking/feeling Age: 6–14 years

(Continued)

Table 12.1 Continued

Measure type	Name	Authors	Method and age group
	Frith–Happé Animations Test	Abell, Happé, and Frith (2000)	Child is shown video clips of two triangles interacting and is asked to describe what is happening. The degree of mental state attribution and appropriateness is scored Age: 8+ years
	Strange Stories	Happé (1994); White et al. (2009)	Child reads (or listens to) short vignettes and is asked to explain why a character says something that is not literally true Age: 7+ years
	Theory of Mind Task Battery (ToMTB)	Hutchins and Prelock (2016)	Short vignettes presented as a storybook to assess a range of theory of mind skills from identifying facial expressions to the ability to infer second-order false beliefs Age: 6+ years
	Theory of Mind Scale	Wellman and Liu (2004)	A developmental scale of measures to assess understanding of diverse desires, diverse beliefs, knowledge-ignorance, false belief, and hidden emotion Age: 3 to 6 years

Seamus was observed at school by the speech and language therapist, who also discussed his strengths and difficulties with his class teacher and the school's inclusion coordinator.

Cognitive assessment using the Wechsler Intelligence Scale for Children, Fifth Edition (Wechsler 2016) revealed an uneven profile of cognitive strengths and weaknesses, with average range Fluid Reasoning and Visual Spatial Index Scores, low average range Verbal Reasoning, and below average range Working Memory and Processing Speed Indices. Seamus scored in the average range for reading subtests requiring phonological and orthographic decoding skills (Word Reading and Pseudoword Decoding from the Wechsler Individual Achievement Test, Third Edition, Wechsler 2017) but struggled with Reading Comprehension, scoring well below the average range and significantly lower than his other attainments. It was observed that Seamus struggled to understand nonliteral language in the text, and to make inferences based on the context of the story or the motivations and viewpoints of the characters.

Speech and language therapist assessment using the Clinical Evaluation of Language Fundamentals (Wiig, Semel, and Secord 2013) revealed that Seamus's expressive language scored within the average range, but in line with his somewhat weak verbal reasoning, his language understanding was significantly weaker. To the surprise of his parents and teacher, his often 'grown-up' use of vocabulary and somewhat formal speaking style made him appear verbally more advanced; however, this can stem from a strong memory and tendency to rely on functional use of scripted speech. Taken together, it was hypothesised that Seamus's weaker language comprehension, working memory, and slow processing speed, were contributing to his poor literacy and maths performance, with weak mentalising ability also impacting on his reading comprehension.

Formulation

The case vignette highlights some of the common difficulties in social functioning in verbal children. Many of Seamus's difficulties can be linked to weak theory of mind. Seamus tries to obtain the social interaction he desires using a rather limited repertoire of strategies. However, underlying executive functioning challenges make it difficult for Seamus to generate alternative strategies and apply these in a dynamic fashion in response to social feedback, at sufficient speed for neurotypical social communication and interaction. Seamus has not developed neurotypical face-processing and other social perceptual skills that would help him decipher peers' facial expressions to identify their interest level in his topic and does not tend to pay attention to, or know how to interpret, body language and other verbal or nonverbal cues that might tell him how his social initiations are being received, such as tone of voice, or a peer walking away. Seamus's 'black and white' thinking style further impacts on his interpretation of others' responses as 'mean' if they do not share his interests or react in the way he expects or wants.

Seamus's underlying difficulties with social understanding and anxiety were largely accepted by his parents but were not immediately apparent to his teacher, who applied behavioural strategies in response to socially unexpected behaviours in class, for example 'answering back'. Without implementing any coaching or support for Seamus to understand exactly what an 'appropriate' response would look like, behavioural strategies were largely ineffective and led to increased stress and a sense of unfairness for Seamus. A stress cycle was perpetuated by Seamus's difficulties communicating his concerns to his parents, therefore making it difficult to understand the root cause of this behaviour. Children at Seamus's age would often confide in friends, but this did not occur to Seamus, thus further limiting his opportunities for comfort and support.

INTERVENTION AND MANAGEMENT

While there is a wide range of interventions that have been developed for children with social communication difficulties in the context of ASD these could potentially be applied to children with social functioning difficulties stemming from other causes such as acquired brain injury (ABI). Interventions can be thought of in three categories, (1) those which maximise potential of the child, such as targeted social skills coaching,

(2) those which minimise barriers which the child might face, such as technology to assist with communication, and (3) those which maximise the fit between the child and their environment, such as peer-mediated interventions (Lai et al. 2020).

How and when to intervene can be complex and should be formulation driven. Co-occurring conditions could act as a barrier to some interventions; for example children with social anxiety, traumatic or ABI, learning difficulties or attention-deficit/ hyperactivity disorder may struggle with a structured group programme or didactic teaching model, unless adaptations are made. The effectiveness of an intervention could be negatively moderated by the presence of co-occurring conditions. For some, social skills interventions may give an unhelpful implicit message that the person with social challenges must change and 'fit in' with society rather than expecting acceptance and 'reasonable adjustments' from those around them. Careful consideration should be given to how social interventions are introduced, whether the goals of intervention are realistic, and whether the child is in an appropriate environment when developing an intervention plan. Interventions for teachers, peers, and parents that promote acceptance and understanding of a child's social needs could feasibly have greater impact on well-being and social confidence for some children than skills development, although it is likely that some combination of the two approaches is useful for optimal outcome.

Recent reviews have highlighted that many widely used psychosocial interventions have limited or no evidence base according to accepted standards for health care evidence (e.g. Green and Garg 2018; Lai et al. 2020), and few interventions have been able to demonstrate significant effects on social behaviour across different social settings (Gates et al. 2017; Wolstencroft et al. 2018). One review found 87.5% of studies identified had a medium–high risk of bias and reported varying outcomes making direct comparisons difficult (French and Kennedy 2018). Therefore, appraising and translating the evidence base for parents/carers, education providers, and health providers is an important clinical role, given the relatively high level of uncertainty.

Types of Social Intervention

The evidence-base for social interventions is rapidly growing and sourcing up-to-date systematic reviews (e.g. Cochrane reviews) is essential for clinicians to provide expert advice. Below are some examples of key types of intervention with social functioning as a primary outcome in young people with ASD that are also likely to be beneficial to children with ABI.

Joint attention, early play, and communication interventions for younger children (0–6 years) typically involve parent and often educational key-worker training in behavioural and/or developmental approaches, with many also involving direct work with the child. Interventions can be delivered in the home, a clinic, education settings, or in combinations of the above. Programmes can vary significantly in intensity from weekly group sessions to full-time intervention over several years (for a review, see French and Kennedy 2018). The use of video feedback to increase parental sensitivity and responsiveness is used by some to enhance parent training (e.g. Green et al. 2010; Pickles et al. 2016).

Group-based interventions, particularly those that run concurrent parent groups, can lead to improved parent-reported social knowledge of young people on the autism spectrum (Wolstencroft et al. 2018), although these gains did not necessarily translate to changes in social behaviour. Among those with significant effect sizes for social responsiveness were the Program for the Education and Enrichment of Relational Skills (PEERS) programme (Laugeson et al. 2014; Schohl et al. 2014) a 14-session programme of 90-minute group sessions for parents and young people, and summerMAX (Thomeer et al. 2016), an intensive 5-week, 5 days per week programme. One feasibility study by Barrera and Schulte (2009) has shown a group intervention to show promise in children with social difficulties post-brain tumour. The PEERS programme has also been applied to adolescents with brain injuries (Gilmore et al. 2019).

Computer-based/online social skills instruction is developing an evidence base (McCoy et al. 2016). Programmes are designed to be appealing, e.g. The Secret Agent Society (Beaumont 2015) incorporates spy-themed computer games into a multimedia small group parent and child programme. An interesting research field investigates the use of robots in social communication training for children with ASD, although findings are preliminary (Pennisi et al. 2016).

School-based peer interventions develop social communication by training a child's peers as partners to facilitate learning of social skills, by enhancing motivation and increasing integration with group activities. These approaches have been found to show promise (Watkins et al. 2015; Chang and Locke 2016), for example the 'Circle of Friends' (Schlieder et al. 2014).

Psychologists are often called on to develop highly individual strategies for specific social difficulties, and will draw on theory-informed techniques from existing interventions as guidelines. Some 'key ingredients' from current interventions for children with social functioning difficulties are outlined below:

- **Including the child's interests** in the delivery of the intervention can increase engagement and motivation. Examples of interventions based around potentially common interests are LEGO® Therapy (Owens et al. 2008) and 'The Transporters' DVD (Young and Posselt 2012), which uses trains to teach emotion recognition. In practice, children have highly individual and sometimes idiosyncratic interests, and therefore it is important to explore and work with individual motivations and to resist making assumptions about what will be of interest based on age, gender, or autism-related expectations or stereotypes. In addition, sensitivity should be paid to the function of that interest to the child and their consent gained to incorporate it. An interest that brings pleasure and relaxation when under the child's own control could potentially become less fulfilling or spoiled if 'taken over' by teachers or therapists.

- **Behaviour modelling, coaching, and role play** are important components of many interventions (e.g. Gresham et al. 2001; Schohl et al. 2014) with emerging but limited evidence for use of video modelling as a mode of delivery (Nikopoulos and Keenan 2006; McCoy et al. 2016).

- **Visual materials** are particularly important for children with language/auditory processing speed difficulties, for example 'Comic Strip Conversations' (Gray 1994) and help children to explore the thoughts of others.

- **Visual augmentative or alternative communication methods** such as Picture Exchange Communication System can facilitate early communication (Schreibman and Starmer 2016).

- **Child-centred social narratives**, for example Social Stories (Gray 2010) have become a widely used technique to teach a skill, concept, or situation, and can benefit social interaction (Karkhaneh et al. 2010).

- **Parent self-guided reading** on providing structured and planned playdates for their child on a regular basis (Frankel 2010).

Outcome

In addition to the formulation, the multidisciplinary team agreed that a diagnosis of Autism Spectrum Disorder, using the DSM-5 criteria, would be appropriate for Seamus. These outcomes were shared with Seamus's parents, verbally and in a written report, and in simpler format with Seamus himself. Seamus and his parents attended a 6-week psychoeducation group with the assessing team (Psychoeducation Groups for Autism Understanding and Support; Gordon et al. 2015) to increase understanding of autism, to connect with other families facing similar challenges and identify supports, and to foster positive self-concept via identifying and celebrating strengths.

Seamus's strengths, needs, and recommended interventions and accommodations were discussed with relevant school staff. Regular communication and cooperation between parents and school were strongly encouraged, in order to 'nip in the bud' problems that were arising for Seamus from his social cognitive challenges and to facilitate generalisation of skill learning across home and school contexts, as well as to jointly problem-solve and share ideas about how best to support Seamus.

Recommendations for school intervention included mentoring by a trusted key member of school staff, and allocated time with a learning support assistant who would be trained and supported to facilitate playground inclusion, and to use, as needed, resources such as Comic Strip Conversations (Gray 1994), Social Thinking (Garcia Winner 2006), Social Stories (Gray 2010), and emotion regulation strategies such as five-point scales (Dunn Buron and Curtis 2012) and Zones of Regulation (Kuypers 2011). These were used flexibly within the classroom, 'nurture' group and one-to-one mentoring sessions, to help Seamus 'unpick' social situations and problem-solve, to increase his confidence in making conversations and his social repertoire, reduce confusion and anxiety, and increase emotional understanding, recognition, and control. A Circle of Friends was created with Seamus's and his parents' agreement, meeting regularly with a supportive adult, to increase peer understanding and support. Adjustments were made in class to reduce 'sensory overload' (use of ear defenders, providing a quiet workstation with reduced visual clutter, access to regular movement breaks, and a quiet space with sensory toys to 'recharge' when he felt overwhelmed).

Opportunities were created by staff for Seamus to share his vast knowledge of animals with the class and to help others with a class project about wildlife, to boost Seamus's confidence and social standing. His interests were used as much as possible to encourage him to complete work that he was not intrinsically motivated by, because social motivation (e.g. to please the teacher) was a less powerful driver for him.

Additional assistance and preparation for transition to secondary school was recommended, during the final year of primary school, using the Systematic Transition in Education Programme for ASD (STEP-ASD) resource (Murin et al. 2016).

Seamus was referred to a clinical psychologist for help with managing anxiety and to support parents with managing meltdowns and behaviours stemming from anxiety, stress around transitions and new experiences, and with managing the sibling relationship. Clinical psychology sessions focused on teaching Seamus to recognise and label his own emotions, and to recognise when he was feeling anxious and put coping strategies in place before reaching a 'point of no return' (meltdown). His parents were supported to understand which behaviours that challenged them at home were likely to stem from anxiety, and to set up structures to reduce uncertainty and increase relaxation (e.g. visual timetabling, time to 'decompress' in a quiet place after school, time to engage in special interests, scheduled time to go over the events of the day with Seamus and help him interpret them, and problem-solve difficulties). Gradually increasing Seamus's tolerance of uncertainty in manageable ways (using the Coping with Uncertainty in Everyday Situations: CUES approach; Rodgers et al. 2017) was encouraged, and the psychologist liaised with the school to encourage coordination and joint working across home and school contexts with regard to behaviour management and supporting Seamus's emotion regulation and understanding.

Bringing up a child with social cognitive challenges places significant additional demands on parents, which can lead to stress and social isolation, and extra financial burden due to costs of intervention, need for individualised childcare, and reduced parental capacity to work. In recognition of this, avenues of social, emotional, and financial support for parents were identified in the local area and referrals made.

SUMMARY

Seamus's clinical vignette highlights the complexities of neuropsychological assessment for children with social communication differences. Seamus's teachers and parents clearly saw areas in his life where he needed some assistance to function at his best socially; however, his areas of difficulty were nuanced. Careful design of a neuropsychological battery allowed his team to pinpoint areas of strength and weakness, informing further intervention.

It is clear from theory and past research that social interaction difficulties in children on the autism spectrum can arise from various cognitive processes. Genetic factors combined with early socialisation patterns lead to complex interactions between the child's inherent biological makeup and their environment. It is important to consider social functioning concerns within a child's academic, peer, and familial environments. In addition, this chapter highlights the necessity of considering strengths and difficulties from multiple angles (e.g. language, attention). Executive functioning, in particular, may contribute significantly to a child's reciprocal communication challenges. For example identifying a difficulty with thinking flexibly would give a clinician a helpful place to start when designing an intervention. Incorporating a child's strengths and interests is also likely to improve engagement and outcomes.

Going forward, there is growing evidence and clear theoretical reasoning to indicate that early identification and intervention is essential for children who present with concern for social functioning difficulty. Not only does this allow the most comprehensive access to intervention, it helps parents and other caregivers conceptualise the roots of their child's emotions and behaviour from an early age and improves caregiver responsivity. Future directions should continue to evaluate evidence for interventions, as many existing interventions unfortunately have not been adequately evaluated, or do not show robust effect sizes in terms of outcomes. Broadening the range of outcomes measured to include and centre quality of life is important, as is consistency in selected outcome measures between trials, enabling direct comparison of intervention efficacy. Deliberate and carefully selected assessments, combined with efforts to identify efficacious parent, peer, and school interventions, should be a goal to provide the best available clinical support for children with social interaction difficulties.

REFERENCES

Ashton R (2018) Framework for assessment of children's social competence, with particular focus on children with brain injuries. *Applied Neuropsychology: Child* 7(2): 175–186. https://doi.org/10.1080/21622965.2016.1261701.

Baron-Cohen S, Leslie AM, Frith U (1985) Does the autistic child have a 'theory of mind'? *Cognition* 21(1): 37–46.

Barrera M, Schulte F (2009) A group social skills intervention program for survivors of childhood brain tumors. *Journal of Pediatric Psychology* 34(10): 1108–1118.

Beaumont R (2015) The Secret Agent Society social-emotional skills training for children with autism spectrum disorders. *The Australian Clinical Psychologist* 1(2): 27–29.

Blakemore SJ (2018) *Inventing Ourselves: The Secret Life of the Teenage Brain*. London: Doubleday.

Chang Y, Locke J (2016) A systematic review of peer-mediated interventions for children with autism spectrum disorder. *Research in Autism Spectrum Disorders* 27: 1–10.

Dunn Buron K, Curtis M (2012) *The Incredible 5-Point Scale: The Significantly Improved and Expanded Second Edition*. Shawnee Mission, KS: AAPC Publishing.

Farroni T, Csibra G, Simion F, Johnson MH (2002) Eye contact detection in humans from birth. *Proceedings of the National Academy of Sciences of the United States of America* 99: 9602–9605.

Fletcher-Watson S, McConnell F, Manola E, McConachie H (2014) Interventions based on the Theory of Mind cognitive model for autism spectrum disorder (ASD). *The Cochrane Database of Systematic Reviews* 2014(3): CD008785. https://doi.org/10.1002/14651858.CD008785.pub2.

Frankel F (2010) *Friends Forever: How Parents Can Help Their Kids Make and Keep Good Friends*. San Francisco, CA: Jossey Bass.

French L, Kennedy EMM (2018) Annual research review: Early intervention for infants and young children with, or at-risk of, autism spectrum disorder: a systematic review. *The Journal of Child Psychology and Psychiatry* 59(4): 444–456.

Garcia Winner M (2006) *Think Social! A Social Thinking Curriculum for School-Age Students*. San Jose, CA: Think Social Publishing Inc.

Gates JA, Kang E, Lerner MD (2017) Efficacy of group social skills interventions for youth with autism spectrum disorder: A systematic review and meta-analysis. *Clinical Psychology Review* 52: 164–181.

Gilmore R, Sakzewski L, Ziviani J et al. (2019) Multicentre, randomised waitlist control trial investigating a parent-assisted social skills group programme for adolescents with brain injuries: Protocol for the friends project. *BMJ Open* 9: e029587. doi: 10.1136/bmjopen-2019-029587.

Gordon K, Murin M, Baykaner O et al. (2015) A randomised controlled trial of PEGASUS, a psychoeducational programme for young people with high-functioning autism spectrum disorder. *Journal of Child Psychology and Psychiatry* 56(4): 468–476. https://doi.org/10.1111/jcpp.12304.

Gray C (1994) *Comic Strip Conversations: Illustrated Interactions That Teach Conversation Skills to Students with Autism and Related Disorders*. Michigan: Future Horizons.

Gray C (2010) *The New Social Story Book*. Canada: Future Horizons.

Green J, Charman T, McConachie H et al. (2010) Parent-mediated communication-focussed treatment in children with autism (PACT): A randomised controlled trial. *The Lancet* 375: 2152–2160.

Green J, Garg S (2018) Annual research review: The state of autism intervention science: Progress, target psychological and biological mechanisms and future prospects. *The Journal of Child Psychology and Psychiatry* 59(4): 424–443.

Gresham FM, Sugai G, Horner RH (2001) Interpreting outcomes of social skills training for students with high-incidence disabilities. *Exceptional Children* 67(3): 331–344.

Gunther Moor B, van Leijenhorst L, Rombouts SA, Crone EA, Van der Molen MW (2010) Do you like me? Neural correlates of social evaluation and developmental trajectories. *Social Neuroscience* 5(5–6): 461–482. https://doi.org/10.1080/17470910903526155.

Happé F, Frith U (2006) The Weak Coherence account: Detail-focused cognitive style in autism spectrum disorders. *Journal of Autism & Developmental Disorders* 36: 5–25. doi: 10.1007/s10803-005-0039-0.

Happé F, Frith U (2014) Annual review: Towards a developmental neuroscience of atypical social cognition. *Journal of Child Psychology & Psychiatry* 55(6): 553–577.

Karkhaneh M, Clark B, Ospina M, Seida JC, Smith V, Hartling L (2010) Social Stories™ to improve social skills in children with autism spectrum disorder: A systematic review. *Autism* 14(6): 641–662.

Kennedy DP, Adolphs R (2012) The social brain in psychiatric and neurological disorders. *Trends in Cognitive Sciences* 16: 559–572.

Kuypers L (2011) *The Zones of Regulation*. San Jose, CA: Think Social Publishing.

Lai M, Anagnostou E, Wiznitzer M, Allison C, Baron-Cohen S (2020) Evidence-based support for autistic people across the lifespan: Maximising potential, minimising barriers, and optimising the person-environment fit. *Lancet Neurology* 19(5): 434–451.

Laugeson EA, Ellingsen R, Sanderson J, Tucci L, Bates S (2014) The ABC's of teaching social skills to adolescents with autism spectrum disorder in the classroom: The UCLA PEERS® Program. *The Journal of Autism and Developmental Disorders* 44: 2244–2256.

McCoy A, Holloway J, Healy O, Rispoli M, Neely L (2016) A systematic review and evaluation of video modeling, role-play and computer-based instruction as social skills interventions for children and adolescents with high-functioning autism. *Review Journal of Autism and Developmental Disorders* 3: 48–67.

Murin M, Hellriegel J, Mandy W (2016) *Autism Spectrum Disorder and the Transition into Secondary School*. London: Jessica Kingsley.

Nelson EE, Jarcho JM, Guyer AE (2016) Social re-orientation and brain development: An expanded and updated view. *Developmental Cognitive Neuroscience* 17: 118–127.

Nikopoulos C, Keenan M (2006) *Video Modelling and Behaviour Analysis: A Guide for Teaching Social Skills to Children with Autism*. London: Jessica Kingsley.

Owens G, Granader Y, Humphrey A (2008) LEGO® therapy and the social use of language programme: An evaluation of two social skills interventions for children with high functioning autism and Asperger syndrome. *Journal of Autism and Developmental Disorders* 38: 1944–1957.

Pennisi P, Tonacci A, Tartarisco G et al. (2016) Autism and social robotics: A systematic review. *Autism Research* 9(2): 165–183.

Pickles A, Le Couteur A, Leadbitter K et al. (2016) Parent-mediated social communication therapy for young children with autism (PACT): Long-term follow-up of a randomized controlled trial. *The Lancet* 388: 2501–2509. doi: 10.1016/S0140-6736(16)31229-6.

Pierce K, Courchesne E, Bacon E (2016) To screen or not to screen universally for autism is not the question: Why the task force got it wrong. *The Journal of Paediatrics* 176: 182–194. doi: 10.1016/j.jpeds.2016.06.004.

Rodgers J, Hodgson A, Shields K, Wright C, Honey E, Freeston M (2017) Towards a treatment for intolerance of uncertainty in young people with autism spectrum disorder: Development of the Coping with Uncertainty in Everyday Situations (CUES©) programme. *Journal of Autism and Developmental Disorders* 47: 3959–3966. doi.org/10.1007/s10803-016-2924-0.

Rogers SJ, Estes A, Lord C et al. (2019) A multisite randomized controlled two-phase trial of the early start Denver model compared to treatment as usual. *Journal of the American Academy for Child and Adolescent Psychiatry* 58: 853–865.

Richardson H, Lisandrelli G, Riobueno-Naylor A, Saxe R (2018) Development of the social brain from age three to twelve years. *Nature Communications* 9(1): 1027. https://doi.org/10.1038/s41467-018-03399-2.

Schlieder M, Maldonado N, Baltes B (2014) An investigation of 'Circle of Friends' peer-mediated intervention for students with autism. *The Journal of Social Change* 6(1): 27–40.

Schohl KA, Van Hecke AV, Carson AM, Dolan B, Karst J, Stevens S (2014) A replication and extension of the PEERS intervention: Examining effects on social skills and social anxiety in adolescents with autism spectrum disorders. *Journal of Autism and Developmental Disorders* 44(3): 532–545.

Schreibman L, Stahmer AC (2014) A randomized trial comparison of the effects of verbal and pictorial naturalistic communication strategies on spoken language for young children with autism. *Journal of Autism and Developmental Disorders* 44(5): 1244–1251. doi: 10.1007/s10803-013-1972-y.

Thomeer ML, Lopata C, Donnelly JP et al. (2016) Community effectiveness RCT of a comprehensive psychosocial treatment for high-functioning children with ASD. *Journal of Clinical Child & Adolescent Psychology* 7(1): 1–12.

Watkins L, O'Reilly M, Kuhn M et al. (2015) A review of peer-mediated social interaction interventions for students with autism in inclusive settings. *Journal of Autism and Developmental Disorders* 45: 1070–1083. https://doi.org/10.1007/s10803-014-2264-x.

Wolstencroft J, Robinson L, Srinivasan R, Kerry E, Mandy W, Skuse D (2018) A systematic review of group social skills interventions, and meta-analysis of outcomes, for children with high functioning ASD. *Journal of Autism and Developmental Disorders* 48: 2293–2307. https://doi.org/10.1007/s10803-018-3485-1.

Young RL, Posselt M (2012) Using The Transporters DVD as a learning tool for children with autism spectrum disorders (ASD). *Journal of Autism and Developmental Disorders* 42: 984–991.

CHAPTER 13

Disruptive Behaviour

Alice Jones Bartoli and Stuart F White

Presenting Concern

Cameron is 8 years old and has received his third school exclusion/suspension for disruptive and aggressive behaviour. There is current discussion about whether Cameron's education might be better continued outside of mainstream school, although no formal process to change his school has begun yet. Cameron's first formal exclusion occurred 18 months previously due to an incident of violent behaviour towards another child that resulted in physical injury. The second exclusion was as a result of Cameron absconding from school, during which time he caused damage to teachers' cars in the school car park. He was found by police in a park not far away.

Cameron lives with his mother and father. Cameron's maternal grandmother and aunt are also involved in his care, providing afterschool and overnight care for him on a regular basis. His mother says that she struggles to stop him from going out – leaving the house and playing in the local park with children older than him. If she tries to stop him, he is verbally aggressive and has damaged property at home.

At 6 years of age, Cameron sustained a frontal lobe brain injury following a fall from his bicycle while the family were on holiday in Morocco. It was reported that Cameron lost control while travelling at high speed and crashed into a wall. He lost consciousness for several minutes at the site of the accident whilst another child raised the alarm. At the time emergency services arrived, he had a Glasgow Coma Scale score of 9 and recovered within 24 hours, although he remained in hospital for a week. He was unable to attend school for several weeks on his return home, and his parents reported a deterioration in his behaviour in subsequent months.

Cameron's early history includes some late initial language development for which he was referred to community speech and language therapy at a local Children's Centre at age 2 years 6 months. Cameron attended the nursery attached to his primary school from age 3 years, where he was noted to have some difficulties managing emotions, including incidents of interrupting others' activities and physical aggression. Cameron's teachers reported that he does not seem to have any close friends and acts in ways to draw other children's attention towards him. He is not invited to other children's birthday parties or on playdates. His teachers have previously tried to use tools to support his emotion regulation skills, including pictorial representations of emotions, but reported little improvement and use of these eventually tailed off.

Educationally, Cameron is working within the expected level for mathematics, but he is reluctant to read and write. His teacher rates his progress in literacy as being around 2 years behind his peers. He is described as being the root of much of the disruption in the classroom and is frequently out of his seat during class activities. Occasionally, he will leave the classroom, wandering about the school corridors until he is brought back to class. There is suspicion that he is responsible for some graffiti in the school toilets and also possibly stealing from other children's bags and coat pockets. No formal cognitive assessments have been carried out to date, but his attention seems to be poor. Cameron often teases or winds up other children to elicit a reaction, seeming to enjoy seeing others get into trouble with the class teacher. He has been involved in numerous playground skirmishes and is quick to blame others for what happens.

THEORY

Disruptive behaviour disorders, such as conduct disorder or oppositional defiant disorder, are most often an indication of other neuropsychological, environmental, and/or mental health challenges. The behaviours are not uncommon following a moderate to severe acquired or traumatic brain injury and indeed may be part of a premorbid presentation in many children who go on to experience traumatic brain injury (Li and Liu 2013; Vasa et al. 2015). There will also be children who have not had evidence of brain injury, yet show disruptive behaviour. This chapter will use 'disruptive behaviour problems' (DBP) to cover the range of conduct and externalising problems that fall under this large umbrella.

There are many possible routes that lead to the same presentation of DBP. Heterogeneity in the profiles of children presenting with DBP is well-documented. By looking across the neuropsychology and neuroscience evidence base on DBP in childhood and adolescence, we can start to identify different trajectories, and select the most appropriate assessments and interventions for children presenting to the clinic.

While disruptive and antisocial behaviour may be the most pressing presenting issue, it is unusual for there to be no other co-occurring difficulties. This section will provide an overview of common potential individual and contextual risk factors and may work best when considered in conjunction with chapters that consider those in more detail such as Chapter 5 on language, Chapter 6 on speech, and Chapter 11 on executive function, for example.

Executive Function

DBP have been associated with executive dysfunction across several domains, including inhibition and decision-making (Woltering et al. 2016). Inhibition in this context refers to the ability to withhold a response. Imaging studies that have sought to examine what happens in the brain during inhibition tasks appear to report different results depending on whether those with comorbid attention-deficit/hyperactivity disorder (ADHD) are included in the sample or not. Those studies that exclude participants with comorbid ADHD show no difference in the regions typically recruited during inhibition, but those that include participants with ADHD show differences in anterior insula cortex and inferior frontal gyrus – both related to ADHD symptom severity (see Tyler et al. 2019 for an overview). Many of the features of DBP fundamentally reflect poor decisions; this pattern of poor decision-making can also be seen in laboratory measures in young people with DBP. Imaging studies have shown that young people with DBP show reduced response in reward signalling regions (such as striatum and ventromedial prefrontal cortex) during both reward anticipation and reward receipt. Furthermore, these young people also show reduced representation of cues to change behaviour in the anterior insula cortex/inferior frontal gyrus (Blair, Veroude, and Buitelaar 2016). Importantly, the severity of DBP is correlated with the degree of disruption within the anterior insula cortex/inferior frontal gyrus (White et al. 2016). Vitally, executive function impairment appears to be increased under conditions of stress – an important factor to consider when behaviour difficulties may be present in the classroom but perhaps not at home (or other contexts) (Schoorl et al. 2018).

Limited Prosocial Emotions/Callous-Unemotional Traits

Diagnostic and Statistical Manual of Mental Disorders, Fifth Edition (DSM-5) introduced the limited prosocial emotions specifier for conduct disorder, with key characteristics of lack of affective empathy, lack of remorse or guilt, and apparent unconcern with own performance in important activities (APA 2013). These features are referred to in the research literature as 'callous-unemotional traits', which are considered to be a precursor to adult psychopathy and antisocial personality disorder (Frick et al. 2018). Callous-unemotional traits are highly heritable, and DBP in children scoring highly on callous-unemotional traits is also strongly genetically influenced (Moore et al. 2019). Children with elevated callous-unemotional traits typically have difficulties in recognising and responding to fear and sadness in others (Marsh and Blair 2008). Consistent with these emotion recognition deficits, children with DBP and callous-unemotional traits show attenuated amygdala responses to fearful facial and vocal expressions (Jones et al. 2009; Hoyniak et al. 2018). Emerging evidence suggests that this relationship may be moderated by maltreatment history, where young people with elevated callous-unemotional traits who had experienced prior trauma showed increased amygdala responsiveness to fearful expressions, compared to those who did not (Meffert et al. 2018). Emerging work on primary versus secondary variants of callous-unemotional traits will be important to monitor.

Language and Verbal Abilities

One area of development currently receiving more attention in relation to DBP is speech, language, and communication. Many studies note an increased rate of speech, language, and communication difficulties amongst children who show behavioural problems (Mackie and Law 2010), and conversely increased behavioural and emotional difficulties amongst children with diagnosed language impairment (Lindsay, Dockrell, and Strand 2007). It is social/pragmatic language difficulties that are most commonly associated with behavioural difficulties, but structural language concerns have also been reported (Snow and Powell 2004). There is some suggestion from research on incarcerated children and adults that DBP is associated with poorer verbal ability, and verbal ability appears to have an influence on whether an offender is more likely to be arrested (Yun and Lee 2013). However, this relationship is small at best and not consistent across disruptive behaviour disorders (Sanchez de Ribera et al. 2019). It may be the case that children's verbal abilities, as measured by standard IQ tests, are adversely affected by missing out on educational opportunities. There is, so far, an underexamined distinction between language problems and verbal abilities in children with DBP.

Environmental Influences

Compared to other psychiatric conditions, the evidence that DBP are associated with family environment risk factors is robust (Wesseldijk et al. 2018). Harsh and inconsistent parenting, and particularly maltreatment, are all risk factors for DBP. Other environmental influences contributing to DBP include maternal smoking, socio-economic deprivation, and parental adjustment problems (Boden, Fergusson, and Horwood 2010). The specific literature on children with brain injury is similar and shows that parenting styles such as overly permissive, authoritarian, and uninvolved may be associated with increased likelihood of disruptive behaviour alongside parental stress (Chavez-Arana et al. 2019).

ASSESSMENT AND FORMULATION

DBP, particularly in childhood, are rarely seen in isolation. They are probably best thought about as a symptom, with the behaviour communicating that something else needs to be addressed. It is necessary to consider the child alongside their individual and contextual risk factors and comorbid conditions.

One of the most important comorbid conditions in the disruptive behaviour disorders is ADHD. Comorbidity between ADHD and oppositional defiant disorder is substantial with one-third to one-half of children with one disorder also meeting criteria for the other (Nock et al. 2007). Examinations of covariance between ADHD and disruptive behaviour points towards common genetic influences on both sets of symptoms (Brikell et al. 2019).

Other important and co-occurring conditions include internalising disorders. The overlap between conduct disorder and anxiety disorders is significant; including social phobia

(31%), specific phobia (25%), post-traumatic stress disorder (20%), and generalised anxiety disorder (16%) (Nock et al. 2007). It is also possible that these comorbidities may alter the presentation of some of the features typically associated with DBP (Short et al. 2016). There is also emerging evidence of association between DBP and bipolar disorder (Vaudreuil et al. 2019).

A recent comprehensive review of conduct disorder, suggests assessment should occur across four areas: (1) conduct problems and the level of harm and risk to self and others; (2) comorbid conditions, including mental health difficulties, social issues, language and learning difficulties, and medical conditions (including injury and neglect); (3) known individual and contextual risk factors including harsh parenting, executive function difficulties, and emotion dysregulation; and (4) the age of onset and presence or absence of limited prosocial emotions (Fairchild et al. 2019). This method of systematically investigating potential contributory factors to DBP means that hypotheses can be tested using screening tools, and more in-depth assessments can be carried out as indicated.

Understanding the level of harm or risk towards self and others should help to guide treatment intensity and context; some children may require more specialist settings to manage extreme aggression and potential harm to self and others. Screening tools such as the Achenbach System of Empirically Based Assessment (Achenbach 2015) or the Behavior Assessment System for Children, Third Edition (BASC-3; Reynolds and Kamphaus 2015) can provide a norm-referenced overview of multiple areas of adjustment and mental health, which may indicate further follow-up using interview-based tools like the Diagnostic Interview for Children and Adolescents (Reich 2000) or Diagnostic Interview Schedule for Children, Fourth Edition (Shaffer et al. 2000).

Investigating comorbid conditions may rely on tools that screen for specific difficulties, for example speech, language, and communication difficulties (e.g. Children's Communication Checklist, Second Edition; Bishop et al. 2003); ADHD (e.g. Conners-3; Conners 2008) as well as internalising difficulties (Achenbach System of Empirically Based Assessment, BASC-3). Information from both parents and teachers will provide perspectives from different contexts may be useful to clinicians during formulation, providing a richer picture of a child's overall profile.

Individual and contextual risk factors may also be assessed using some of the screening tools outlined above, but alongside these it may also be helpful consider asking about parental stress or conflict (Parenting Stress Index, Fourth Edition; Abidin 2012), and/or observing parent–child interaction and carrying out assessments of cognitive ability and school attainment. Limited prosocial emotions or callous-unemotional traits may be screened for using the Inventory of Callous-Unemotional Traits (Frick 2003) or Child Problematic Traits Inventory (Colins et al. 2014).

Finally, considering DSM-5 subtypes and qualifiers of conduct disorders, reporting on the age of onset of DBP and the extent to which the limited prosocial emotions qualifier is met can be useful in directing treatment. Research in this area is fast emerging, but it seems that interventions that promote the use of reward strategies and reductions in punishment; promote executive function and empathy-building skills; and focus on increasing positive aspects of parenting, including the children in parenting treatment, are likely to be useful (Hawes, Price, and Dadds 2014). A focus on problem-solving has been identified as potentially offering benefit to reduce behavioural difficulties (Wade et al. 2011) and of particular note are adaptations using online interventions for children with brain injury and their families (Wade et al. 2018).

In Cameron's case, it is necessary to think about multiple factors that are contributing to his behaviour. It will be important to revisit his speech and language development, particularly his social use of language. Given his traumatic brain injury, an assessment of his cognitive ability and attainment would also be helpful to help target intervention happening at school and to understand his behaviour. It will be necessary to think about how the home and school environments are also contributing to, or maintaining, disruptive behaviour. For example observations of interactions between Cameron and his mother or Cameron at school may be helpful for understanding antecedents and consequences of challenging behaviour. From Cameron's case study, we can tell little about his understanding about emotions, but there are hints that this is an area of concern, and that he may be quite fearless in his behaviour; it may be useful to include a brief screen for limited prosocial emotions.

INTERVENTION AND MANAGEMENT

Interventions for DBP need to be tailored to the specific individual and contextual risk factors, and/or presenting comorbidities. However, parenting interventions have also been shown to be a cost-effective and fairly time-efficient method of treatment – particularly focused in early and middle-childhood, yielding large effect sizes in meta-analyses of treatment (Michelson et al. 2013), including children with acquired brain injury (Brown et al. 2014) and chronic illness (Law et al. 2019). We know that parenting may act as a mediator and moderator for individual and environmental risk factors, and so using a parenting programme as a first-line intervention is likely to mitigate the impact of some of the risk factors identified during assessment. Parenting programmes have also been shown to improve maternal mental health, ADHD symptoms, and reduce child abuse – all potential risk factors for conduct problems (Furlong et al. 2012). Parenting programmes, such as Triple P or the Incredible Years, are designed to improve parenting style and also promote positive parent–child relationships. It is, however, important to note that initial uptake of parenting programme interventions can be low for families of children with DBP, and drop-out rates can be up to 40% (Koerting et al. 2013). These rates are even less favourable for families experiencing multiple economic and social hardships, where barriers include time constraints and other practical problems, stigma, distrust, and misconception of services (see Koerting et al. 2013 for a comprehensive review). Facilitators to participation include 'soft entry' to the service, via taster sessions or coffee mornings; tailored interventions to families' own main concerns and developing a positive group experience (Koerting et al. 2013).

Alongside parenting programmes, there is also evidence that social problem-solving training and interventions focusing on developing self-regulation are helpful for children and families, following both therapist-administered and self-guided approaches (Kaminski and Claussen 2017; Kurowski et al. 2020). Interventions such as problem-solving skills training focus on teaching children explicit social problem-solving strategies. These interventions use role-plays and other techniques to allow children with DBP to practise social skills to achieve their social goals in a prosocial manner. Such a multimodal approach allows the development and consolidation of skills and relationship-building across children and their parents.

For adolescents, these parenting programmes may be less effective, although parenting still forms an important part of the recommended interventions for young people presenting with DBP. Multi-component interventions, like multi-systemic therapy, work intensively with the young person and family in the home to improve family functioning, parenting, and the young person's own skills for managing emotions and problem situations. Moreover, the multi-systemic therapy provider actively works with the family to access resources and support from the broader community. There is good evidence for the effectiveness of multi-systemic therapy (van der Stouwe et al. 2014), although one UK-based trial failed to find any enhanced long-term effect over standard services (Fonagy et al. 2018).

In some cases, particularly when there is clear comorbidity, psychopharmacological interventions may prove helpful. For those with comorbid ADHD, medium to large effect sizes of psychostimulants such as methylphenidate have been found for conduct problems in children and adolescents with DBP (Pringsheim et al. 2015). For other comorbid conditions, modular treatments that combine psychotherapy that is focused on depression or anxiety disorders with parenting and skills training for DBP have been shown to improve outcomes for children (Weisz 2012).

Treatments that offer opportunities for skills and relationship building are key, and so perhaps it is unsurprising that there is limited evidence for the efficacy of harsh or punitive methods of intervention. There is limited support for other punitive or fear-based interventions. Importantly, 'boot camps' and 'scared straight' interventions have been demonstrated to actually increase DBP symptoms (Petrosino et al. 2013), so it is important to be guided by the evidence base.

Outcome

Prior to the assessment, Cameron's mother and class teacher completed a number of screening questionnaires to help guide the initial assessment meeting. Cameron was also observed in school, and standardised tests were used to obtain an idea about his cognitive ability and academic attainment. Cameron's full-scale IQ was within the average range, but his attainment score in literacy was one standard deviation below what would be expected given his ability. Responses from his mother and teacher on the BASC-3 also indicated that Cameron had difficulties with attention, social skills, and functional communication, which were also echoed by the Children's Communication Checklist, Second Edition (Bishop 2003). Referral to the speech and language team resulted in consultation with school about supporting Cameron in the classroom, and working on developing comprehension, conversation, and narrative skills. At school, Cameron was also being supported to work with other children in the classroom and started to develop several positive social relationships. Fewer incidents of walking out of class occurred in the following months.

Educational material was offered to Cameron's mother about traumatic brain injury and she was offered feedback following many of the principles described in Chapter 25. She was offered a place on a local parenting programme run within Cameron's school, which used the Triple P intervention. The mother was able to access support both from the parenting group leader and also a new peer group of parents within the school. The clinician who carried out the assessment also spoke with the parenting group leader and advised them on Cameron's history of brain injury and the challenges that his parents reported at home prior to the assessment. She reported feeling more positive in her approach to parenting, using fewer reactive and punitive strategies. Cameron's mother reports that he is less angry and verbally aggressive at home, and that she started to seek new activities for him that will distract him from wanting to go back to hanging out with older children in the park. She says that she feels less overwhelmed by his oppositional behaviour and is starting to enjoy parenting.

SUMMARY

Disruptive behaviours come with a large financial and social strain. Despite this, they often go under-recognised or untreated, even though there is clear scope for both assessing and providing early intervention with the young person and their family. This can occur within and beyond the occurrence of traumatic or acquired brain injury. It is likely that mental health provisions in contexts where DBP are more likely to be seen, including schools and in the criminal justice system (Williams et al. 2018), will be important to getting children and adolescents the support that they need. In addition to better understanding comorbidities with mental health conditions, there is also a lack of research on physical health in those with DBP. There is much we still need to untangle in relation to the antecedents of disruptive behaviours. Due to the heterogeneity in presentation, it is necessary for us to be able to detail the different pathways that contribute towards DBP: genetic, neuropsychological, and environmental. Prospective longitudinal studies, starting prenatally, should allow us to better understand individual and contextual risk factors – and allow for more effective targeted prevention and early intervention.

REFERENCES

Achenbach TM (2015) Achenbach System of Empirically Based Assessment (ASEBA). In RL Cautin and SO Lilienfeld, *The Encyclopedia of Clinical Psychology* (eds). Wiley and Sons. https://doi.org/10.1002/9781118625392.wbecp150.

American Psychiatric Association (2013) *Diagnostic and Statistical Manual of Mental Disorders,* Fifth Edition. Arlington, VA: American Psychiatric Association.

Boden JM, Fergusson DM, Horwood LJ (2010) Risk factors for conduct disorder and oppositional/defiant disorder: Evidence from a New Zealand birth cohort. *Journal of the American Academy of Child & Adolescent Psychiatry* **49**(11): 1125–1133. https://doi.org/10.1016/j.jaac.2010.08.005.

Brown FL, Whittingham K, Boyd RN, McKinlay L, Sofronoff K (2014) Improving child and parenting outcomes following paediatric acquired brain injury: A randomised controlled trial of Stepping Stones Triple P plus Acceptance and Commitment Therapy. *J Child Psychol Psychiatry* **55**(10): 1172–1183. https://doi.org/10.1111/jcpp.12227.

Chavez-Arana C, Catroppa C, Yáñez-Téllez G et al. (2019) How do parents influence child disruptive behavior after acquired brain injury? Evidence from a mediation model and path analysis. *J Int Neuropsychol Soc* **25**(3): 237–248. doi: 10.1017/S1355617718001236.

Fairchild G, Hawes DJ, Frick PJ et al. (2019) Conduct disorder. *Nature Reviews Disease Primers* **5**(1): 1–25. https://doi.org/10.1038/s41572-019-0095-y.

Fonagy P, Butler S, Cottrell D et al. (2018) Multisystemic therapy versus management as usual in the treatment of adolescent antisocial behaviour (START): A pragmatic, randomised controlled, superiority trial. *The Lancet Psychiatry* **5**(2): 119–133. https://doi.org/10.1016/S2215-0366(18)30001-4.

Frick PJ, Robertson EL, Clark JE (2018) Callous–unemotional traits. In *Developmental Pathways to Disruptive, Impulse-Control and Conduct Disorders.* New York: Academic Press, pp. 139–160.

Furlong M, McGilloway S, Bywater T, Hutchings J, Smith SM, Donnelly M (2012) Behavioural and cognitive-behavioural group-based parenting programmes for early-onset conduct problems in children aged 3 to 12 years. *Cochrane Database of Systematic Reviews* **2**: CD008225. https://doi.org/10.1002/14651858.CD008225.pub2.

Hawes DJ, Price MJ, Dadds MR (2014) Callous-unemotional traits and the treatment of conduct problems in childhood and adolescence: A comprehensive review. *Clinical Child and Family Psychology Review* **17**(3): 248–267. https://doi.org/10.1007/s10567-014-0167-1.

Hoyniak CP, Bates JE, Petersen IT, Yang C-L, Darcy I, Fontaine NMG (2018) Reduced neural responses to vocal fear: A potential biomarker for callous-uncaring traits in early childhood. *Developmental Science* **21**(4): e12608. https://doi.org/10.1111/desc.12608.

Jones AP, Laurens KR, Herba CM, Barker GJ, Viding E (2009) Amygdala hypoactivity to fearful faces in boys with conduct problems and callous-unemotional traits. *American Journal of Psychiatry* **166**(1): 95–102. https://doi.org/10.1176/appi.ajp.2008.07071050.

Kaminski JW, Claussen AH (2017) Evidence base update for psychosocial treatments for disruptive behaviors in children. *Journal of Clinical Child & Adolescent Psychology* **46**(4): 477–499. https://doi.org/10.1080/15374416.2017.1310044.

Koerting J, Smith E, Knowles MM et al. (2013) Barriers to, and facilitators of, parenting programmes for childhood behaviour problems: A qualitative synthesis of studies of parents' and professionals' perceptions. *European Child & Adolescent Psychiatry* 22(11): 653–670. https://doi.org/10.1007/s00787-013-0401-2.

Kurowski BG, Taylor HG, McNally KA et al. (2020) Online Family Problem-Solving Therapy (F-PST) for executive and behavioral dysfunction after traumatic brain injury in adolescents: A randomized, multicenter, comparative effectiveness clinical trial. *J Head Trauma Rehabil* 35(3): 165–174. doi: 10.1097/HTR.0000000000000545.

Law E, Fisher E, Eccleston C, Palermo TM (2019) Psychological interventions for parents of children and adolescents with chronic illness. *Cochrane Database Syst Rev* 18(3): CD009660. https://doi.org/10.1002/14651858.CD009660.pub4.

Li L, Liu J (2013) The effect of pediatric traumatic brain injury on behavioral outcomes: A systematic review. *Dev Med Child Neurol* 55(1): 37–45. https://doi.org/10.1111/j.1469-8749.2012.04414.x.

Lindsay G, Dockrell JE, Strand S (2007) Longitudinal patterns of behaviour problems in children with specific speech and language difficulties: Child and contextual factors. *British Journal of Educational Psychology* 77(4): 811–828. https://doi.org/10.1348/000709906X171127.

Mackie L, Law J (2010) Pragmatic language and the child with emotional/behavioural difficulties (EBD): A pilot study exploring the interaction between behaviour and communication disability. *International Journal of Language & Communication Disorders/Royal College of Speech & Language Therapist* 45: 397–410. doi: 10.3109/13682820903105137.

Marsh AA, Blair RJR (2008) Deficits in facial affect recognition among antisocial populations: A meta-analysis. *Neuroscience & Biobehavioral Reviews* 32(3): 454–465. https://doi.org/10.1016/j.neubiorev.2007.08.003.

Meffert H, Thornton LC, Tyler PM et al. (2018) Moderation of prior exposure to trauma on the inverse relationship between callous-unemotional traits and amygdala responses to fearful expressions: An exploratory study. *Psychological Medicine* 48(15): 2541–2549. https://doi.org/10.1017/S0033291718000156.

Michelson D, Davenport C, Dretzke J, Barlow J, Day C (2013) Do Evidence-based interventions work when tested in the 'real world?' A systematic review and meta-analysis of parent management training for the treatment of child disruptive behavior. *Clinical Child and Family Psychology Review* 16(1): 18–34. https://doi.org/10.1007/s10567-013-0128-0.

Moore AA, Blair RJ, Hettema JM, Roberson-Nay R (2019) The genetic underpinnings of callous-unemotional traits: A systematic research review. *Neuroscience & Biobehavioral Reviews* 100: 85–97. https://doi.org/10.1016/j.neubiorev.2019.02.018.

Nock MK, Kazdin AE, Hiripi E, Kessler RC (2007) Lifetime prevalence, correlates, and persistence of oppositional defiant disorder: Results from the National Comorbidity Survey Replication. *Journal of Child Psychology and Psychiatry* 48(7): 703–713. https://doi.org/10.1111/j.1469-7610.2007.01733.x.

Petrosino A, Turpin-Petrosino C, Hollis-Pee, ME, Lavenberg JG (2013) 'Scared Straight' and other juvenile awareness programs for preventing juvenile delinquency. *Cochrane Database of Systematic Reviews* 4: CD002796. https://doi.org/10.1002/14651858.CD002796.pub2.

Pringsheim T, Hirsch L, Gardner D, Gorman DA (2015) The Pharmacological management of oppositional behaviour, conduct problems, and aggression in children and adolescents with attention-deficit hyperactivity disorder, oppositional defiant disorder, and conduct disorder: A systematic review and meta-analysis. Part 1: Psychostimulants, Alpha-2 agonists, and atomoxetine. *The Canadian Journal of Psychiatry* 60(2): 42–51. https://doi.org/10.1177/070674371506000202.

Sanchez de Ribera O, Kavish N, Katz IM, Boutwell BB (2019) Untangling intelligence, psychopathy, antisocial personality disorder, and conduct problems: A meta-analytic review. *European Journal of Personality* 33(5): 529–564. https://doi.org/10.1002/per.2207.

Schoorl J, van Rijn S, de Wied M, van Goozen S, Swaab H (2018) Boys with oppositional defiant disorder/conduct disorder show impaired adaptation during stress: An executive functioning study. *Child Psychiatry & Human Development* 49(2): 298–307. https://doi.org/10.1007/s10578-017-0749-5.

Short RM, Adams WJ, Garner M, Sonuga-Barke EJ, Fairchild G (2016) Attentional biases to emotional faces in adolescents with conduct disorder, anxiety disorders, and comorbid conduct and anxiety disorders. *Journal of Experimental Psychopathology* 7(3): 466–483. https://doi.org/10.5127/jep.053915.

Snow P, Powell M (2004) Developmental language disorders and adolescent risk: A public-health advocacy role for speech pathologists? *Advances in Speech Language Pathology* 6(4): 221–229. https://doi.org/10.1080/14417040400010132.

Tyler PM, White SF, Thompson RW, Blair RJR (2019) Applying a cognitive neuroscience perspective to disruptive behavior disorders: Implications for schools. *Developmental Neuropsychology* 44(1): 17–42. https://doi.org/10.1080/87565641.2017.1334782.

van der Stouwe T, Asscher JJ, Stams GJJM, Deković M, van der Laan PH (2014) The effectiveness of Multisystemic Therapy (MST): A meta-analysis. *Clinical Psychology Review* 34(6): 468–481. https://doi.org/10.1016/j.cpr.2014.06.006.

Vasa RA, Suskauer SJ, Thorn JM et al. (2015) Prevalence and predictors of affective lability after paediatric traumatic brain injury. *Brain Inj* 29(7–8): 921–928. doi: 10.3109/02699052.2015.1005670.

Vaudreuil CAH, Faraone SV, Di Salvo M et al. (2019). The morbidity of subthreshold pediatric bipolar disorder: A systematic literature review and meta-analysis. *Bipolar Disorders* 21(1): 16–27. https://doi.org/10.1111/bdi.12734.

Wade SL, Narad ME, Shultz EL et al. (2018) Technology-assisted rehabilitation interventions following pediatric brain injury. *J Neurosurg Sci* 62(2): 187-202. doi: 10.23736/S0390-5616.17.04277-1.

Wade SL, Walz NC, Carey J et al. (2011) Effect on behavior problems of teen online problem-solving for adolescent traumatic brain injury. *Pediatrics* 128(4): e947-953. doi: 10.1542/peds.2010-3721.

Weisz JR (2012) Testing standard and modular designs for psychotherapy treating depression, anxiety, and conduct problems in youth: A randomized effectiveness trial. *Archives of General Psychiatry* 69(3): 274. https://doi.org/10.1001/archgenpsychiatry.2011.147.

Wesseldijk LW, Bartels M, Vink JM et al. (2018) Genetic and environmental influences on conduct and antisocial personality problems in childhood, adolescence, and adulthood. *European Child & Adolescent Psychiatry* 27(9): 1123–1132. https://doi.org/10.1007/s00787-017-1014-y.

White SF, Tyler PM, Erway AK, Botkin ML, Kolli V, Meffert H, Blair JR (2016) Dysfunctional representation of expected value is associated with reinforcement-based decision-making deficits in adolescents with conduct problems. *Journal of Child Psychology and Psychiatry* 57(8): 938–946.

Williams WH, Chitsabesan P, Fazel S et al. (2018) Traumatic brain injury: A potential cause of violent crime?. *The Lancet. Psychiatry* 5(10): 836–844. https://doi.org/10.1016/S2215-0366(18)30062-2.

Woltering S, Lishak V, Hodgson N, Granic I, Zelazo PD (2016) Executive function in children with externalizing and comorbid internalizing behavior problems. *Journal of Child Psychology and Psychiatry* **57**(1): 30–38. https://doi.org/10.1111/jcpp.12428.

Yun I, Lee J (2013) IQ and delinquency: The differential detection hypothesis revisited. *Youth Violence and Juvenile Justice* **11**(3): 196–211. https://doi.org/10.1177/1541204012463410.

CHAPTER 14

Literacy

Valerie Muter and Margaret Snowling

Presenting Concern

Alex was referred at age 11 years by her parents on the recommendation of teachers at her secondary school where she had been a pupil for 6 months. Alex had a history of significant speech and language delay, and had received intensive speech and language therapy as a preschooler. Her language problems had not resolved by the time she started primary school and it was soon evident that she was falling well behind her peers in educational, especially literacy, development. Alex underwent a statutory assessment at age 8 years and was diagnosed with a severe language disorder. Alex went on to attend a special school for children with language disorder. During her 2 years there, she received intensive speech and language therapy such that by the time she returned to mainstream schooling at age 10 years, most of her speech and language difficulties had resolved. However, she continued to present with severe problems accessing printed words, which formed the basis for the present referral. It was suspected that Alex might have higher order language difficulties, which were affecting her ability to access an increasingly demanding school curriculum. Alex had consistently presented as stronger in maths than literacy. Her parents and teachers reported that there were no behavioural deficits, social problems, or difficulties with attention control, but Alex herself reported low self-esteem, especially in academic settings. There was a family history of dyslexia paternally, with Alex's father having been a late reader and experiencing spelling difficulties, even as an adult.

THEORY

In order to understand why some children fail to learn to read accurately, fluently, and with understanding, it is necessary to have an appreciation of the processes involved in typical reading development. Word recognition and reading comprehension are built on two relatively separate foundations. Word level reading largely depends on the child's development of phonological awareness (their sensitivity to the sound structure of words) and letter knowledge; together these skills assessed at age 5 years account for 90% of the variance in word reading, specifically decoding print, at age 6 years (Muter et al. 2004). In essence, learning to read depends on creating 'mappings' between letter strings of printed words (orthography) and phonology, which become increasingly consolidated and automatised during the elementary school years. However, in order to read with meaning, decoding is only the first step. The development of reading comprehension skills depends largely on broader oral language abilities including vocabulary knowledge, sentence comprehension, and the ability to make inferences (Cain 2010).

When the development of word level decoding skills is disrupted, as it is in 3% to 7% of children, the term dyslexia is commonly employed (Snowling 2009). According to Diagnostic and Statistical Manual of Mental Disorders, Fifth Edition (DSM-5) (American Psychiatric Association 2013), dyslexia is an alternative term for specific learning disorder with impairment in reading, although it usually also affects spelling accuracy. Although the term is used as a diagnosis, it varies along a dimension of mild to severe and has variable manifestation. It should also be noted that around 7% to 10% of children who read accurately have difficulties understanding what they read (Nation et al. 2004); such children almost invariably have broader language difficulties including weaknesses in oral comprehension, expressive vocabulary, and grammar; some have English as an additional language. The importance of educational history is critical in determining the clinical picture and it should be borne in mind that inadequate teaching may be a sufficient explanation for some children's poor reading skills.

Many children with dyslexia experience problems of reading fluency and spelling that persist into adulthood despite intervention. Dyslexia commonly co-occurs alongside other developmental difficulties, such as developmental language disorder (Bishop et al. 2017), mathematical problems, attention-deficit/hyperactivity disorder, or motor difficulties. Our case study is an 11-year-old girl with a history of preschool speech and language difficulties who went on to present with significant and persisting literacy problems.

Case Study – Alex

It is well established that children with language difficulties are at high risk of reading problems (Bishop and Snowling 2004). Given that Alex had preschool language difficulties, this may provide an explanation for her severe dyslexia. On the other hand, Alex has a family history of dyslexia; many children at family-risk of dyslexia who later develop literacy problems experience preschool language difficulties (Snowling and Melby-Lervåg 2016), suggestive of a shared genetic risk. However, the home literacy environment is likely to be a strong mediator of genetic differences, such that parents with dyslexia who themselves read less frequently will create less rich home literacy environments for their children. In addition, children who have a genetic disposition for dyslexia may prefer activities other than reading and hence experience low levels of exposure to print. These are powerful examples of passive and active gene–environment correlation. More generally, young people with dyslexia often present with low self-esteem in relation to their academic skills, avoidance of reading, and attentional and emotional difficulties (Snowling et al. 2007).

The case of Alex demonstrates that literacy disorders run in families and family members of someone with dyslexia are at high risk of developing the condition. The genetics of dyslexia is complex with many gene variants, each with small effect, acting together through the environment to produce behavioural outcomes that also reflect the operation of protective factors. It is these influences working together that determine whether an individual child will go on to develop dyslexia (Avon Longitudinal Study of Parents and Children [ALSPAC]; Golding et al. 2002). In turn, the genetic variations associated with dyslexia act to influence the development of brain regions involved in learning to read and the connections between these regions. In dyslexia, there is some evidence of both structural and functional differences in the left hemispheric brain regions involved in reading; the most robust finding is smaller brain volume in individuals with dyslexia, with the left perisylvian and occipitotemporal regions mostly (but not always) implicated (Ramus et al. 2018). However, there is an important issue to be addressed regarding the causal significance of such findings. A promising approach is to investigate the neural correlates of dyslexia in children born to families with a high risk of dyslexia and then determine if measures of brain activity in the earliest stages of development are predictive of later reading skill. Saygin et al. (2013) found that the phonological awareness performance of 40 preschoolers at risk for dyslexia correlated positively and significantly with the volume of the left arcuate fasciculus which is an area known to connect the anterior and posterior language regions of the brain – those regions that are involved in the translation of print to sound. Both the preschool phonological awareness scores and the brain volumes predicted the children's reading scores after they had started school.

It is now well established that the proximal cause of dyslexia in the cognitive system is an underlying weakness in the phonological system of language, which is persistent and compromises the development of the mappings required from phonology to orthography and vice versa. This weakness is indicated by poor performance from preschool onwards on a wide range of phonological tasks, such as deleting specified phonemes from words, speeded (rapid) naming of letters or numbers, and repeating nonwords (Snowling et al. 2019). Difficulties in processing, memorising, and analysing speech segments in words invariably results in problems learning to decode words in children with dyslexia. The most direct means of investigating this decoding deficit is to ask children to read nonwords like 'tig' and 'floob'. Children with dyslexia typically have great difficulty reading nonwords, compared with younger children without dyslexia.

The development of *reading comprehension* depends on broader oral language skills, such as the knowledge of word meanings and the ability to understand sentences, make inferences where appropriate, and remember what was read in order to create an integrated and cohesive sense of the text (Cain 2010). In contrast to children with dyslexia, poor reading comprehenders perform well on tests of phonological skills (see Castles, Rastle, and Nation 2018 for review). They do, however, experience problems with a wide range of language-related tasks that assess oral language (vocabulary, grammar, and oral expression), higher level language skills (including narrative and use of figurative language), metacognitive processes (integration and inference making, knowledge of story conventions and structures), and executive processes (verbal working memory, suppression, and inhibition). Nation et al. (2010) carried out a longitudinal study of poor reading comprehenders from age 5 to 8 years; the children assessed as having reading comprehension difficulties at age 8 years showed oral language problems that were present at school entry 3 years earlier. Such findings suggest that language problems, such as those Alex demonstrated, are likely to be causally related to later reading comprehension difficulties. It is highly probable therefore that she will not only have problems with reading and spelling accuracy but also with reading comprehension.

In dyslexia, the severity of the child's phonological deficit will influence the extent of their reading and spelling difficulties. However, other cognitive risk factors also play a role; these include lower nonverbal ability, weaknesses in auditory processing, and short-term verbal memory limitations. Indeed, there is growing evidence that a phonological deficit is one of a number of risk factors for dyslexia that accumulate towards a threshold which characterises the disorder (Pennington et al. 2012). In considering the co-occurrence of dyslexia, language disorder, and speech sound disorders, Pennington and Bishop (2009) conclude that there are some risk factors that are general to all three disorders, especially difficulties in acquiring phoneme awareness. However, there are also risk factors that are specific to particular disorders; a deficit in rapid naming is specific to children with dyslexia, but is not always evident in children with speech and language disorders.

ASSESSMENT AND FORMULATION

Most children with literacy disorders are referred for assessment in the middle school years. However, there is increasing recognition of the importance of early identification before the child has fallen behind educationally and begins to experience declining levels of motivation and confidence. Since early screening batteries have tended to have low validity, a review for the UK government (Rose 2009) recommended the identification of 'at risk' children via close monitoring of their response to reading instruction during the first 2 years at school (e.g. Snowling et al. 2011). Children who fail to progress sufficiently in response to mainstream, differentiated and additional literacy support require further assessment for likely dyslexia or reading comprehension disorder. More recent studies have suggested that being at family risk for dyslexia can provide an indication from a relatively early age (age 3 years 6 months) whether a child is likely to experience later reading difficulties (Thompson et al. 2015). Poor language development is an additional risk factor particularly if speech and language difficulties do not resolve by school entry. Early screening and identification of at risk children can lead to advice as to how parents could best support their child's early reading development, bearing in mind that a home literacy environment rich in books and print-related interactions is associated with a good start in word decoding and comprehension. More generally, children who enter school with poor language skills are at high risk of dyslexia. However, screening at an earlier stage is not always productive because some children resolve these difficulties without intervention.

A brief assessment for dyslexia should include tests of single word and nonword reading and spelling alongside assessments of phonological awareness, rapid naming, and verbal short-term memory. Recent research suggesting that vocabulary growth does not keep pace with development in children who do not read, indicates that including a measure of vocabulary would also be useful. Furthermore, given the high degree of co-occurrence, a standardised test of arithmetic is a useful addition (Landerl and Moll 2010). If, as the result of this brief assessment, it is suspected that a child has broader language difficulties, then tests of sentence and nonword repetition can confirm whether referral to a speech and language therapist is necessary. If required, a short-form IQ test makes it possible to determine whether the child has other learning difficulties that need to be taken into account when planning intervention.

More comprehensive assessment of literacy to aid in the development of an intervention plan needs to recognise that not all components of literacy will be equally impaired in a given child. Reading is a multi-componential skill and the tests administered to a given child will need to cover a broad range of subskills (see Table 14.1). For the child

Table 14.1 Skills and subskills that comprise a comprehensive assessment of literacy

Construct	Test
Reading attainment	
Decoding	Single word reading
	Nonword reading
Fluency	Single words and continuous text
Reading comprehension	Text reading and comprehension
Spelling	Single word spelling
	Spelling in free writing
Writing	Narrative structure and organisation
	Writing quality and speed
Mathematic attainment	Mental arithmetic
	Mathematical reasoning
Phonological skills	Phoneme awareness
	Rapid naming
	Nonword repetition
Language skills	Vocabulary
	Sentence repetition
	Grammar and morphology
	Verbal memory

with reading comprehension difficulties, it is important to evaluate oral language skills and text comprehension strategies. Finally, in view of the common co-occurrence of developmental disorders, the assessment needs to determine whether additional difficulties are affecting behaviour or school adjustment. Hypotheses of which co-occurring difficulties are likely to be present in an individual child can be based on parent and school information, observations during the course of the assessment and screening measures. Given time constraints, standardised questionnaires that assess, for instance, attention or language difficulties can be used to determine whether further investigation of these difficulties is warranted.

The 'diagnosis' of dyslexia is not straightforward because, as discussed above, it is a dimensional disorder with no clear cut-off and variation over time is to be expected given the availability or otherwise of compensatory resources both within the child and through intervention. Moreover, different terminology is in use, including reading disorder, specific learning disorder, and, in the UK, specific learning difficulty. DSM-5 suggests that for a diagnosis of 'dyslexia' levels of reading and spelling attainment should be significantly below age expectation, but the precise criteria will vary according to context and criteria will normally be agreed by local professional authorities.

INTERVENTION AND MANAGEMENT

There is a growing body of evidence on effective interventions for reading and language development (Hulme and Melby-Lervåg 2015). It is important to match the form of intervention to the individual child's needs. The form of intervention chosen will depend not only on the child's profile of difficulty but also on their age and stage of development. Early intervention for dyslexia might include helping parents, who themselves have experienced literacy difficulties, to support their children's prereading skills. Activities should include learning to name and write letters but formal reading instruction is not needed during preschool. More generally, sharing books and being exposed to 'book language' (rather than conversations) is important since activities such as these are the foundation of reading comprehension.

At the core of school-based reading intervention programmes is work on phonological skills; depending on the age of the child, this will include work on letter-sound correspondences, phoneme awareness, and linking the two together to provide effective phonic decoding strategies. A comprehensive survey of such approaches which encourage structured, multisensory interaction with printed books is provided by Brooks (2016). However, reading intervention needs to go beyond phonics if fluency is to be acquired (Castles et al. 2018). Importantly, teaching children to read does not guarantee that spelling will improve and separate interventions will be required. Spelling presents a particular challenge for children with dyslexia. Even children who progress well in reading in response to phonological and phonic-based interventions tend to have long-term spelling difficulties. Compared with reading, we know much less about the efficacy of spelling intervention; however, good practice suggests that systematic introduction to the orthographic (spelling) patterns of English is helpful. Such interventions may need to emphasise orthographic units including grammatical morphemes (such as -ed) and aspects of derivational morphology (e.g. -tion, -ery) (Nunes and Bryant 2009).

Preliminary evidence suggests that successful intervention in children with dyslexia results in behavioural improvements that are also accompanied by changes in brain structure and function. For instance in a voxel-based morphometry study of 11 children with dyslexia (Krafnik et al. 2011), grey matter volume in four brain regions (left anterior fusiform gyrus/hippocampus, left precuneus, right hippocampus, and right anterior cerebellum) increased during an 8-week structured intervention in which children made progress in learning to read. However, to date, studies are small scale and in need of replication.

A smaller evidence base has shown that reading comprehension difficulties can be ameliorated by suitable interventions that boost vocabulary, broader oral language, and text comprehension skills (Snowling and Hulme 2011). Preschool programmes aimed at strengthening the foundations of literacy (specifically oral language skills and phoneme awareness) can also have positive effects on reading comprehension (Fricke et al. 2013).

It is natural for interventions to focus on remediating the child's difficulties. However, there is a place for encouraging children to draw on their cognitive strengths so that they can develop compensatory strategies. For example the verbally able child with dyslexia encountering an unfamiliar word may be taught to supplement their (imperfect) attempt at decoding by using vocabulary knowledge. As children get older, their needs extend beyond direct teaching of reading and spelling to include instruction in the use of information technology (computers, spell checks, and voice-activated software) and techniques for improving organisational skills and assessment arrangements (typically extra time in examinations but also possibly being supplied with a 'reader' or scribe).

Understandably, the teaching of children with dyslexia has focused largely on remediating reading and spelling problems; however, co-occurring difficulties need to be addressed in their own right. Management programmes should not be limited to literacy instruction but should also consider the individual child's need for speech and language therapy, occupational/physiotherapy, medication or behavioural programmes for attention deficits, and additional maths/spellings support.

Finally, many parents are attracted to 'alternative' or complementary therapies; not infrequently, these aim to target the biological or neurological basis of developmental learning disorders. Such treatments are rarely subjected to robust evaluation and the evidence for their efficacy is lacking (Bishop 2013).

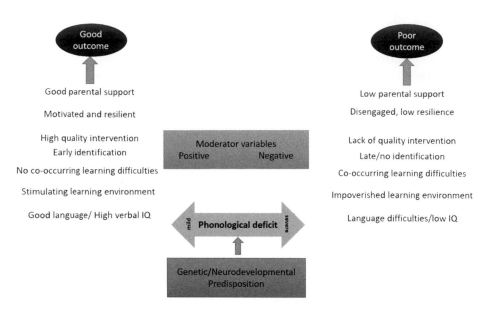

Figure 14.1 Moderator variables that can lead to good and poor outcomes for individuals with literacy disorders

The long-term outcome for individuals with literacy disorders varies enormously. Whether it is broadly positive or negative depends on the underlying severity of the phonological deficit, the presence of co-occurring difficulties (which complicate both presentation and intervention), when the disorder is identified, the quality, frequency, and intensity of intervention, and educational and broader environmental experiences. Such 'moderator' variables influence the outcome, which may be positive or negative as described in Figure 14.1. The verbally able child with mild dyslexia and no co-occurring difficulties and/or who has access to good intervention from an early age may well go on to have a successful schooling experience and reach higher education. Nonetheless, in the workplace, dyslexia can still cause problems especially in occupations which demand high levels of literacy. The child with more severe dyslexia and those with co-occurring language or attentional problems may have a more challenging educational experience and a poorer outcome. This will be especially true if there is a failure to identify the problem and provide appropriate intervention and support.

Outcome

Alex was highly cooperative during testing and demonstrated excellent concentration and high levels of motivation. Her IQ assessment showed that she is a young girl of average intelligence with definite strengths (and indeed above average scores) on nonverbal scales of ability. In contrast, her verbal abilities are at best low-average. The discrepancy between the verbal and nonverbal indices is statistically significant and is in the direction and size expected for a child with a pre-school diagnosis of specific language disorder. Educational attainment testing revealed that Alex's mathematical abilities are well developed and far in advance of her literacy skills, which are very weak. Reading fluency and spelling are especially compromised. Alex performed at a below average level on the reading comprehension measures, and her written narrative skills are poor. Diagnostic testing revealed severe phonological processing and short-term verbal memory limitations, which have impaired the development of decoding skills. On a sentence repetition test, often regarded as a 'marker' for language disorder, she obtained a very low score.

Alex has severe dyslexia co-occurring in the context of developmental language delay. She has poor phonological skills, which are known to be a shared 'risk' for these disorders. These, in turn, have resulted in problems learning to decode, thus preventing her reading and spelling skills from developing at an expected level. Alex has shown significant improvements in her oral language in response to intensive speech and language therapy, while progress in response to literacy intervention has been much slower. Her reading comprehension difficulties are likely explained in part by her poor reading accuracy and fluency but could also be attributed to her long-standing language impairment.

Recommendations for intervention and management of Alex's difficulties should include:

- ✓ access to a structured multisensory phonological/phonic-based literacy intervention scheme that specifically targets phonological awareness, phonic decoding, and spelling conventions within a flexible teaching framework that includes reading books at an appropriate level of difficulty;
- ✓ provision of an integrated language and reading comprehension programme that promotes vocabulary and higher order language skills, together with specific text-based strategies such as comprehension monitoring, rereading, and highlighting key points, questioning, and summarising;
- ✓ encouragement to take advantage of the editing and spellcheck facilities that technology offers and permission to submit a significant proportion of her course work in word processed form;
- ✓ being permitted time accommodations, access to a reader and provision of a scribe or use of a laptop computer in formal written examinations;
- ✓ curricula and classroom accommodations such as exemption from taking a foreign language, being provided with photocopied notes, and having access to a mentor who can support the development of improved study and organisational skills.

Alex's outcome will undoubtedly be impacted by her having severe dyslexia occurring in the context of marked language delay and disorder. Whilst this might be considered predictive of a generally poor long-term outcome in many individuals, Alex has experienced a significant number of positive moderators – including early identification and intensive intervention for her language disorder, having good nonverbal skills that might provide some compensatory resources and contribute to her stronger maths ability, a supportive home environment, and good levels of psychological adjustment and motivation, which would be expected to improve her outcome. With continued targeted intervention, curricula and examination accommodations, access to technology, and high levels of teacher and parent support, it would be well within the realms of possibility for Alex to obtain school-based qualifications and to then proceed to further education courses which reflect her relative strengths within the nonverbal and mathematical domains of ability.

SUMMARY

Literacy disorders are recognised as dimensional, with no clear cut-off between typical and impaired reading; it has been proposed that the term 'dyslexia' may be most appropriate for children with persisting difficulties who make a slower than expected response to targeted intervention. Disorders of reading accuracy stemming from phonological (speech sound processing) difficulties are partially independent from disorders of reading comprehension which are associated with broader oral language impairments. Dyslexia is a genetically based disorder associated with demonstrable structural and functional differences in the left hemispheric regions of the brain that underlie language and literacy; these differences are predictive of variations in reading skill in children with dyslexia and have been shown to be modifiable with targeted intervention. Literacy disorders tend to co-occur alongside other learning difficulties (e.g. maths and written expression disorders, visuomotor problems, and attention difficulties). Literacy skills are multi-componential, a fact that needs to be reflected in the tests administered at assessment; these should cover a broad range of subskills that go beyond basic reading accuracy to include decoding ability, spelling, writing skills, phonological processing, and verbal short-term memory. Different forms of literacy disorder require different interventions; there is an evidence-base of effective interventions to promote phonological skills and for treatments that foster language (especially vocabulary) development. Protective factors play an important part in improving the outcome for children with literacy disorders. These protective factors include early identification and high-quality intervention, the child's ability to maintain attention and motivation, fostering high levels of print exposure, encouragement to engage in activities in which the child might excel, and family support. Children who have severe and complex literacy problems (treatment nonresponders) will need intensive and high-quality treatment, learning support, and appropriate accommodations that are sustained into the teenage years and beyond. Amongst the biggest challenges and indeed questions still to be answered is how best to improve the outcome for children who make a poor response to standard interventions and, allied to that, how to motivate older children to read more and develop greater resilience.

REFERENCES

American Psychiatric Association (2013) *Diagnostic and Statistical Manual of Mental Disorders*, 5th edition. Arlington, VA: American Psychiatric Association

Bishop DV (2013) Neuroscientific studies of intervention for language impairment in children: Interpretive and methodological problems. *Journal of Child Psychology and Psychiatry, and Allied Disciplines* 54: 247–259.

Bishop DV, Snowling MJ (2004) Developmental dyslexia and specific language impairment: Same or different? *Psychological Bulletin* 130(6): 858–886.

Bishop DV, Snowling MJ, Thompson PA et al. (2017) Phase 2 of CATALISE: A multinational and multidisciplinary Delphi consensus study of problems with language development: Terminology. *Journal of Child Psychology and Psychiatry* 58(10): 1068–1080.

Brooks G (2016) *What Works for Children and Young People With Literacy Difficulties? The Effectiveness of Intervention Schemes*, 5th edition. Sheffield: Dyslexia-SpLD Trust.

Cain K (2010) *Reading Development and Difficulties*. Oxford: Wiley-Blackwell.

Castles A, Rastle K, Nation K (2018) Ending the reading wars: Reading acquisition from novice to expert. *Psychological Science in the Public Interest* **19**(1): 5–51.

Fricke S, Bowyer-Crane C, Haley AH, Hulme C, Snowling MJ (2013) Efficacy of language intervention in the early years. *Journal of Child Psychology & Psychiatry* **54**: 280–290.

Golding J, Pembrey M, Jones R, ALSPAC Team (2002) ALSPAC – The Avon longitudinal study of parents and children. *Paediatric and Perinatal Epidemiology* **15**: 74–87.

Hulme C, Melby-Lervåg M (2015) Educational interventions for children's learning difficulties. In: Thapar A, Pine D, Leckman J et al. editors, *Rutter's Child and Adolescent Psychiatry.* Chichester: Wiley, pp. 533–544.

Krafnik A, Flowers D, Napoliello E, Eden G (2011) Gray matter volume changes following reading intervention in dyslexia children. *NeuroImage* **57**: 733–741.

Landerl K, Moll K (2010) Comorbidity of learning disorders: Prevalence and familial transmission. *Journal of Child Psychology and Psychiatry* **51**(3): 287–294.

Muter V, Hulme C, Snowling M, Stevenson J (2004) Phonemes, rimes, vocabulary and grammatical skills as foundations of early reading development: Evidence from a longitudinal study. *Developmental Psychology* **40**: 663–681.

Nation K, Clarke P, Marshall CM, Durand M (2004) Hidden language impairments in children. *Journal of Speech, Language, and Hearing Research* **47**: 199–211.

Nation K, Cooksey J, Taylor J, Bishop DV (2010) A longitudinal investigation of the early language and reading skills in children with reading comprehension impairment. *Journal of Child Psychology & Psychiatry* **51**(9): 1031–1039.

Nunes T, Bryant P (2009*) Children's Reading and Spelling: Beyond the First Steps.* Oxford: Wiley-Blackwell.

Pennington BF, Bishop D (2009) Relations among speech, language, and reading disorders. *Annual Review of Psychology* **60**: 283–306.

Pennington BF, Santerre-Lemmon L, Rosenberg J et al. (2012) Individual prediction of dyslexia by single versus multiple deficit models. *Journal of Abnormal Psychology* **121**: 212–224.

Ramus F, Altarelli I, Jednorog K, Zhao J, Scotto di Covella L (2018) Neuroanatomy of developmental dyslexia: Pitfalls and promise. *Neuroscience and Biobehavioural Reviews* **84**: 434–452.

Rose J (2009) *Identifying and teaching children and young people with dyslexia and literacy difficulties.* An independent report from Sir Jim Rose to the Secretary of State for Children, School and Families. Nottingham: DCSF.

Saygin Z, Norton E, Osher D et al. (2013) Tracking the roots of reading ability: White matter volumes and integrity correlate with phonological awareness in prereading and early reading kindergarten children. *Journal of Neuroscience* **33**: 13251–135258.

Snowling MJ (2009) Changing concepts of dyslexia: Nature, treatment and co-morbidity. *Journal Child Psychology & Psychiatry*. Virtual Issue. http://www.wiley.com/bw/vi.asp?ref=0021-9630&site=0021#0436.

Snowling MJ, Duff F, Petrou A, Schiffeldrin J, Bailey AM (2011) Identification of children at risk of dyslexia: The validity of teacher judgements using 'Phonic Phases'. *Journal of Research in Reading* **34**(2): 157–170.

Snowling MJ, Hulme C (2011) Evidence-based interventions for reading and language difficulties: Creating a virtuous circle. *British Journal of Educational Psychology* **81**(1): 1–23.

Snowling MJ, Melby-Lervåg M (2016) Oral language deficits in familial dyslexia: A meta-analysis and review. *Psychological Bulletin* **142**(5): 498–545.

Snowling MJ, Muter V, Carroll JM (2007) Children at family risk of dyslexia: A follow-up in adolescence. *Journal of Child Psychology and Child Psychiatry* **48**: 609–618.

Snowling MJ, Nash HM, Gooch DC, Hayiou-Thomas M, Hulme C (2019) Developmental outcomes for children at high risk of dyslexia and children with developmental language disorder. *Child Development* **90**(5): 1–17.

Thompson PA, Hulme C, Nash HM, Gooch D, Hayiou-Thomas E, Snowling MJ (2015) Developmental dyslexia: Predicting individual risk. *Journal of Child Psychology & Psychiatry* **56**: 976–987.

CHAPTER 15

Handwriting

Mellissa Prunty and Emma Sumner

Presenting Concern

Aydin is a 9-year-old boy who is in his second to last year of primary school in the UK. Next year, his writing in English lessons will be formally assessed by his class teacher. In order for Aydin to be working at the expected standard for English (Department for Education 2018) he will need to write effectively for a range of purposes and audiences. He will need to select language that shows good awareness of the reader and use vocabulary and grammatical structures that reflect what the writing requires. His writing should demonstrate his ability to use verb tenses correctly and consistently whilst implementing a range of punctuation (e.g. inverted commas). In addition, he will need to spell most words correctly and maintain legibility in joined handwriting when writing at speed.

Whilst Aydin is a bright and capable boy, he has significant difficulties with handwriting and spelling driven by his dual diagnoses of developmental coordination disorder (DCD) and dyslexia. Aydin is aware that his handwriting is not as good as his peers and it is impacting on his motivation to write. These difficulties are likely to have a significant impact on his writing outcomes, as handwriting and spelling are foundational skills, both of which have been shown to predict compositional quality in school-aged children (Limpo, Alves, and Connelly 2017). Aydin's teacher reports that he has difficulty forming his letters (an outcome he should have achieved 3 years ago) and writing at speed. Looking at his class workbooks, his letters are formed incorrectly and the size of his letters are inconsistent. He reverts to an unjoined style of handwriting when under pressure to either write quickly or generate and produce the content of the text independently. In terms of reading and spelling ability, he is underachieving in comparison to his peers and, in these areas, school-based assessments suggest that he is performing similar to children who are 2 years behind him. Specifically, Aydin demonstrates insecure phonics knowledge and a difficulty with spellings that contain split digraphs (a digraph is a combination of two letters that represent one sound, for example 'ie' representing the long 'i' vowel sound in 'pie'; split digraphs are where the two letters are split between a consonant, for example the long vowel sound 'i-e' in 'bike'), initial consonant blends (such as 'bl', 'br'), and more complex vowel and consonant digraphs (e.g. 'ai' representing the long 'a' sound; 'wh' in 'what'). His teacher is increasingly concerned about his handwriting performance in particular and is wondering what can be done to address his writing productivity. She has made a referral to occupational therapy and the school's specialist teacher to see what can be done.

THEORY

Handwriting and spelling are crucial components of the overall task of *writing*. Neuroimaging studies investigating the neural correlates of handwriting are presented with challenges in disentangling the networks recruited specific to handwriting (motor) execution and those that engage the language systems for orthographic selection (see Planton et al. 2013); yet note the left-hemisphere network and the frontal and parietal superior areas to be crucially involved in handwriting tasks. Theoretical models of writing recognise how handwriting and spelling are intertwined and are grouped together as *'transcription* skills', which are the first skills to be learned in young writers (Berninger and Amtmann 2003). These lower level skills in children can be so laboured that they consume substantial working memory resources when writing. As a result, the child has fewer resources available to devote to producing and developing the written text, which impacts not only on the amount of text that they produce but also the quality of the text (i.e. vocabulary used, organisation, sentence structure, cohesion, grammar, punctuation, etc.) (Berninger and Amtmann 2003).

The learning of spelling and handwriting is complex. The initial stages of learning to spell involve developing an awareness of the sounds within words (phonology), the relationships between sounds and letters (phoneme–grapheme correspondences), and the grammatical units of language (morphology) (Siegel 2008 – also see Chapter 14 on Literacy for further information). At the same time, when learning handwriting, children need to be able to map the sounds of a letter to the visual representation (the letter form) followed by retrieving and executing the correct patterns (allograph) from memory (Van Galen 1991). They also need to be able to control the movement of the pen to form the letters and often to produce letters at speed. According to the Simple View of Writing model (Berninger and Amtmann 2003), which was developed based on 6- to 15-year-olds, it is not until these 'transcription' skills become more automatic that higher level processes can be attended to. Indeed, working memory resources are central to the model as it is these resources that are redirected to higher-level processes once transcription skills are developed. Whilst in most children these skills advance with experience and practice, children with spelling and/or handwriting difficulties may struggle to progress with their writing.

In Aydin's case we know that he has difficulties in motor skill and spelling and, as such, the mechanisms driving his handwriting difficulties are complex. Van Galen's (1991) psychomotor model of handwriting is a useful theoretical framework for considering Aydin's difficulties. The hierarchical model (Fig. 15.1) outlines the cognitive processes that occur before and during the production of handwriting. According to the model the writer must first activate the intention to write and start to generate ideas about content. They then translate the ideas into language (semantic retrieval) and construct the sentence (syntactical construction) that they wish to write using the correct grammar/phrases. It is at the next level of spelling where the handwriting processes start to engage as the sounds of the letters are mapped to the visual representations (the grapheme) followed by a set of instructions (allograph) being generated for the letter. It is also at

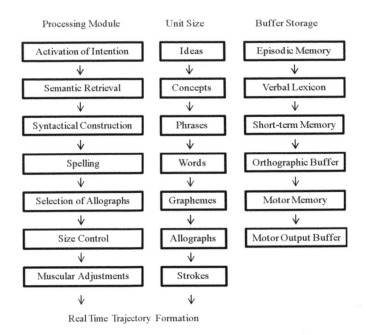

Figure 15.1 The process modules from Van Galen's (1991) Psychomotor Model of Handwriting.

the allograph level where the *style* of handwriting (joined, unjoined) is programmed. Once the set of instructions for the letter are generated they need to be programmed for size (size control) and speed (how fast it needs to be produced). Following this, the command is sent from the brain to the muscles resulting in muscular adjustment and the real time movement of the pen. A difficulty at any one of these levels could impact on handwriting production, and it is therefore important to consider whether there is a difficulty at these levels when assessing a child's handwriting. In this case, the primary concern is Aydin's handwriting, but any improvement in his handwriting production would likely have a positive impact up the chain in the higher-level processes of writing (ideas and content generation).

ASSESSMENT AND FORMULATION

In Aydin's case both his spelling and motor impairment are impacting on his handwriting production and Van Galen's (1991) model serves as a useful framework for considering assessment.

The Level of 'Spelling'

First, we know that Aydin has difficulties with spelling as a result of his dyslexia. Research on handwriting in children with dyslexia has found that spelling difficulties

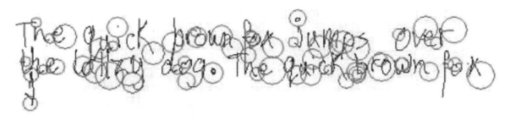

Figure 15.2 Sample of text from a 10-year-old boy with dyslexia – pauses (circles) occur within words due to the challenges experienced with fluent spelling.

alone can result in slower production of text. For example Sumner, Connelly, and Barnett (2014) examined handwriting production in children with dyslexia who did not have co-occurring motor difficulties. They found that they produced fewer words per minute than their typically developing peers. Using digital writing tablets to examine the real-time movement of the pen, Sumner and colleagues (2014) found that the group with dyslexia had a tendency to pause within misspelled words, which slowed down the production of handwriting. Figure 15.2 shows a sample of text from a 10-year-old boy with dyslexia compared to a typically developing peer of the same age. Whilst the handwriting is readable, the circles on the text illustrate *pauses* during writing (captured by the digital writing tablet technology). The authors argued that the high proportion of pauses observed within-words was an indicator of a lack of automaticity in retrieving and producing spelling information by hand. Note for the typically developing writer (Fig. 15.3) few pauses occur within words, which is an indication of skill. Whilst it is beyond the scope of this chapter to cover spelling assessments in great detail, given the impact of spelling difficulties on handwriting, spelling should be considered using observations from class workbooks or administration of informal (e.g. common high frequency words, subject specific word lists, the spelling lists shown in the national curriculum [Department for Education 2013] etc.) or formal (standardised) spelling tests.

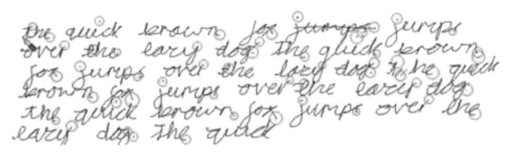

Figure 15.3 Typically developing 10-year-old boy: pauses (circles) occur between words only is indicative of typical, age-appropriate writing ability.

Level of the 'Allograph' (Letter Formation)

Aydin's difficulties with motor skill pose an additional challenge in the context of his handwriting. Studies on handwriting performance in children with this have revealed difficulties at the level of letter formation, that is the allograph level. Using similar methods to Sumner et al. (2013, 2014), Prunty et al. (2013, 2014) examined handwriting performance in children with DCD in the absence of reading and spelling difficulties. Temporal analyses of their handwriting using writing tablet technology revealed that children with DCD have a tendency to pause for a greater percentage of writing tasks compared to typically developing peers (Prunty et al. 2013). In particular, they have a tendency to pause within illegible words (Prunty et al. 2014). Prunty and Barnett (2017) examined letter formation in children with DCD in detail by replaying the children's handwriting in real time and coding their letters for errors. For example letters were deemed to have errors in their formation if they were started in the incorrect place, were formed with strokes in the wrong direction, were missing strokes, had added strokes, or were reversed. The study revealed that children with DCD produced a higher percentage of errors in letter formation compared to the typically developing group (Prunty and Barnett 2017). The most common errors included incorrect start position and strokes completed in the wrong direction. These letter formation errors indicate difficulties at the allograph level. In Aydin's case his teacher has noticed that he tends to produce letters in a way that would not be taught in the school system. This can be assessed through informal observation (watching the child form their letters) or captured using an assessment of handwriting legibility such as the Handwriting Legibility Scale (Barnett, Prunty, and Rosenblum 2018). Figure 15.4 illustrates an example of handwriting from a 10-year-old boy with DCD.

Level of Size Control and Speed

Size control is the second mechanism at play in the handwriting of children with DCD. It seems that when children with DCD are required to speed up or handwrite whilst

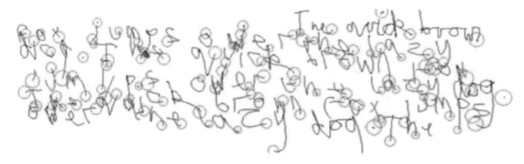

Figure 15.4 Boy aged 10 years with DCD: many pauses (circles) within words due to poor and incorrect letter formation.

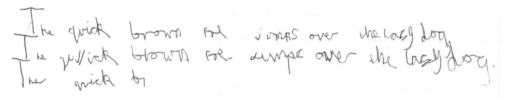

Figure 15.5 Boy aged 10 years with DCD – Copy Best Task from the DASH.

generating content, the size of their handwriting increases. Figures 15.5 and 15.6 illustrate this during two copying tasks. In Figure 15.5 the boy with DCD copied the sentence in his best handwriting (Copy Best Task from the Detailed Assessment of Speed of Handwriting [DASH]; Barnett et al. 2007). In this case the handwriting is joined (he programmes joined letters at the allograph level) and his handwriting is even and consistently sized. However, in Figure 15.6 he copies the same sentence again, but this time as quickly as possible (Copy Fast Task from the DASH). Here his handwriting is no longer joined (he programmes unjoined letters at the allograph level), and his size is distinctly different. Size of handwriting can be considered using an assessment of handwriting legibility.

Handwriting speed in Van Galen's (1991) model refers to the speed of the pen when it is in motion. This is not a contributor to handwriting difficulties in children with dyslexia or DCD as they are able to move the pen just as quickly as their typically developing peers (Prunty et al. 2013; Sumner et al. 2013). However, handwriting speed by way of the amount of text a child can produce (usually measured on a timed task where the number of letters or words produced per minute is recorded) is particularly important for Aydin as he approaches the end of primary school. Indeed, the number of words a child can produce per minute has been shown to predict not only text length but also the quality of written composition (how good the text is) (Puranik and Alotaiba 2011). This underpins many models of writing including Berninger and Amtmann's (2003) Simple View of Writing model described in the section on theory where transcription (spelling ability and handwriting speed) skills predict compositional quality. As such, the ability to write at speed is a very important component of handwriting skill.

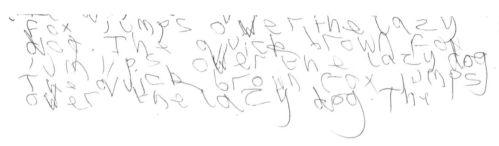

Figure 15.6 Boy aged 10 years with DCD – Copy Fast Task from the DASH.

Several tests of handwriting speed are available including the DASH (Barnett et al. 2007) which considers handwriting speed using a variety of different tasks (copying, writing the alphabet from memory, and free writing) and conditions (best handwriting vs writing at speed). Figures 15.5 and 15.6 illustrate the importance of looking across tasks when assessing a child for a handwriting difficulty as there is an obvious difference in legibility between them. However, in the context of speed, looking across tasks can yield important information. For example if a child can copy a sentence at speed but cannot write quickly during a free writing task then this may indicate difficulties with combining handwriting speed with higher-level writing processes (idea generation, language, etc.). Equally, if a child cannot write the alphabet quickly from memory but can copy a sentence at speed this may indicate difficulties in retrieving letter forms independently without a visual prompt. By looking across a range of tasks, a comprehensive picture of the child's handwriting speed can be formed. This will enable a more person-centred plan for intervention.

INTERVENTION AND MANAGEMENT

Whilst explicit support and on-paper practice is essential for improving handwriting, these strategies alone will not improve handwriting in the classroom particularly when there is a spelling difficulty involved, as linked to the Van Galen model. In Aydin's case his handwriting is also impacted by difficulties with spelling (see previous sections) and so careful consideration should also be given to this. In a meta-analysis on spelling instruction, Graham and Santangelo (2014) demonstrated that increasing the amount of spelling instruction above what is typically offered in the classroom has a positive impact on spelling development. Harris and colleagues (2017) suggest that spelling instruction may focus on the systematic study of spelling patterns that the child needs to learn. Strategies could include weekly spelling lists, contrasting/different spelling patterns in the weekly word lists, tracing and visualisations, practice, repetition and generalisation, or word study (morphology – understanding the root word and how the word changes once prefixes/suffixes are added). In the case example, Aydin demonstrates insecure phonics knowledge, therefore specialist support with teaching systematic phonics would be appropriate alongside spelling instruction. Spelling activities designed around detecting all phonemes within words and identifying their corresponding letter(s) would be useful (e.g. initial consonant blends: 'bl', 'br'), as well as developing Aydin's awareness of alternative ways of spelling phonemes (e.g. split digraphs, alternative long /a/ sounds; 'ay', 'ai', 'ae'). Whilst strategies to support spelling for children with literacy difficulties have been reported by Brooks (2016), for someone with Aydin's profile both handwriting and spelling would need to be considered together in order to support development in both. Using spelling practice to inform and compliment handwriting practice would be a useful strategy in this case.

Individual Differences

In order to implement the most effective intervention to support Aydin, it is essential to assess his handwriting for both speed and legibility (as outlined above) as a focus on only one aspect of handwriting could mean that a difficulty with the skill goes undetected. Studies have looked at variability in the handwriting profiles of children with DCD by looking across measures such as legibility, speed, percentage of pausing, and letter formation errors (Prunty and Barnett 2017; Prunty and Barnett 2019). They found that whilst most children in the DCD group had difficulties with global legibility, others had difficulties with speed only, whilst others struggled with letter formation. These individual differences are key informants when it comes to selecting appropriate assessments and interventions.

Intervention for Handwriting

In order to address Aydin's difficulties with handwriting, pen-on-paper practice is essential (Hoy et al. 2011; Santangelo and Graham 2016). The international clinical practice recommendations for DCD advocate a focus on 'activity' based interventions rather than trying to remediate the underlying motor difficulties (Blank et al. 2019). However, whilst pen-on-paper practice is crucial, it also needs to be accompanied by specific instructions for handwriting. Children with DCD are able to learn motor skills, but it takes them longer to learn, and they require explicit instruction. In particular, interventions that involve self-evaluation and problem-solving have been shown to be effective and therefore recommended (i.e. the Cognitive Orientation to Daily Occupational Performance, Polatajko and Mandich 2004; Blank et al. 2019). By helping the child problem-solve their difficulties with handwriting it engages them in the process of letter formation (i.e. it makes them think through the steps involved in producing a letter) in a way that they will remember.

One way of engaging the child in problem-solving is to avoid 'telling' them how to form a letter at the level of the allograph. Instead, the therapist/teacher could prompt the child through the use of questions. For example rather than telling Aydin to place his letters 'on the line' the therapist/teacher could rephrase this in the form of a question such as 'I noticed that your letter 'a' is floating off the line, what could you do differently to ensure it is placed *on* the line next time?' This engages the child in thinking about what they could do differently when forming the letter rather than being told what to do by the therapist/teacher. The evidence suggests that the child should be encouraged to think for themselves and self-evaluate as much as possible when working on an activity such as handwriting (Blank et al. 2019). In terms of teaching strategies for use in the classroom, the use of technology (digitising writing tablets to provide feedback on letter production) and demonstrating/modelling correct letter formation have both been found to be effective strategies for improving handwriting (Santangelo and Graham 2016). These interventions target the level of the allograph as research has shown that difficulties at this level (correct letter formation) in children with DCD has an impact on fluency of writing and ultimately speed (Prunty and Barnett 2017; Prunty and Barnett 2019).

Outcome

One school term later Aydin is making progress with his letter formation. Explicit teaching surrounding correct letter formation and additional input on spelling has meant that Aydin is able to maintain correct letter formation within sentences that are easy to spell. When asked to speed up or produce more difficult spellings, Aydin still resorts to some of his old habits. However with practice combining both handwriting and spelling his new letter formations will become more stable.

SUMMARY

Children have difficulties with handwriting for all sorts of reasons. In this chapter, Van Galen's (1991) model was used to illustrate how impairments in attention, language, spelling, or motor skill can all impact on handwriting production in their own way. The model serves as a useful tool for considering handwriting difficulties in children as it can serve as a framework for clinicians to consider the possible mechanisms at play. This chapter focused on a boy with a dual diagnosis of DCD and dyslexia and it outlined why a focus on the handwriting difficulty in isolation would not be enough to improve production. Indeed, the difficulties with spelling would also need to be addressed given the role of spelling in the writing process. For more information and resources for handwriting visit the National Handwriting Association's website at https://nha-handwriting.org.uk or www.Canchild.ca.

REFERENCES

Berninger VW, Amtmann D (2003) Preventing written expression disabilities through early and continuing assessment and intervention for handwriting and/or spelling problems: Research into practice. In Swanson HL, Harris KR, Graham S (Eds.) *Handbook of learning disabilities*. New York: The Guilford Press, pp. 345–363.

Blank R, Barnett A, Cairney J et al (2019) International clinical practice recommendations on the definition diagnosis assessment intervention and psychosocial aspects of developmental coordination disorder. *Developmental Medicine and Child Neurology* **61**(3): 242–285. doi: 10.1111/dmcn.14132.

Brooks G (2016) *What Works for Children and Young People With Literacy Difficulties?* Fifth edition. Frensham: Dyslexia-SpLD Trust.

Department for Education (2013) *National curriculum in England English programmes of study: Key stages 1 and 2*. Retrieved from https://assetspublishingservicegovuk/government/uploads/system/uploads/attachment_data/file/335186/PRIMARY_national_curriculum_-_English_220714pdf [Accessed January 2019].

Department for Education (2018) *National curriculum assessments: Teacher assessment frameworks at the end of Key Stage 2*. Retrieved from https://assetspublishingservicegovuk/government/uploads/system/uploads/attachment_data/file/740345/2018-19_teacher_assessment_frameworks_at_the_end_of_key_stage_2_WEBHOpdf [Accessed January 2019].

Graham S, Santangelo T (2014) Does spelling instruction make students better spellers reader and writing? A meta-analytic review. *Reading and Writing* 27: 1703–1743. doi.org/101007/s11145-014-9517-0.

Hoy MMP, Egan MY, Feder KP (2011) A systematic review of interventions to improve handwriting. *Canadian Journal of Occupational Therapy* 78: 13–25. https://doi.org/10.2182/cjot.2011.78.1.3.

Limpo T, Alves R, Connelly V (2017) Examining the transcription-writing link: Effects of handwriting fluency and spelling accuracy on writing performance via planning and translating in middle grades. *Learning and Individual Differences* 53: 26–36. https://doi.org/10.1016/j.lindif.2016.11.004.

Planton S, Jucla M, Roux F-E, Démonet F (2013) The 'handwriting brain': A meta-analysis of neuroimaging studies of motor versus orthographic processes. *Cortex* 49(10): 2772–2787. doi: 10.1016/j.cortex.2013.05.011.

Polatajko H, Mandich M (2004) *Enabling Occupation in Children: Occupational Performance (CO-OP) Approach.* Ottawa: CAOT Publications ACE.

Prunty M, Barnett AL (2017) Understanding handwriting difficulties: A comparison of children with and without motor impairment. *Cognitive Neuropsychology* 34(3/4): 205–218. doi: 10.1080/02643294.2017.1376630.

Prunty M, Barnett AL, Wilmut K, Plumb M (2013) Handwriting speed in children with developmental coordination disorder: Are they really slower? *Research in Developmental Disabilities* 34(9): 2927–2936. doi: 10.1016/j.ridd.2013.06.005.

Prunty M, Barnett AL, Wilmut K, Plumb M (2014) An examination of writing pauses in the handwriting of children with developmental coordination disorder. *Research in Developmental Disabilities* 35(11): 2894–2905. doi: 10.1016/j.ridd.2014.07.033.

Prunty M, Barnett AL (2019) Accuracy and consistency of letter formation in children with developmental coordination disorder: An exploratory study. *Journal of Learning Disabilities* 53(2): 120–130. https://doi.org/10.1177/0022219419892851.

Puranik C, Alotaiba S (2011) Examining the contribution of handwriting and spelling to written expression in kindergarten children. *Reading and Writing: An Interdisciplinary Journal* 25: 1523–1546.

Santangelo T, Graham S (2016) A comprehensive meta-analysis of handwriting instruction. *Educational Psychology Review* 28: 225–265. doi: 10.1007/s10648-015-9335-1.

Siegel LS (2008) Morphological awareness skills of English language learners and children with dyslexia. *Topics in Language Disorders* 28: 15–27. doi.org/10.1097/01.adt.0000311413.75804.60.

Sumner E, Connelly V, Barnett A (2013) Children with dyslexia are slow writers because they pause more often and not because they are slow at handwriting execution. *Reading & Writing* 26(6): 991–1008. doi: 10.1007/s11145-012-9403-6.

Sumner E, Connelly V, Barnett AL (2014) The influence of spelling ability on handwriting production: Children with and without dyslexia. *Journal of Experimental Psychology: Learning Memory and Cognition* 40(5): 1441–1447. doi: 101037/a0035785.

van Galen GP (1991) Handwriting: Issues for a psychomotor theory. *Human Movement Science* 10: 165–191. https://doi.org/10.1016/0167-9457(91)90003-G.

PART 2

Factors Influencing Clinical Formulation

CHAPTER 16

Prenatal Exposure to Medicines and Chemicals

Rebecca Bromley and Jennifer Shields

Presenting Concern

Oscar is a 7-year-old boy referred by a clinical geneticist who is seeking an opinion as to whether Oscar's neurodevelopmental difficulties are consistent with exposure to sodium valproate in the womb. Oscar was exposed to 1000mg daily of sodium valproate prescribed to treat seizures in his mother throughout gestation. The family have been concerned for some time that Oscar's difficulties may be attributable to this exposure, as they have met other families with similar experience. The clinical geneticist notes that Oscar does not have a major congenital malformation but did present with a wide nasal bridge, anteverted nostrils, and a high-formed forehead – typical dysmorphic facial features for fetal valproate spectrum disorder (Clayton-Smith et al. 2019). Oscar also presented with joint laxity.

Oscar was born at full term. Early motor development was roughly on time, but he had difficulty with his speech development and had speech and language therapy from the age of 3 to 5 years. Oscar took a long time to settle into the school environment and required one-to-one support for academic and 'emotional' reasons, which was offered informally by the school. He struggled socially. At home there were challenges with daily living tasks such as dressing, which leads to difficulty getting ready in the mornings when time is limited. His family background is unremarkable and both parents completed postgraduate education. Genetic testing (microarray comparative genomic hybridisation) did not find a cause for Oscar's developmental difficulties. The primary concerns from the family surround his cognitive, emotional, and social functioning.

THEORY

In this chapter we introduce the concept of a teratogen: exposure to certain chemicals, medications, or maternal diseases can increase the risk of abnormal fetal development. These are termed 'teratogens'. Higher frequencies of spontaneous abortions, alterations in fetal growth, or structural malformations (birth defects) occur depending on the exposure type. Additionally, more minor physical alterations can be induced such as dysmorphic facial features or digit abnormalities that are exposure specific (Jones and Carey 2011). Thus, a characteristic pattern of physical symptoms specific to the exposure type can be observed. Maternal illness with rubella (Freij et al. 1988) and Zika viruses (Moore et al. 2017), for example are associated with a higher risk of abnormal physical symptoms. Similarly, a number of medications are known to be teratogenic including isotretinoin, thalidomide, and sodium valproate (Rasmussen 2012) – there are a number of medicine exposure syndromes listed in the International Classification of Diseases, 11th Revision (ICD-11; https://icd.who.int). Lifestyle choices such as smoking and alcohol consumption also have a longstanding association with altered fetal development and are widely known.

Pertinent to the paediatric neuropsychologist is considering the impact of exposure to chemicals, illness, and medicines on the process of brain development and function. During the embryonic–fetal period complex processes create an effective and reliable neuroarchitecture that supports developing cognitive, social, motor, and behavioural function. These developmental processes of neurogenesis, synaptogenesis, neuronal migration, and programmed cell loss, along with glial development, are all susceptible to alteration (Thompson et al. 2009). Such alterations may have no consequence but, if significant enough, may influence postnatal child functioning in a wide range of domains.

As with the physical effects of a teratogen, the possible impact on the developing fetal brain is on a continuum ranging from substantial brain malformations such as observable cortical malformations (e.g. schizencephaly) through to a disruption of postnatal functioning hypothesised to be underpinned by more subtle alterations to the neuronal architecture (Vorhees 1986; Adams et al. 2000). The former can be identified on neuroimaging, however in the majority of cases cognitive and behavioural difficulties are more frequently seen in the absence of visible abnormalities on neuroimaging (Adams et al. 2000; Thompson et al. 2009).

Fetal Alcohol Spectrum Disorder and Other Common Conditions

One of the most commonly used prenatal developmental toxins is alcohol, with an estimated 41% of pregnancies in the UK exposed at some point during gestation; 15% to significant quantities (Popova et al. 2017; Abernethy et al. 2018). Fetal alcohol spectrum disorder (FASD; Andrew 2011) is a condition caused by exposure to alcohol in pregnancy. Alcohol leads to risk of major physical malformations and minor aberrations. Facial characteristics of FASD include short palpebral fissures, a smooth philtrum, a thin upper lip, low nasal bridge, flat mid-face, and micrognathia (Wattendorf and Muenke 2005); however, these are only evident in approximately 10% of affected children (Andrew 2011).

Alcohol exposure disrupts developmental processes within the fetal brain, the neuropsychological consequences being variable due to individual patterns of exposure and dose throughout gestation (Mattson et al. 2019). Low general intellectual ability with scores one standard deviation below the mean but not necessarily in the intellectual disability range are common (Mattson et al. 2019). Language, memory, visuospatial functioning, attention, and motor skills can also be below age expectations. However, executive functioning is most commonly a core difficulty with deficits greater in FASD than conditions such as attention-deficit/hyperactivity disorder (Khoury and Milligan 2016). A caveat on our understanding of the risk of confounding factors associated with diagnosing FASD are discussed in a recent review (Schölin et al. 2021).

Other known prenatal brain development disruptors include maternal diabetes, maternal hypothyroidism, maternal Zika virus, nicotine, marijuana, isotretinoin, lead, and mercury. Isotretinoin, a treatment for severe cystic acne, has deleterious effects on the fetal brain leading to substantial postnatal neuropsychological deficits, affecting visual spatial functioning in particular (Adams and Lammer 1993). Thalidomide, with its infamous effect on limb development, is also documented to increase the rates of autism spectrum disorder (Strömland et al. 1994). Table 16.1 displays the child outcomes of a number of known human developmental neurotoxicants and demonstrates that the effects can be widespread, substantial, and in most cases lifelong.

What Conditions Lead to an Impact on Development?

Not all chemicals, medications, and maternal diseases are disruptive or pose a risk to the development of the fetal brain and even when such exposures are considered to convey an increased risk, not every child will be affected (Brent 2004). A series of principles were outlined to explain the variability of symptoms and severity across individuals (Vorhees 1986).

- The susceptibility to a certain exposure varies across individuals and across different fetal tissue types within an individual.
- The gestational timing of the exposure dictates the pattern of susceptibility across the body systems.
- The duration of the exposure may mediate severity, with longer exposures leading to greater impairment.
- The dose of the exposure is critical, with higher doses conveying greater levels of risk and severity of disruption.
- Functional difficulties, such as neuropsychological abilities, could be induced at doses lower than that required for physical symptoms (i.e. malformations).

To be altered, a particular fetal tissue type would need to be susceptible to that specific exposure, the dose would need to be high enough, and only organs under development at the time of exposure could be altered. A fetus exposed to a chemical in the second

Table 16.1 Medications, chemicals, and diseases that impact the brain

	Associated major congenital malformations	Associated minor congenital malformations	Neuropsychological deficits
Medications			
Isotretinonin (Adams and Lammer1993; Adams 2010)	Orofacial Brain	Ear abnormalit es Dysmorphic features: depressed nasal bridge, hypertelorism Facial nerve pa sy	13% IQ <70, 30% IQ <80 Significant impact on nonverbal reasoning, visual spatial, and visual motor integration abilities Relative preserving of verbal abilities in >60%
Valproate (Moore et al. 2000; Bromley et al. 2014; Weston et al. 2016; Clayton-Smith et al. 2019)	Spina bifida Cardiac Limb Skeletal Orofacial	Dysmorphic features: flat philtrum, thin upper lip, full everted lower lip, short anteverted nose, small mouth, epicanthic folds, neat arched, eyebrows, broad nasal roct	Reduction in IQ; verbal indices most notably impacted upon but in some cases a global lowering of ability is seen History of poorer early language development and motor skills Social difficulties and increased rates of autistic spectrum disorder
Thalidomide (Strömland et al. 1994; Miller et al. 2005; Cornelius et al. 2012)	Limb Cardiac Skeletal Gastrointestinal Genitourinary	Ear abnormalities Cranial nerve abnormalities Opthalmice abnormalities Digit abnormalities	Increased rate of autism spectrum disorders
Lifestyle			
Alcohol (Andrew 2011; Mattson et al. 2019)	Brain Heart Kidneys Liver	Microcephaly Dysmorphic features: short palpebral fissures, smooth philtrum, thin upper lip	Reduction in IQ spanning low average, borderline, or extremely low IQ and intellectual disability range Significant impairment in executive functioning Significant impairment in adaptive functioning (not correlated with cognition)

	Associated major congenital malformations	Associated minor congenital malformations	Neuropsychological deficits
	Gastrointestinal tract Endocrine system	Musculoskeletal anomalies: camptodactyly, clinodactyly, hypoplastic nails Otitis media Cleft lip/palate Ptosis Retinal malformation Strabismus	Impaired language skills, particularly comprehension Marked sensory differences Marked attentional difficulties (particularly switching or everyday attention) Attention deficit Memory difficulties Academic and social difficulties
Nicotine (Cornelius et al. 2012)	Orofacial clefts	X	Increased difficulties with attention and hyperactivity Increased behavioural difficulties including increased rates of aggression, rule breaking, and social difficulties
Cannabis (Sharapova et al. 2018)	X	X	Preschool children demonstrate poorer language and memory skills where use in pregnancy was frequent (several times per week) School-aged children with daily exposure have reduced levels of verbal reasoning/IQ Attention deficits and impulsivity difficulties
			Maternal diseases
Zika (Moore et al. 2017; Wheeler, 2018)	Brain Skeletal	Microcephaly Eye abnormalities	Moderate to severe early developmental difficulties effecting motor, cognitive, and language development Longer-term outcomes are unclear due to the relatively recent Zika outbreak
Hypothyroidism (Korevaar et al. 2016)	X	Unclear	Reduced IQ in cases of severe hypothyroidism Treatment reduces risk of neuropsychological deficits There is inconsistent evidence that the offspring of females with borderline levels are at risk of language developmental difficulties

X = no currently established pattern.

trimester only would not be at a higher risk of physical structural malformations as the period of organogenesis is complete, but the exposure could place that child at risk of altered neuronal development, as the susceptible period for the brain spans the entire gestational period (Vorhees 1986; Adams et al. 2000; Rice and Barone 2000). Considering this, developmental neurotoxicological effects of exposure will therefore co-occur with physical markers but may also occur in isolation (Adams et al. 2000).

Certain prenatal developmental neurotoxins may slow the developmental trajectory but then a period of catch up occurs. Alternatively, the deficits in neuropsychological functioning may be lifelong (Vorhees 1986) and may evolve over time. A pattern of 'emerging deficits' (Anderson et al. 2011), whereby a child fails to make the expected developmental progress in one or more areas of neuropsychological functioning, is most frequently seen in the profiles of children with a history of a teratogen exposure.

ASSESSMENT AND FORMULATION

Research indicates that clinicians should enquire about and consider prenatal exposures in formulations as potential causes of neuropsychological deficits. When asked in an understanding manner, it is our experience that mothers open up about their health, diet, medication, and lifestyle experiences during pregnancy. There are a number of reasons potentially risky exposures occur: mothers may have been unaware that they were pregnant, and they may not have been provided with clear information or understood the risks their diet, medication, lifestyle, or illness posed. For others a careful risk–benefit decision balancing both maternal health and medication may have been made in difficult or unavoidable circumstances.

Children presenting without significant physical symptoms (e.g. congenital malformations) may not have been reviewed by a clinical geneticist or paediatrician, which is thought to be a key aspect of their care. There is no single diagnostic test for fetal teratogen syndromes and diagnoses are made by excluding other potential influencers on development, including genetic test results (Jackson et al. 2020) so multidisciplinary working is key to understanding the broader formulation of the child's neuropsychological strengths and needs.

Important information to be gathered as part of the background history includes the type of exposure, the dose or level of the exposure, and the duration (i.e. sporadic use or consistent throughout). Attention to early developmental milestones is important as often developmental trajectories deviate from peers early in development, and regression of previously obtained skills would require consideration of another influencing factor. Family developmental and academic history is important context.

A neuropsychological assessment should be based on current and up-to-date literature. If there is evidence that the exposure in question is a teratogen, a detailed understanding of the pattern of symptoms commonly seen should be gained to guide assessment. The UK Teratology Information Service (https://www.medicinesinpregnancy.org/Medicine-pregnancy/) and the US-based Mother to Baby webpages (https://mothertobaby.org) have useful summaries, which are updated regularly on a wide range of exposures. The neuropsychological assessment should be broad covering the core skills of IQ, memory, language, attention, processing speed, visuospatial skills, executive function, and importantly, adaptive functioning. For some exposures there may be a distinct cognitive profile and additional testing should be guided by this to build a detailed picture of the child's strengths and weaknesses. It is often vital to include assessments by allied health professionals such as speech and language therapists and occupational therapists to elicit difficulties with language or motor skills that could also impact on daily functioning and quality of life. Further, information collected from teachers and school observations will also bring useful information to the formulation, particularly if academic difficulties are present.

Case Study – Assessment

Oscar was exposed to sodium valproate in the womb. He did not have any major birth defects, but he did present with a characteristic facial presentation and joint laxity, which are part of the clinical diagnosis for fetal valproate spectrum disorder (Clayton-Smith et al. 2019). The clinical geneticist referred Oscar to understand whether the pattern of neuropsychological functioning was in keeping with a diagnosis of fetal valproate spectrum disorder, in which deficits with cognitive, social, and motor development are characteristic (Meador et al. 2009; Bromley et al. 2010; Cohen et al. 2011). In school-aged children the symptoms include low IQ, specifically weak verbal reasoning (Nadebaum et al. 2011a; Meador et al. 2013; Baker et al. 2015; Huber-Mollema et al. 2020), although there may be global deficits in children exposed to high doses of sodium valproate. The associated impact on the brain may be greater in the presence of the physical symptoms of the exposure (Bromley et al. 2019). Language functioning is vulnerable and the need for speech and language therapy is frequent (Moore et al. 2000; Nadebaum et al. 2011b). Poorer memory abilities are observed. Children exposed to sodium valproate are reported to experience difficulty with the encoding and retrieval of verbal and visual stimuli (Barton et al. 2018; Cohen et al. 2019). Following the research in this area, Oscar's neuropsychological assessment covered many neuropsychological domains and in particular verbal and auditory skills.

The assessment results revealed a pattern of performance consistent with that commonly observed in fetal valproate spectrum disorder (Clayton-Smith et al. 2019), weaknesses in verbal and language skills, alongside relative strengths in nonverbal skills. Oscar's auditory working memory and processing speed abilities were significantly impaired. He was strong in his word reading but experienced significant difficulty in reading comprehension. His fine motor skills, although not assessed formally, also appeared to be below age expectations (e.g. writing ability, ability to do and undo buttons). Parental ratings on the Behavior Rating Inventory of Executive Function, Second Edition and observations during the assessment indicated significant executive functioning difficulties including task focus, initiation, switching, and inhibition difficulties.

Observation in the classroom found Oscar to spend long periods of time off task and he had difficulty holding in mind instructions and implementing directions given.

The risks associated with sodium valproate, as with other teratogens, are dose dependent (Bromley et al. 2014). Oscar was exposed to 1000mg daily, which is high enough to pose an increased risk to cognitive functioning. In a UK study, the level of associated IQ reduction was almost halved if the dose of sodium valproate was ≤800 mg daily versus a mean 9.7 IQ point reduction for daily doses above this (Baker et al. 2015). Importantly, the prescribed doses of medication may not represent the blood level accurately (Johannessen Landmark et al. 2017), resulting in cases where a severe syndrome may be apparent at a moderate dose level.

Formulation

A detailed understanding of the child's neuropsychological profile should be gained to understand the exposure's potential relevance within the child's formulation. For exposures where risk or safety is still to be determined, the exposure should be included in the formulation as a 'possible but yet unknown influencer'. Other medical diagnoses, family, and educational contexts should also be considered in the formulation, as they would for childhood brain injuries or neurological conditions, and sometimes these factors may be more pertinent to the neuropsychological difficulties than the exposure history.

Case Study – Formulation

In Oscar's case there were no other identifiable causes of his difficulties and although not exclusive to fetal valproate spectrum disorder, his neuropsychological profile was consistent with this diagnosis. The fact that he displayed expected physical markers made the diagnosis more probable. In collaboration with the clinical geneticist a formulation and diagnosis was presented to the family which identified the exposure as the probable cause of Oscar's difficulties and a diagnosis of fetal valproate spectrum disorder was made.

Additional assessment and formulation was needed specifically around Oscar's behavioural challenges. In-depth parental and teacher interviews along with direct observation highlighted that Oscar becomes frustrated easily, particularly when task demands were high or time was limited. He struggled to shift from one activity to another; initiation of academic tasks took time and guidance and structure from an adult was often required. Further, an uneven cognitive profile with good attainment in single word reading skills, led to overly high expectations in other academic areas. Thus, the environment and expectations of Oscar within the environment were out of sync with his ability levels. Here the formulation contained the exposure as a contextual factor, which drove a focus on environmental adaptations, along with an increased understanding that a number of things, including emotional regulation, would be more challenging for Oscar than his chronological age would suggest.

INTERVENTION AND MANAGEMENT

There are currently no specialist intervention packages for the neuropsychological sequelae to exposures to teratogens and neuropsychologists should follow typical intervention procedures led by the child's individual strengths and needs. Sensitive handling of whether an exposure is associated with an altered neuropsychological profile is needed. A discussion with parents on their own can provide a space to enquire about the impact of a diagnosis on them and the offer to signpost to adult psychological services can be helpful. For Oscar's parents, they had already extensively researched sodium valproate exposure in utero and the diagnosis was a relief from uncertainty and provided a framework within which they could view Oscar's challenges.

Outcome

The formulation identified that environmental changes would be required as Oscar had cognitive difficulties that were associated directly with academic performance but also to the behavioural challenges, through increased levels of frustration. A number of modifications to support Oscar both in the classroom and in other environments were made:

✓ Visual timetables;

✓ A visual guide for tasks that required sequencing such as dressing;

✓ Recommendations to shorten task instructions;

✓ To provide adult support to plan approach to academic tasks and to 'check-in' frequently to ensure Oscar remained on task;

✓ Shorter periods to work, interspersed with small breaks;

✓ To increase hobbies and tasks he enjoyed, got a sense of achievement from, and to provide social opportunities;

✓ Revisiting previous topics to increase consolidation in small group and one-to-one settings.

The support required was recorded in an application for formal educational support. Sharing a formulation that highlighted the contribution of the cognitive difficulties to Oscar's ability to be independent in daily living tasks and regulate his behaviour created a new shared understanding about Oscar's strengths and weaker areas. Consistent guidelines across home and school were developed to reduce the demands on Oscar. Oscar's parents had raised concerns that his social skills were less well developed than his peers and difficulties in reading the intentions of others were reported by his teaching assistant. Difficulties with social understanding and functioning (Huber-Mollema et al. 2019) are areas of weakness in children exposed to sodium valproate and there is an increased risk of autism spectrum disorder in this population (Bromley et al. 2013; Christensen et al. 2013). The pros and cons of a referral to the local autism assessment pathway were discussed, but this was not something the family felt would be useful at that time.

The modifications in the environment helped to reduce the demands placed on Oscar and an almost immediate reduction in outbursts was witnessed in school. A bespoke timetable helped to balance his unique balance of academic and daily living learning tasks and a small supportive social group was formed by the school. The family and teachers reported an increased understanding around his difficulties and actively sought to problem-solve difficult situations with Oscar's difficulties in mind.

Advancing the Area

For many exposures, even those which commonly occur in pregnancy, evidence of risk or safety are not known, and this is the case for both chemicals and medications. It has taken on average 27 years to determine whether newly approved medication poses a risk to the developing fetus (Adam et al. 2011). Given the central nature of neuropsychological deficits in teratogen syndromes, neuropsychologists have an important role in generating the evidence base. As well as undertaking research, it is important that when assessing a child with neuropsychological difficulties in the context of a medication exposure in utero that this is reported to the medicines regulator. In the UK, this is the Medicines and Healthcare Products Regulatory Agency's Yellow Card scheme (https://yellowcard.mhra.gov.uk) and in the US through the Food and Drug Administration (https://www.fda.gov/drugs). You do not have to be the prescriber to report and you are not required to provide identifiable patient information or be certain of causality. These spontaneous reports form the cornerstone of how regulators investigate safety of medications in pregnancy currently.

SUMMARY

Enquiries regarding any pertinent prenatal exposures should be a key query in the neuropsychological interview. The risks to typical neuropsychological functioning from certain exposures can be significant and carry lifelong implications for the child and family. Dose, timing, and duration of the exposure are all important considerations. Providing the child's family and professionals involved in their care (and if developmentally appropriate the child themselves) with an understanding of the condition and their individual neuropsychological strengths and weaknesses is a key intervention in itself and standard management strategies for other neurological conditions are applicable to those exposed to developmental neurotoxins.

REFERENCES

Abernethy C, McCall K, Cooper G et al. (2018) Determining the pattern and prevalence of alcohol consumption in pregnancy by measuring biomarkers in meconium *Archives of Disease in Childhood – Fetal and Neonatal Edition* **103**: F216–F220.

Adam MP, Polifka JE, Friedman JM (2011) Evolving knowledge of the teratogenicity of medications in human pregnancy. *American Journal of Medical Genetics, Part C: Seminars in Medical Genetics* **157**(3): 175–182.

Adams J (2010) The neurobehavioral teratology of retinoids: A 50-year history. *Birth Defects Res A Clin Mol Teratol* **88**: 895–905.

Adams J, Barone S, Lamantia A et al. (2000) Workshop to identify critical windows of exposure for children's health: Neurobehavioral work group summary. *Environ Health Perspect* **108**: 535–544.

Adams J, Lammer E (1993) Neurobehavioral teratology of isotretinoin. *Reproductive Toxicology* **7**: 175–177.

Anderson V, Spencer-Smith M, Wood A (2011) Do children really recover better? Neurobehavioural plasticity after early brain insult. *Brain* **134**: 2197–2221.

Andrew G (2011) Diagnosis of FASD: An overview. In: Riley EP, Weinberg SCJ, Jonsson E, editors, *Fetal Alcohol Spectrum Disorders: Management and Policy Perspectives of FASD*. Weinheim: Wiley-Blackwell, pp. 127–148.

Baker GA, Bromley RL, Briggs M et al. (2015) IQ at 6 years after in utero exposure to antiepileptic drugs: A controlled cohort study. *Neurology* 84: 382–390.

Barton S, Nadebaum C, Anderson VA, Vajda F, Reutens DC, Wood AG (2018) Memory dysfunction in school-aged children exposed prenatally to antiepileptic drugs. *Neuropsychology* 32: 784–796.

Brent RL (2004) Environmental causes of human congenital malformations: The pediatrician's role in dealing with these complex clinical problems caused by a multiplicity of environmental and genetic factors. *Pediatrics* 113: 957–968.

Bromley R, Weston J, Adab N et al. (2014) Treatment for epilepsy in pregnancy: Neurodevelopmental outcomes in the child. *Cochrane Database Syst Rev* 10: Cd010236.

Bromley RL, Baker GA, Clayton-Smith J, Wood AG (2019) Intellectual functioning in clinically confirmed fetal valproate syndrome. *Neurotoxicol Teratol* 71: 16–21.

Bromley RL, Mawer G, Love J et al. (2010) Early cognitive development in children born to women with epilepsy: A prospective report. *Epilepsia* 51: 2058–2065.

Bromley RL, Mawer GE, Briggs M et al. (2013) The prevalence of neurodevelopmental disorders in children prenatally exposed to antiepileptic drugs. *J Neurol Neurosurg Psychiatry* 84: 637–643.

Christensen J, Gronborg TK, Sorensen MJ et al. (2013) Prenatal valproate exposure and risk of autism spectrum disorders and childhood autism. *JAMA* 309: 1696–1703.

Clayton-Smith J, Bromley R, Dean J et al. (2019) Diagnosis and management of individuals with fetal valproate spectrum disorder; a consensus statement from the European Reference Network for Congenital Malformations and Intellectual Disability. *Orphanet Journal of Rare Diseases* 14: 180.

Cohen MJ, Meador KJ, Browning N et al. (2011) Fetal antiepileptic drug exposure: Motor, adaptive, and emotional/behavioral functioning at age 3 years. *Epilepsy and Behavior* 22(2): 240–246.

Cohen MJ, Meador KJ, May R et al. (2019) Fetal antiepileptic drug exposure and learning and memory functioning at 6 years of age: The NEAD prospective observational study. *Epilepsy Behav* 92: 154–164.

Cornelius MD, Goldschmidt L, Day NL (2012) Prenatal cigarette smoking: Long-term effects on young adult behavior problems and smoking behavior. *Neurotoxicology and Teratology* 34: 554–559.

Freij BJ, South MA, Sever JL (1988) Maternal rubella and the congenital rubella syndrome. *Clin Perinatol* 15: 247–257.

Huber-Mollema Y, Oort FJ, Lindhout D, Rodenburg R (2019) Behavioral problems in children of mothers with epilepsy prenatally exposed to valproate, carbamazepine, lamotrigine, or levetiracetam monotherapy. *Epilepsia* 60: 1069–1082.

Huber-Mollema Y, Van Iterson L, Oort FJ, Lindhout D, Rodenburg R (2020) Neurocognition after prenatal levetiracetam, lamotrigine, carbamazepine or valproate exposure. *Journal of Neurology* 267: 1724–1736.

Jackson A, Ward H, Bromley RL et al. (2020) Exome sequencing in patients with antiepileptic drug exposure and complex phenotypes. *Archives of Disease in Childhood* 105: 384–389.

Johannessen Landmark C, Burns ML, Baftiu A et al. (2017) Pharmacokinetic variability of valproate in women of childbearing age. *Epilepsia* 58: e142–e146.

Jones KL, Carey JC (2011) The importance of dysmorphology in the identification of new human teratogens. *Am J Med Genet C Semin Med Genet* **157**: 188–194.

Khoury JE, Milligan K (2016) Comparing executive functioning in children and adolescents with fetal alcohol spectrum disorders and ADHD: A meta-analysis. *Journal of Attention Disorders* **23**: 1801–1815.

Korevaar TI, Muetzel R, Medici M et al. (2016) Association of maternal thyroid function during early pregnancy with offspring IQ and brain morphology in childhood: A population-based prospective cohort study. *Lancet Diabetes Endocrinol* **4**: 35–43.

Mattson SN, Bernes GA, Doyle LR (2019) Fetal alcohol spectrum disorders: A review of the neurobehavioral deficits associated with prenatal alcohol exposure. *Alcohol Clin Exp Res* **43**: 1046–1062.

Meador KJ, Baker GA, Browning N et al. (2009) Cognitive function at 3 years of age after fetal exposure to antiepileptic drugs. *New England Journal of Medicine* **360**: 1597–1605.

Meador KJ, Baker GA, Browning N et al. (2013) Fetal antiepileptic drug exposure and cognitive outcomes at age 6 years (NEAD study): A prospective observational study. *Lancet Neurol* **12**: 244–252.

Miller MT, Stromland K, Ventura L, Johansson M, Bandim JM, Gillberg C (2005) Autism associated with conditions characterized by developmental errors in early embryogenesis: A mini review. *Int J Dev Neurosci* **23**: 201–219.

Moore CA, Staples JE, Dobyns WB et al. (2017) Characterizing the pattern of anomalies in congenital Zika syndrome for pediatric clinicians. *JAMA Pediatr* **171**: 288–295.

Moore SJ, Turnpenny P, Quinn A et al. (2000) A clinical study of 57 children with fetal anticonvulsant syndromes. *Journal of Medical Genetics* **37**: 489–497.

Nadebaum C, Anderson V, Vajda F, Reutens D, Barton S, Wood A (2011a) The Australian brain and cognition and antiepileptic drugs study: IQ in school-aged children exposed to sodium valproate and polytherapy. *Journal of the International Neuropsychological Society* **17**: 133–142.

Nadebaum C, Anderson V, Vajda F, Reutens D, Barton S, Wood A (2011b) Language skills of school-aged children prenatally exposed to antiepileptic drugs. *Neurology* **76**: 719–726.

Popova S, Lange S, Probst C, Gmel G, Rehm J (2017) Estimation of national, regional, and global prevalence of alcohol use during pregnancy and fetal alcohol syndrome: A systematic review and meta-analysis. *The Lancet Global Health* **5**: e290–e299.

Rasmussen SA (2012) Human teratogens update 2011: Can we ensure safety during pregnancy? *Birth Defects Res A Clin Mol Teratol* **94**: 123–128.

Rice D, Barone S Jr (2000) Critical periods of vulnerability for the developing nervous system: Evidence from humans and animal models. *Environ Health Perspect* **108**(3): 511–533.

Schölin L, Mukherjee R, Aiton N et al. (2021) Fetal alcohol spectrum disorders: an overview of current evidence and activities in the UK. *Archives of Disease in Childhood* **106**: 636–640.

Sharapova SR, Phillips E, Sirocco K, Kaminski JW, Leeb RT, Rolle I (2018) Effects of prenatal marijuana exposure on neuropsychological outcomes in children aged 1–11 years: A systematic review. *Paediatric and Perinatal Epidemiology* **32**: 512–532.

Strömland KNV, Miller M, Akerström B, Gillberg C (1994) Autism in thalidomide embryopathy: A population study. *Developmental Medicine and Child Neurology* **36**: 351–356.

Thompson B, Levitt P, Stanwood G (2009) Prenatal exposure to drugs: Effects on brain development and implications for policy and education. *Nature Reviews Neuroscience* **10**: 303–310.

Vorhees CV (1986) Principles of behavioral teratology. In Riley EP, Vorhees CV, editors, *Handbook of Behavioral Teratology*. New York: Plenum Press, pp. 23–48.

Wattendorf DJ, Muenke M (2005) Fetal alcohol spectrum disorders. *Am Fam Physician* **72**: 279–285.

Weston J, Bromley R, Jackson CF et al. (2016) Monotherapy treatment of epilepsy in pregnancy: Congenital malformation outcomes in the child. *Cochrane Database Syst Rev* **11**: Cd010224.

Wheeler AC (2018) Development of infants with congenital Zika syndrome: What do we know and what can we expect? *Pediatrics* **141**: S154–S160.

CHAPTER 17

Early Adversity

Bettina Hohnen and Jane Gilmour

Presenting Concern

Linnéa, aged 8 years, was referred to a Child and Adolescent Mental Health Service as her adoptive parents were struggling to cope with her behaviour at home. Linnéa was adopted at 3 years 2 months along with her 18-month-old sister. She had lived with her birth family until she was almost 2 years old, moving frequently, then was placed in foster care for 16 months. Linnéa experienced emotional and physical neglect from her birth parents in her early years. There was a history of chaos, domestic violence, multiple visits to hospital with burns and bumps, and likely in utero exposure to drugs and alcohol. The precise nature of the effects on the developing brain of prenatal drug exposure is complex (e.g. Thompson et al. 2009; also see Chapter 16) but it is highly likely it had a negative impact for Linnéa. This picture of extremely poor parenting in the early years amounts to toxic stress and has a well-established effect on many aspects of development, including neuropsychological (e.g. Shonkoff et al. 2012).

Details of Linnéa's developmental history were slim, although when adopted her language (expressive and receptive) and motor skills (gross motor such as ability to climb stairs and fine motor such as use of knife and fork) were delayed. When adopted, Linnéa was strongly attached to her sister and took a while to adjust to her new home and adoptive parents (hereafter 'parents'). Within months, she developed a strong bond with her parents, but there continued to be vulnerabilities in her attachment style. She had separation anxiety day and night, which was ongoing, and her behaviour was highly variable. While she could be calm and gentle, she had periods of intense rage and aggression at home or was distressed and tearful without any obvious precursor. She enjoyed playing LEGO®, making up imaginative stories, and cooking with her mother. She made friends in the early years of school, but in the year leading up to the referral she was not integrating well with her peers, often being 'left out' with reports of bullying. Linnéa was uncertain about new places, did not enjoy being in large groups, and reluctantly attended events like birthday parties.

Educationally, Linnéa was one of the last in her class to learn her letters and was slow to attain reading fluency. Her teachers noticed she did not process verbal instructions well. Linnéa had become increasingly anxious before school, with frequent somatising symptoms (stomach aches) and decreasing school attendance. At school, she was often highly emotional, lashing out at her mother, and was frequently tearful. Small homework tasks such as reading or writing were highly stressful, and there were daily battles with her mother who was finding it hard to cope. The mother was concerned she was failing her daughter because Linnéa seemed so unhappy.

THEORY

It is well documented that early-life stressors lead to a cascade of biological effects on the neuroendocrine system (McCarty 2016), immune system (Danese and Lewis 2017), and brain development (McCrory and Viding 2015). Both environmental and genetic factors impact brain development, and it is important to consider both with this case.

Effect of Early Maltreatment – Experience

In the past decade, neurocognitive differences have been associated with maltreatment in the early years (see Gerin et al. 2019 for a review). Two well-established and important cognitive biases are found in this group. First, individuals who have been maltreated show privileged processing of negative events and hypervigilance. At times of stress, the activated brain networks include several limbic regions (e.g. amygdala, anterior cingulate cortex, and hippocampus) and cortical regions (e.g. the prefrontal cortex). For example children who have experienced institutional neglect show greater neural activity in the left amygdala and hippocampus when viewing fearful faces and in the absence of typical patterns of parental caregiving (which act to dampen amygdala response over time), reactivity in the amygdala remains heightened (Callaghan and Tottenham 2016). McCrory et al. (2013) also showed that this heightened amygdala response to angry faces is apparent pre-attentively showing it is not under conscious regulatory control. This neural adaptation is thought to offer short-term functional advantages, as hypervigilance to threat may confer protection, but there are potentially long-term costs such as causing problems negotiating both adult and peer relationships and affecting allocation of attention resources otherwise needed for normative aspects of educational engagement (Gerin et al. 2019).

The second neural adaptation related to extreme stress caused by maltreatment is in autobiographical memory (memories of episodes or events). Individuals who have experienced maltreatment tend to overgeneralise memories, which means that they struggle to recall details whether positive or negative (Valentino, Toth, and Cicchetti 2009). This adaptation to the cognitive system may be protective in the short-term, allowing individuals to push away difficult memories, but long-term this reduces the ability to draw on past experience to negotiate novel stressors and adapt in social situations. During recall of positive events, maltreated children showed reduced activity in the hippocampus, and during recall of negative events they show increased amygdala activation (McCrory et al. 2017). Moreover, children who have been maltreated favour negative memories over positive. McCrory and colleagues (2017) link this finding to an increased likelihood of negative rumination, which has been found in individuals with a history of abuse (Wright, Crawford, and Del Castillo 2009).

Latent Vulnerability of Early Neural Changes

McCrory and Viding (2015) propose that these neural adaptations confer latent vulnerability, predisposing such individuals to future mental health problems, mediated by social functioning difficulties. The direct effects of the neurocognitive changes associated with maltreatment include difficulties with emotional regulation, which means everyday stresses will tax an individual who has experienced early adversity more than those who have not (Tottenham and Gabard-Durnam 2017) – the so-called *stress susceptibility* route. There is a second mechanism at play, increasing vulnerability further. Such individuals may also act in a way to increase the likelihood of stressful events occurring (*the stress generation route*) for example small interpersonal misunderstandings become major rifts (Gerin et al. 2019). The third mechanism of vulnerability may be through a process of 'social thinning'. The 'latent' effect of maltreatment, which has a lasting impact on a person's threat-processing system (Hein and Monk 2017), may compromise social functioning by increasing a person's vigilance to threat, leading to over attribution of threat cues (Lee and Hoaken 2007), affecting their ability to sustain positive relationships. Indeed, data show that individuals who have experienced adversity do not have the degree of social support that the general population have because of cognitive differences described (Sperry and Widom 2013). Reduced social support is a well-established 'buffer' against stressful life events (e.g. Cohen and Hoberman 1983). Social learning theory (Bandura 1973) is also relevant here, where problematic interaction strategies that were previously positively reinforced are repeated, adding to social stress.

The daily consequences of these neurocognitive patterns are evident from early on in a young person's experience. Young people who have been maltreated are more likely to be ranked in the bottom 10% for social competence by their teachers. Longitudinal studies have shown independent associations between early adversity and social competence at each developmental stage (e.g. Raby et al. 2018). Moreover, young people with a history of maltreatment have an increased likelihood of rejection and victimisation by peers (Benedini, Fagan, and Gibson 2016). The social and emotional issues described in this population reflect many of Linnéa's presenting problems.

Underlying Neurocognitive Profile – Biology

With Linnéa's presentation, it is important to consider the possibility of genetically transmitted biological neurodiversity in addition to the above. Many of the difficulties described by Linnéa's parents and teachers are consistent with developmental dyslexia (slow to learn the alphabet, poor phonological processing, auditory processing difficulties, and slow to gain fluency in reading and spelling) (Shaywitz and Shaywitz 2003; also see Chapter 14). Developmental dyslexia is a common neurodevelopmental disorder (prevalence 5–17%) (Shaywitz and Shaywitz 2003) primarily affecting the development of reading and spelling fluency and accuracy. It is strongly heritable and there are convincing candidate genes (Paracchini, Scerri, and Monaco 2007). Brain studies show reduced left parieto-temporal activation and increased activation in frontal and right hemispheric regions (Shaywitz, Mody, and Shaywitz 2006) in this condition, quite distinct from those affected by adversity.

Early adversity may also result in reduced language exposure contributing to language delay (Hough and Kaczmarek 2011) and at the same time it is well accepted that developmental dyslexia and language difficulties have common roots (Bishop and Snowling 2004) so either or both these routes to language delay are possible and need to be discerned through cognitive assessment.

ASSESSMENT AND FORMULATION

Linnéa's presentation is complex, requiring an understanding of potential environmental and genetic contributions. For a child with a significant adverse early history, psychotherapy is often the first line of intervention, but it is important to be thorough and cautious and consider underlying biological vulnerability, possibly exacerbated by epigenetic effects (Smith 2011). It is essential to measure cognitive functioning in the initial stages of a case work up, to establish if there are general limitations in ability. Neuropsychological assessment can confirm or rule out a specific learning difficulty by testing competing hypotheses about a child's profile, which is important in a case like Linnéa where there are emotional and behavioural issues at school and in relation to school work.

It is important to use a developmental framework. One can also consider the question of *why now* to inform the hypothesis. At 8 years old, there is a shift to more formal educational tasks that will reveal weaknesses in core academic skills. Friendships become more complex, language based, and less structured and mediated by adults. This too, might reveal difficulties that have been previously masked.

A broad neuropsychological battery of assessments was administered. Linnéa's overall intellectual ability measured on the Wechsler Intelligence Scale for Children, Fifth Edition was within the average range (Full Scale IQ – 104) without atypical variation between verbal and nonverbal reasoning abilities. She showed a relative weakness in breadth of vocabulary (Vocabulary subtest, 16th percentile) and was slow at processing verbal instructions and verbal expression. Her working memory and processing speed were below average (5th and 10th percentile respectively). There was a significant discrepancy between Linnéa's core intellectual scores and her achievement measured on the Wechsler Individual Achievement Test, Third UK Edition, particularly in the area of literacy (Word Reading, 1st percentile; Pseudoword decoding 5th percentile). Moreover, her performance on cognitive-based 'marker' tests for developmental dyslexia, phonological awareness, and rapid naming, measured by the Comprehensive Test of Phonological Processing, Second Edition, were significantly impaired and discrepant from reasoning (7th and 2nd percentile respectively). In contrast, Linnéa performed at an age-appropriate level in numeracy and math reasoning (47th and 45th percentile respectively). Linnéa's manual dexterity measured on the Beery-Buktenica Developmental Test of Visual-Motor Integration was an area of weakness (5th percentile) in line with her slow processing speed.

There were no observations of inattention, restlessness, or impulsivity during testing; however, validated screening tools such as the Conners Rating Scales from multiple informants (parent and teacher) are recommended in the assessment of attention-deficit/hyperactivity disorder (NICE 2016; also see Chapter 8 for further detailed evaluations). Linnéa scored in the clinical range for hyperactivity/impulsivity on teacher report with no clinical symptoms indicated in the home environment.

Symptoms of reactive attachment disorder and autism spectrum disorder overlap (McKenzie and Dallos 2017) and it was important to establish whether there were underlying markers of social communication difficulties. The Autism Diagnostic Observation Schedule, Second Edition (ADOS-2®), and the Developmental Dimensional and Diagnostic Interview were administered. Linnéa scored well below clinical threshold on the ADOS-2®, showing fluent and responsive communication and social reciprocity, good imaginative play, with no evidence of restricted or repetitive behaviours. She scored below clinical threshold in all four areas on the ADOS-2®, and the Developmental Dimensional and Diagnostic Interview (social reciprocity, communication, nonverbal communication, and restricted/repetitive behaviours).

Occupational therapy assessment recorded fine motor dyspraxia along with sensory processing disorder with particular hypersensitivity to noise (see Chapter 3 for a comprehensive overview).

Case Study – Formulation

Linnéa is a girl of average intellectual ability with a relative weakness in verbal skills. She presents with developmental dyslexia affecting word decoding, spelling, written expression, and reading comprehension. Possible alternative neurodevelopmental conditions (autism spectrum disorder and attention deficit hyperactivity disorder) were formally assessed and excluded. The neurocognitive changes resulting from her early maltreatment are understood to be impacting on social relationships at home and school including hypervigilance to threat and negative rumination. The exacerbation of symptom presentation at this time was hypothesised to be a response to the increased academic challenges at school, intensifying the impact of her specific learning difficulty, which was overwhelming to her and her parents. Linnéa's parents need help to understand her cognitive profile and support her at home.

INTERVENTION AND MANAGEMENT

Social/Peer Intervention

McCrory and Viding (2015) call for preventative interventions for children who have experienced neglect and maltreatment and their families to offset their risk of later difficulties. Strengthening social competence is important for long-term good mental health across the population, even when reactive attachment disorder and autism spectrum disorder have been ruled out, and this was a focus of the work with Linnéa's parents alongside sensitive parenting. There is an association between reduced social support and an increased risk of anxiety and depression in adulthood (van Harmelen 2016) and so increasing social competence is likely to reduce the risk of later mental health problems in individuals with a history of maltreatment. Linnéa was already showing some peer relationship difficulties and this was a key area of intervention using structured play dates based on work by Frankel (2010).

Anxiety Intervention and Parenting

There is a strong evidence base for treatment of anxiety disorders using a cognitive behavioural approach (Higa-McMillan et al. 2016). The chosen programme should be developmentally appropriate (i.e. for primary school-aged children). A programme that includes a family skills component would be helpful in this case so Linnéa's mother could practise on a daily basis at home, using appropriate reinforcement strategies. It would also be helpful to use a programme that focuses on making friends and building social networks, so addressing some of the preventative social competence work she is likely to need given her profile.

A recent meta-analysis showed parenting interventions to effectively increase sensitive parenting, decrease dysfunctional discipline, and improve parenting knowledge and understanding (Schoemaker et al. 2019). The 20-week Circle of Security Parenting programme was administered with the parents and the paediatric neuropsychologist, which has been shown to improve parental emotional function (Huber, McMahon, and Sweller 2015).

Interventions for Developmental Dyslexia

If left untreated, developmental dyslexia is a significant barrier to educational achievement and opportunities and can have a spiralling effect on self-esteem, emotions, and behaviour (Shaywitz and Shaywitz 2003). Such a profile in the context of early adversity, without being addressed, is likely to have a more significant impact and so intervention in school with support from home is essential. See Chapter 14 for a discussion of effective treatments for developmental dyslexia.

Outcome

Linnéa's parents were highly engaged with the interventions offered, which were generally for-mulation driven. One of the most important aspects of the formulation was that it gave them a framework to understand Linnéa's behaviour. Her behavioural difficulties, anxiety, and social vulnerability might be best understood as a reflection of her social neurocognitive differences, vulnerable attachment pattern (given her early parenting), and her aversive experiences attaining literacy, one of the earliest milestones in school. Understanding these multiple processes meant that her parents were empowered and less likely to feel to blame for Linnéa's difficulties. At the same time, the interventions increased parental sensitivity, provided tools of positive disciplining, and reduced parental stress.

Six months after referral, Linnéa's anxiety and somatising behaviour had decreased significantly. The cognitive behavioural programme gave Linnéa and her parents the tools to understand anxiety and its clinical presentation. Linnéa's parents were better equipped to manage her intense emo-tions before attending school and during literacy activities at home. She was praised by her parents if she described, in words, a worry. They had confidence to support her calmly and steer her away from using safety behaviours (a behavioural response to a difficult feeling that provides short-term release but maintains the behaviour in the long-term) such as avoiding sleeping in her own bed. With growing confidence, Linnéa demonstrated increasing independence at home, settled to sleep well in her own bed, and coped with more demanding social events, such as birthday parties. Linnéa's parents were able to 'read' her behaviours, supporting and encouraging her need to explore the world and providing a safe haven for her to return to their safe 'hands' when needed. She was engaged with individualised literacy support sessions. Another classmate with a dyslexic profile joined the teaching session and the two children developed a firm friendship. Her wider peer relationships improved too, in part reflecting her increased confidence, calmer demeanour, and her developing understanding of her personal history and learning needs.

SUMMARY

A complex environmental picture such as extreme early adversity can 'dominate' the formulation. However, it is important to review systematically and exclude other possible explanations for presenting problems (such as emotional and behavioural difficulties at home or school in this case). Where neurodevelopmental conditions with a genetic basis (like developmental dyslexia) are established, the dual impact of these conditions and a child's environmental experiences must be considered as they will both impact on a child's presentation, learning experience, and family response. Family and school staff are likely to need considerable and ongoing input to support children with such complex needs as the child's presentation will evolve as the demands of their social, emotional, and academic world develop.

REFERENCES

Bandura A (1973) *Aggression: A Social Learning Analysis.* Englewood Cliffs, NJ: Prentice Hall.

Benedini KM, Fagan AA, Gibson CL (2016) The cycle of victimization: The relationship between childhood maltreatment and adolescent peer victimization. *Child Abuse & Neglect* **59**: 111–121. doi: 10.1016/j.chiabu.2016.08.003.

Bishop DVM, Snowling MJ (2004) Developmental dyslexia and specific language impairment: Same or different? *Psychological Bulletin* **130**(6): 858–886. http://dx.doi.org/10.1037/0033-2909.130.6.858.

Callaghan BL, Tottenham N (2016) The neuro-environmental loop of plasticity: A cross-species analysis of parental effects on emotion circuitry development following typical and adverse caregiving. *Neuropsychopharmacology* **41**: 163–176. doi: 10.1038/npp.2015.204.

Cohen S, Hoberman HM (1983) Positive events and social supports as buffers of life change stress. *Journal of Applied Social Psychology* **13**(2): 99–125. http://dx.doi.org/10.1111/j.1559-1816.1983.tb02325.x.

Danese A., Lewis SJ (2017) Psychoneuroimmunology of early-life stress: The hidden wounds of childhood trauma? *Neuropsychopharmacology* **42**(1): 99–114. doi: http://dx.doi.org.libproxy.ucl.ac.uk/10.1038/npp.2016.198.

Frankel F (2010) *Friends Forever: How Parents Can Help Their Kids Make and Keep Good Friends.* San Francisco, CA: Jossey Bass.

Gerin MI, Hanson E, Viding E, McCrory EJ (2019) A review of childhood maltreatment, latent vulnerability and the brain: Implications for clinical practice and prevention. *Adoption & Fostering* **43**(3): 310–328. doi: 10.1177/0308575919865356.

Hein TC, Monk CS (2017) Research review: Neural response to threat in children, adolescents, and adults after child maltreatment – A quantitative meta-analysis. *Journal of Child Psychology and Psychiatry* **58**: 222–230. doi: 10.1111/jcpp.12651.

Higa-McMillan, Francis SE, Rith-Najarian L, Chorpita BF (2016) Evidence base update: 50 years of research on treatment for child and adolescent anxiety. *Journal of Clinical Child & Adolescent Psychology* **45**(2): 91–113. doi: 10.1080/15374416.2015.1046177.

Hough SD, Kaczmarek L (2011) Language and reading outcomes in young children adopted from Eastern European orphanages. *Journal of Early Intervention* **33**(1): 51–74. https://doi.org/10.1177/1053815111401377.

Huber A, McMahon C, Sweller N (2015) Improved child behavioural and emotional functioning after Circle of Security 20-week intervention. *Attachment and Human Development* **17**(6): 547–569.

Lee V, Hoaken PNS (2007) Cognition, emotion, and neurobiological development: Mediating the relation between maltreatment and aggression. *Child Maltreatment* **12**: 281–298. doi: 10.1177/1077559507303778.

McCarty R (2016) Learning about stress: Neural, endocrine and behavioral adaptations. *Stress* **19**(5): 449–475. doi: 10.1080/10253890.2016.1192120.

McCrory EJ, De Brito S, Kelly PA et al. (2013) Amygdala activation in maltreated children during pre-attentive emotional processing. *The British Journal of Psychiatry* **202**(4): 269–276.

McCrory E, Puetz V, Maguire E et al. (2017) Autobiographical memory: A candidate latent vulnerability mechanism for psychiatric disorder following childhood maltreatment. *British Journal of Psychiatry* **211**(4): 216–222. doi: 10.1192/bjp.bp.117.201798.

McCrory EJ, Viding E (2015) The theory of latent vulnerability: Reconceptualizing the link between childhood maltreatment and psychiatric disorder. *Developmental Psychopathology* **27**(2): 493–505.

McKenzie R, Dallos R (2017) Autism and attachment difficulties: Overlap of symptoms, implications and innovative solutions. *Clinical Child Psychology and Psychiatry* **22**(4): 632–648.

National Institute for Health and Clinical Excellence (NICE) (2016) *Attention Deficit Hyperactivity Disorder: Diagnosis and Management (CG72).* London: The British Psychological Society and The Royal College of Psychiatrist.

Paracchini S, Scerri T, Monaco AP (2007) The genetic lexicon of dyslexia. *Annual Review of Genomics and Human Genetics* **8**(1): 57–79.

Raby KL, Roisman GI, Labella MH, Martin J, Fraley RC, Simpson JA (2018) The legacy of early abuse and neglect for social and academic competence from childhood to adulthood. *Child Development* **90**(5): 1684–1701. doi: 10.1111/cdev.13033.

Shaywitz SE, Mody M, Shaywitz BA (2006) Neural mechanisms in dyslexia. *Current Directions in Psychological Science* **15**(6): 278–281. https://doi.org/10.1111/j.1467-8721.2006.00452.x.

Shaywitz SE, Shaywitz BA (2003) Dyslexia (specific reading disability). *Pediatr Rev* **24**: 147–153.

Shonkoff JP, Garner AS, Siegel BS et al. (2012) The lifelong effects of early childhood adversity and toxic stress. The committee on psychosocial aspects of child and family health, committee on early childhood, adoption and dependent care and section on developmental and behavioural pediatrics. *Pediatrics* **129**(1): e232–e246. doi: 10.1542/peds.2011-2663.

Schoemaker N, Wentholt W, Goemans A, Vermeer H, Juffer F, Alink L (2019) A meta-analytic review of parenting interventions in foster care and adoption. *Development and Psychopathology* **32**(3): 1149–1172. doi: 10.1017/S0954579419000798.

Smith SD (2011) Approach to epigenetic analysis in language disorders. *Journal of Neurodevelopmental Disorder* **3**(4): 356–364.

Sperry DM, Widom CS (2013) Child abuse and neglect, social support, and psychopathology in adulthood: A prospective investigation. *Child Abuse and Neglect* **47**: 175–176.

Thompson BL, Levitt P, Stanwood GD (2009) Prenatal exposure to drugs: Effects on brain development and implications for policy and education. *Nature Reviews. Neuroscience* **10**(4): 303–312. doi: 10.1038/nrn2598.

Tottenham N, Gabard-Durnam LJ (2017) The developing amygdala: A student of the world and a teacher of the cortex. *Current Opinion in Psychology* **17**: 55–60.

Valentino K, Toth SL, Cicchetti D (2009) Autobiographical memory functioning among abused, neglected, and nonmaltreated children: The overgeneral memory effect. *Journal of Child Psychology and Psychiatry*, **50**: 1029–1038.

van Harmelen AL, Gibson JL, St Clair MC et al. (2016) Friendships and family support reduce subsequent depressive symptoms in at-risk adolescents. *PLoS One* **11**(5): e0153715. doi: 10.1371/journal.pone.0153715.

Wright MO, Crawford E, Del Castillo D (2009) Childhood emotional maltreatment and later psychological distress among college students: The mediating role of maladaptive schemas. *Child Abuse Negl* **33**(1): 59–68. doi: 10.1016/j.chiabu.2008.12.007. Epub 2009 Jan 23.

CHAPTER 18

School and Education

Rebecca Ashton and Helen Jackson

Presenting Concern

Joseph is a 15-year-old student who attends a mainstream school. In his early years, Joseph was noted to be a very active boy, 'into everything', and found it hard to be still. Through primary school, difficulties with attention became more apparent. Joseph had extensive assessments to rule out hearing loss, language difficulties, and general learning difficulties, before the paediatrician diagnosed attention-deficit/hyperactivity disorder (ADHD) at the age of 10 years.

Joseph was prescribed medication for ADHD and had in-class academic support provided by school. He followed a mainstream curriculum. The family had received years of psychological guidance and training on the structures and supports needed for a child with ADHD but relationships were still challenging at home.

Joseph met with his parents and the learning support teacher regularly to review his Individual Education Plan. They attempted to incorporate into the plan advice from the advisory teacher and clinical psychologist, who were external to the school.

Cognitive test results from assessment with Joseph at 14 years of age included verbal reasoning in the very high range, with fluid reasoning and visuospatial skills in the high average range; working memory was average, as were visual and verbal memory skills; processing speed was low average. On the basis of these scores, staff assumed that Joseph should be able to access the curriculum as there were no areas of learning difficulty.

Over the preceding 2 years, Joseph's learning had plateaued and his behaviour was becoming increasingly challenging. His family were worried about how he would cope on leaving school at 18 years. The school had put into place a number of intensive interventions that were not working to improve the situation, and everyone was frustrated that Joseph was not achieving his predicted grades. The school therefore requested input from an educational neuropsychologist to help refocus everyone's efforts.

THEORY

Executive Function

Executive functioning is a complex construct, with differing views about its composition. However, most authors would agree that, 'executive function is a process used to effortfully guide behaviour toward a goal, especially in nonroutine situations' (Banich 2009). Harvard University's Center on the Developing Child (2011) provides a useful analogy of executive functions as the air traffic control systems of the brain: they are needed to organise and coordinate other skills (see Chapter 11 for further information on executive function).

ADHD is seen primarily as a disorder of executive functioning (Pennington and Ozonoff 1996; Barkley 1997), although with wide heterogeneity in which executive functions are most affected for each individual (Kofler et al. 2018). Most of the evidence points towards deficits in 'cool' (cognitive rather than 'hot' emotional) executive functioning, specifically vigilance, working memory, inhibition, and planning (Willcutt et al. 2005; Rubia 2011).

The neuroscience data also supports the idea that ADHD is a complex issue with many neural areas involved, key amongst them being hypoactivation in the frontoparietal networks which underpin executive functioning (Cortese et al. 2012). Shaw, Gogtay, and Rapoport (2010) have shown that cortical development, particularly of the prefrontal cortex, is delayed in young people with ADHD. Some people go on to 'catch up' with their neural development and show remission of symptoms as they grow older, whilst others continue to experience ADHD into adulthood.

Social Inclusion

Young people with ADHD often have difficulties socialising with their peers, leading to them being more frequently rejected by the peer group by the time they reach secondary school (de Boer and Pijl 2016). These difficulties are underpinned by the cognitive executive function difficulties at the core of ADHD, as the person is less able to adapt their behaviour to the social situation and to inhibit their impulses, so their peers may see them as unpredictable, egocentric, and irritating.

Students with slower processing speeds, alongside their executive functioning/ADHD characteristics, may find the pace of peer interactions too rapid, the verbal interchanges too swift, and their own contributions too slow in response time. This can lead to further discomfort/humiliation and feelings of inadequacy.

Education System at This Key Developmental Stage

Adolescence is a key developmental stage for executive functioning (Blakemore and Choudhury 2006). It is during these years that most people advance their executive skills towards adult levels, and therefore the differences between individuals with ADHD and without become more pronounced.

In most countries, the education system includes a step-change from primary to secondary schools just as puberty begins. Young people have to manage a change of educational environment, new relationships with staff and peers, and a more complex daily routine, alongside the developmental tasks of adolescence and the biological changes in hormones and neural organisation.

Students in secondary school are usually expected to move around to different classrooms and teachers for different subjects, to organise their own equipment, and to solve problems more independently. For most students, executive functions develop during their secondary school career such that they are able to cope with becoming more independent at school. Indeed, the more complex environment may be a factor in helping students develop their executive skills. However, for young people with executive function difficulties such as those seen in ADHD, secondary school presents a much greater challenge than primary school. Executive difficulties therefore become much more problematic at this stage of education.

Getting the Right Provisions in Place

Most developed countries have systems of assessment and criteria that need to be met in order to direct resources towards children with additional needs in education. In some systems, diagnoses or labels are key to accessing these resources, while in others a more descriptive, needs-led approach is taken.

For common disabilities and difficulties, there is sometimes a shared understanding about what approaches might help and what resources will be required. For example even though there will be a wide range of individual presentations, issues such as hearing impairment or dyslexia usually feature in assessment frameworks and will be recognised as needing specific support. However, executive function difficulties are much harder to classify in terms of educational categories and usually have to be fitted into headings such as cognition, emotional/behavioural, physical/sensory, or communication difficulties.

Children may have a clinical assessment using medical or psychiatric terminology, but this does not always translate easily into educational practice. For example in Joseph's case he had a clinical diagnosis of ADHD, but this label would not necessarily attract specific educational resources or help school staff know what to do differently for him. Recent efforts are being made to bring together educational approaches with clinical diagnosis frameworks (Norwich 2016).

A Tiered Approach to Assessment and Intervention

In the education field, even the most complex cases are often managed in terms of a staged approach to assessment and intervention. For example in the UK this is known as the graduated approach (Department for Education 2015), and in the USA it is usually called the multitiered system of support (National Association of School Psychologists 2016).

Both the UK's and USA's systems for educational support have two key elements: assess-plan-do-review cycles and stages of intervention depending on the outcome of these cycles (known in the USA as RTI: Response to Intervention). Both countries use virtually identical three tier models for this process: Tier 1 (universal) typically refers to provision for all students; Tier 2 (targeted) involves support available to some students identified as having some additional needs; Tier 3 (intensive) are highly specialised interventions for a small number of individuals. With the passing of Every Student Succeeds Act in the USA in 2015, the same three-tiered model comes into effect on a statutory basis for student need identification.

In the clinical field, a paediatric neurocognitive interventions (PNI) model can be used to guide rehabilitation following brain injury (Limond et al. 2014). This PNI model also takes a staged approach, although here the successive stages are based on developmental and cognitive needs rather than the intensity of intervention required (Fig. 18.1).

We would argue that the PNI levels provide a useful structure within Tier 3 of the multitiered system of support/graduated response, as the focus is on adjustments and interventions tailored to an individual, even if those interventions are systemic in nature. For example psychoeducation for a whole class about a particular psychological or neurological condition would probably be undertaken only if it were relevant to a student

Level	Cognitive Impairments	Intervention Aim	Examples of Interventions
D	Specific cognitive skills e.g. episodic memory, visual processing, language skills	Compensatory strategies to be used independently	Training in the use of e.g.; elaborative encoding, retrieval strategies, visual compensations
C	Evaluative skills e.g. metacognition, supervisory processes, and reasoning	Training to support general cognitive functioning	Training of e.g. goal management skills, prospective reminding, "stop and think"
B	Core skills e.g. working memory, inhibitory control, processing speed, and sequencing	Remediation of skills	Intensive practice e.g. working memory, attention process , and speed training
A	Semantic knowledge, adaptive functioning and specific cognitive skills (e.g. episodic memory)	Compensatory strategies, cued and supported by others	Providing techniques such as precision teaching, errorless learning, elaborative encoding and rehearsal

Pyramid levels (left side): Level D Skills & Interventions; Level C Skills & Interventions; Level B Skills & Interventions; Level A Skills & Interventions; Psychosocial and Systemic Foundations

Psychosocial and Systemic Foundations - Supporting health needs, sensory impairments, pragmatic and social care issues (e.g. visual processing, diet, exercise, financial, and practical resources). Addressing systemic factors (e.g. family chaos). Ensuring positive behavioral support for challenging behavior. Accessing parenting skills training to ensure development of emotional competence. Providing psychotherapy for mood disorders.

Figure 18.1 Paediatric neurocognitive interventions model. Reproduced from Limond, Adlam, and Cormack (2014).

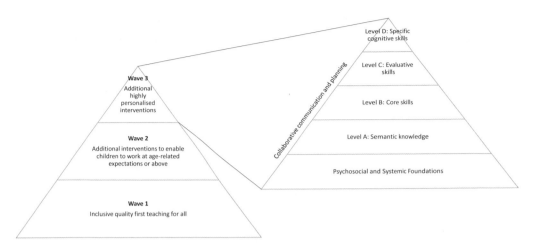

Figure 18.2 Tiered system of educational support with paediatric neurocognitive intervention levels nested within the top tier.

in that class, hence the PNI base layer, 'psychosocial and systemic foundations', sits within Tier 3 of the education framework (Fig. 18.2).

ASSESSMENT AND FORMULATION

Much was already known about Joseph before the assessment described here. At this point a sound formulation was required, bringing together the information available in a framework that could help direct what further data was needed and target intervention more effectively.

Educational neuropsychology assessment took a holistic view of Joseph's situation as well as focusing specifically on his current executive skills. Observations were carried out in order to see what was happening in lessons and how staff were differentiating for Joseph's needs. Joseph, his mother, and his teacher were all individually consulted to gather their views and to assess relevant factors including sleep, diet, exercise, emotional well-being, and social functioning. Social adjustment was also directly assessed using sociometry with the whole tutor group (Ashton 2018).

While executive skills testing has ecological validity issues (Wallisch et al. 2018), it can be helpful especially when the data are triangulated with questionnaires that assess everyday functioning. Joseph therefore undertook subtests from the Delis-Kaplan Executive Function System (Delis et al. 2001) and the Rey Complex Figure Test (Meyers and Meyers 1995). His mother and teacher both completed a Behavior Rating Inventory of Executive Function, Second Edition (Gioia et al. 2015).

Executive function difficulties in planning, organisation, task initiation, inhibition, and flexibility were evident in test, school, and home settings. If the task was highly structured, with step-by-step instructions, Joseph could often complete it. However, at this level of education students were often given open-ended tasks or a set of work to complete during the session, and Joseph frequently produced very little. Joseph had begun to lie to adults about his work and his task completion. He forgot materials, even for courses, such as drama, that he enjoyed. Joseph under- or overestimated how long tasks would take, so frequently failed to finish or did a rushed job that was not the best quality he could produce. At the age of 15 years, it was unclear whether Joseph's ADHD symptoms would remit over time or persist into adulthood (Shaw et al. 2010), but at this point in time there was a big gap between Joseph's executive skills and those expected for his age group.

School had provided a laptop for writing, which made no difference to the structure of what he wrote; indeed the range of software available often distracted Joseph from the task in hand. The situation was frustrating for everyone, as they knew Joseph understood the concepts and was capable of a good standard in a range of subjects.

Weekly goal-setting for lessons and for after school work was done between Joseph and his teacher, but the goals were rarely met. He showed good intentions but was unable to manage himself during the week to achieve his goals.

Joseph felt that he had no real friends, which bothered him. He had found his place within the peer group that reinforced his reputation as what he termed a 'hard man', being defiant with adults and not engaging with learning. Other students either avoided him as they feared his unpredictability and impulsivity or enjoyed watching Joseph get into trouble. This description was consistent with the sociometry measure, which identified him as a 'controversial' member of the group (high number of both 'likes' and 'dislikes' from other students).

In terms of school systems, the learning support teacher liaised well with the professionals outside school, and worked closely with Joseph and his family. However, in secondary education the bulk of the teaching is done by subject teachers and the internal communication between school staff was not so effective. The learning support teacher would write the plans for Joseph and distribute them to subject teachers, who may or may not read or act upon them. Lesson observations showed that there was wide variation in teaching approaches, with some staff following the strategies in Joseph's individual plan and others unaware that the plan existed. In addition, the external professionals rarely came together, each liaising separately with the school.

Family dynamics were affected by all the executive function deficits, with parents wanting to encourage and support his increased independence into adulthood, leading to frustration when he could not remember to bring his materials to school or lost items. The level of support and scaffolding Joseph required raised the parents' fears about his ability to function independently outside the safety of the school and home environments. His parents also felt guilty when they showed their anger at Joseph lying to cover up his executive function errors.

For Joseph, it was important to return to more basic skills and adaptations that had not been consolidated. Parents and staff were expecting a lot from Joseph, especially given his good performance on cognitive testing, but his executive difficulties meant that he could not utilise these skills effectively in complex or unfamiliar situations.

It was helpful to think about Joseph as a student with specific learning difficulties – in this case, difficulties with executive functioning and with slower processing speed. His ADHD medication was helping him to direct and maintain his attention, but Joseph was still struggling with other executive skills such as planning, organisation, task initiation, inhibition, and flexibility. His social situation could be construed as a result of these executive functioning difficulties and as a way of coping with them.

Using the tiered models to help guide formulation, Joseph's educational plan had become focused on higher levels of intervention, with complex and specific interventions in place at the expense of solid foundations. With this structure in mind, the team were able to review the interventions currently in place. Most of them were agreed to be ineffective because they required skills that Joseph just did not have yet or a support system that was not yet in place.

INTERVENTION AND MANAGEMENT

For specialist professionals working on a complex case from outside a school setting, there is a temptation to move quickly from neuropsychological assessment to recommending interventions, often at intensive levels (Tier 3 and level C or D within that). Whilst such advanced interventions may well be appropriate, it is equally essential to consider what systemic and specific interventions have previously been implemented and evaluated for success. Such work is complicated and requires the effective and frequent communication of all professionals, as well as the family and the student. Typically, this tiered system of intervention would have taken place prior to any referral for neuropsychological or psychiatric assessment and should therefore be included in the formulation.

With the ADHD diagnosis and parallel intervention plans in place (medication, individualised goal-setting, use of laptop for writing), Joseph was already considered a student at the Tier 3 stage of intervention. However, the PNI model helped the team to think about interventions at different developmental levels and to prioritise what needed to be put into place at this point.

In Joseph's case, a whole range of interventions were suggested by the educational psychologist, clinical psychologist, and school support teacher. It was then discussed where they would fit within the PNI levels. While it was difficult for some of the team to 'back down' and accept that their idea was at too high a level for Joseph at this time, this process was very important for developing a coherent plan that was not too overwhelming for him as an individual. A record of all the ideas was kept, as they could well be helpful for Joseph at a later stage.

Psychosocial and Systemic Foundations

- *Functional Behavioural Assessment* in the classroom – leading to better antecedent management of behaviour, triggers, motivators, and positive and negative consequences.
- *Family work*
  - *Parenting support* – the family had received previous training but Video Interaction Guidance (Kennedy, Landor, and Todd 2011) may provide a more positive approach to implementing the strategies they have learned.
  - *Family therapy* – therapeutic intervention by a specialist well-versed in ADHD and family systems therapy, to help repair relationships and give Joseph a more emotionally secure base.
- *Psycho-education* – staff and parent
  - *Executive functions* and how difficulties with these affect Joseph – projectlearnet.org has excellent resources.
  - *Diagnosis* – parent and staff education about the diagnosis of ADHD and what it means for Joseph.
  - *Medical therapy* – parents and staff education regarding the role of medication in ADHD treatment, how it may help with some aspects of difficulty but not others.
  - *Consistent approach* – annual brief meeting of staff teaching Joseph to share formulation and strategies, from which a more collective plan could be written.
- Use of assessment information to make the case that Joseph has specific learning difficulties in the domain of executive functioning – this could then be used to apply for *additional resources*. Often the more 'basic' level interventions require a high level of resources as they need to be delivered in everyday situations all the time, rather than confined to specific scheduled sessions.

Level A: Skills and Interventions

- *Social skills training* – done with prompts to use the skills in the moment, and with work done with the peer group to understand and accept the young person (Mikami et al. 2017).
- *Environmental and instructional considerations* for the student – negotiating with the student with the intention to move some of the strategies to Level D for independent use.
  - Consider task duration
  - Immediate feedback on accuracy and quality of work

- Timers for work completion
- Location for independent work with reduced distractions
- To-do lists that break down the task into smaller steps
- Timetable adjustments to enable movement breaks, ideally with physical activity
- Consideration of a daily schedule with academic-heavy classes in the morning given evidence of increased on-task behaviour in the morning
- Carefully structured lessons with key information clearly identified visually and verbally
- Frequent but nonobtrusive rule reminders and visual cues
- Agreement of nonverbal cues for on-task behaviour or task initiation
- *Precision teaching* – to help consolidate key knowledge to fluency so that it is available to Joseph without having to work it out each time.

Level B: Skills and Interventions

- *Training of specific executive skills* – there is some evidence that skills training can improve individual areas of cognitive weakness, although the skills may need more support to be generalised and utilised effectively in everyday situations (e.g. Diamond 2012).
  - Working memory
  - Attention processes
  - Inhibitory control

Level C: Skills and Interventions – Focused on Developing Insight and Self-Awareness

- *Individualised therapy for the student* – such as motivational interviewing or narrative therapy; the premise being that once he feels that change is possible and desirable, he will be more open to Level D work.
- *Psycho-education for the student* – further exploration of Joseph's own learning profile, executive functions, and the role of medication.
- *Peer group support* – for example Circle of Friends (Newton and Wilson 2003) to help Joseph understand how others see him and for them to support him in the moment.

Level D: Skills and Interventions

- *Executive functioning coaching* – individualised goal-setting and review, requiring a high level of metacognition as part of becoming more independent.

- *Independent strategies* – for Joseph to use himself, for example
  - Self-talk
  - Developing his own to-do lists
  - Setting and responding to his own mobile phone reminders
  - Organising key information visually, for example using mind maps and colour coding
- *Token economy system* or response cost program – consequence rather than antecedent management.

Key to the success of any systematic approach to intervention is interdisciplinary communication and planning. In this case, the school had previously been presented with lengthy diagnostic reports concluding with myriad recommendations prescribed by external professionals. At this point, it was essential to spend the time getting together and planning with clear goals and strategies (Dunsmuir et al. 2009). It was important for everyone involved to be part of the planning as equal partners and to agree what should go into the plan for the current time as well as what should be stopped, paused, or modified.

We would therefore suggest that the PNI model could be enhanced with the explicit addition of ongoing interdisciplinary planning across all levels of intervention in Tier 3, here described as 'collaborative communication and planning'. No professional can work effectively with a child at this level of complexity without being part of a team who strive towards a holistic understanding of the child's situation and needs, and who plan together so that the child gets a coherent package of intervention. While this joined-up approach is implied in the article by Limond et al. (2014), we feel it is important to give collaboration greater prominence as it is vital, but not always implemented.

Outcome

In Joseph's case, refocusing his intervention package on foundation/Level A approaches was very helpful. The multidisciplinary team were able to share their thoughts and coordinate their work towards a small number of agreed goals, rather than each professional pursuing their own programme separately. The adults around Joseph saw him in a new light, as someone with executive functioning difficulties rather than as a lazy or naughty boy. They were quickly able to adjust how help was offered, so that Joseph had a much greater experience of success with tasks at home and at school. The assessment information was successful in helping to make the case for additional resources.

These resources were used to provide the daily little inputs that Joseph needed, for example an adult to write down the steps needed to complete a task, as the teacher was explaining it. The same adult ran a social skills group, and was then able to prompt all the students to use what they had been learning when a relevant situation arose in class.

The family were able to hire a home-based tutor to support Joseph with homework and revision, and he was involved in recruiting the individual. This tutor's role was to help keep Joseph on task and moving forward with each homework assignment. The tutor was instructed to cue Joseph to attend (using a signal determined by Joseph), write down his goals for the session, and then ask scaffolding questions such as 'What will you need?', 'What's next?', and 'Are you on track?'

Joseph was very pleased to eliminate the weekly goal-setting sessions that had been nothing but disappointing for him, because these were at Level D and therefore he was not ready to benefit from them. Instead he started to see why managing himself had been so hard for him and to understand the ways in which adults were now structuring things for him. This awareness was encouraging as it laid the foundations for Joseph to think about doing some of that structuring for himself. Joseph even started to see a student from his social skills group outside of school, which he considered his first real friendship.

SUMMARY

Joseph's case highlights the need for case formulation to be considered within a context and for interventions to be prioritised using a tiered approach.

It is all too easy for neuropsychologists to conduct assessments in a vacuum, without careful analysis of the system and the individual within the system, both in terms of formulation and intervention planning. The temptation of a 'prescription' approach is strong but is unlikely to generate universally desirable outcomes. An integrated analysis requires ongoing/regular professional discussion and dialogue. Limited time may be better spent consulting with relevant people and noting down key points and agreed actions, rather than writing lengthy reports. This joined-up work will allow for appropriate, data-driven identification of specific goal areas and progress, with a realistic view of what might be useful at a particular point in time.

A tiered approach is particularly useful in neuropsychology work because the cases are often so complex, involving neurological, cognitive, physical, emotional, and social aspects. There can be many possible targets for intervention, at different developmental/cognitive levels, so the tiered approach helps to organise the team's thinking about what to prioritise at each point in time. In this case, Joseph was having Level C/D interventions, which were not working because the foundations were not yet in place. A more productive approach for him was to formulate together, generating a shared understanding of Joseph's needs. With this in mind, the team could agree to drop these higher-level interventions and refocus efforts on foundation/Level A support.

The notion of a developmentally driven tiered system of interventions within the top tier of educational support has not yet been explored in the literature but is worthy of evaluation. The integration of the multitiered system of support and PNI models, with the addition of collaborative communication and planning, offers a promising systematic approach to intervention planning and implementation.

REFERENCES

Ashton R (2018) Framework for assessment of children's social competence, with particular focus on children with brain injuries. *Applied Neuropsychology: Child* 7(2): 175–186.

Banich MT (2009) Executive function: The search for an integrated account. *Current Directions in Psychological Science* **18**(2): 89–94.

Barkley RA (1997) Behavioral inhibition, sustained attention, and executive functions: Constructing a unifying theory of ADHD. *Psychological Bulletin* **121**(1): 65–94.

Blakemore SJ, Choudhury S (2006) Development of the adolescent brain: Implications for executive function and social cognition. *Journal of Child Psychology and Psychiatry* **47**(3–4): 296–312.

Center on the Developing Child at Harvard University (2011) Building the Brain's 'Air Traffic Control' System: How Early Experiences Shape the Development of Executive Function: Working Paper No. 11. http://www.developingchild.harvard.edu.

Cortese S, Kelly C, Chabernaud C et al. (2012) Toward systems neuroscience of ADHD: A meta-analysis of 55 fMRI studies. *American Journal of Psychiatry* **169**(10): 1038–1055.

de Boer A, Pijl SJ (2016) The acceptance and rejection of peers with ADHD and ASD in general secondary education. *The Journal of Educational Research* **109**(3): 325–332.

Department for Education (2015) Special educational needs and disability code of practice: 0 to 25 years. DFE-00205-2013.

Diamond A (2012) Activities and programs that improve children's executive functions. *Current Directions in Psychological Science* **21**(5): 335–341.

Dunsmuir S, Brown E, Iyadurai S, Monsen J (2009) Evidence-based practice and evaluation: From insight to impact. *Educational Psychology in Practice* **25**(1): 53–70.

Kennedy H, Landor M, Todd L (2011) *Video Interaction Guidance*. London: Jessica Kingsley.

Kofler MJ, Irwin LN, Soto EF et al. (2018) Executive functioning heterogeneity in pediatric ADHD. *Journal of Abnormal Child Psychology* **47**(2): 273–286.

Limond J, Adlam AR, Cormack M (2014) A model for pediatric neurocognitive interventions: Considering the role of development and maturation in rehabilitation planning. *The Clinical Neuropsychologist* **28**(2): 181–198.

Mikami AY, Smit S, Khalis A (2017) Social skills training and ADHD—what works? *Current Psychiatry Reports* **19**(12): 93.

National Association of School Psychologists (2016) *Building capacity for student success: Every student succeeds act opportunities: Multitiered systems of support*. Available from: from https://www.nasponline.org/research-and-policy/policy-priorities/relevant-law/the-every-student-succeeds-act/essa-implementation-resources/essa-and-mtss-for-school-psychologists [Accessed 4 February 2020].

Newton C, Wilson D (2003) *Creating Circles of Friends*. Nottingham: Russell Press.

Norwich B (2016) Conceptualizing special educational needs using a biopsychosocial model in England: The prospects and challenges of using the International Classification of Functioning framework. *Frontiers in Education* **1**: 5.

Pennington BF, Ozonoff S (1996) Executive functions and developmental psychopathology. *Journal of Child Psychology and Psychiatry* **37**(1): 51–87.

Rubia K (2011) 'Cool' inferior frontostriatal dysfunction in attention-deficit/hyperactivity disorder versus 'hot' ventromedial orbitofrontal-limbic dysfunction in conduct disorder: A review. *Biological Psychiatry* **69**(12): e69–e87.

Shaw P, Gogtay N, Rapoport J (2010) Childhood psychiatric disorders as anomalies in neurodevelopmental trajectories. *Human Brain Mapping* **31**(6): 917–925.

Wallisch A, Little LM, Dean E, Dunn W (2018) Executive function measures for children: A scoping review of ecological validity. *OTJR: Occupation, Participation and Health* **38**(1): 6–14.

Willcutt EG, Doyle AE, Nigg JT, Faraone SV, Pennington BF (2005) Validity of the executive function theory of attention-deficit/hyperactivity disorder: A meta-analytic review. *Biological Psychiatry* **57**(11): 1336–1346.

CHAPTER 19

Mental Health

Megan Eve and Fiona McFarlane

Presenting Concern

Sakura, a 15-year-old girl with longstanding epilepsy, was referred for neuropsychological assessment due to concerns raised by her parents and teachers that her academic performances had noticeably dropped over the past year. She lived with her parents: a dentist and a marketing manager. Her older brother lived away from the family home studying economics at university. Sakura's early developmental history was unremarkable, with the exception that, in the toddler years, her speech had been difficult for those outside the family to understand.

At 6 years of age, Sakura developed epilepsy. Magnetic resonance imaging scan of her brain showed no structural abnormalities, but electroencephalogram investigations showed that the seizures had a left frontal focus with secondary generalisation. For many years the control of Sakura's seizures with medication had been variable. However, for the past 18 months, Sakura had been seizure free on a combination of two antiseizure medications (ASMs; levetiracetam and lamotrigine).

Sakura's school attendance at primary school was variable as she needed to sleep following seizures and also had to attend frequent medical appointments. She had additional learning support to keep her safe when she had seizures and to help her to catch up on missed work. Sakura's parents had paid for private tutoring in Year 6 and Sakura had achieved expected academic targets at the end of her primary education. Sakura settled in well at secondary school, but over the course of the past year, her grades had fallen, and there were concerns that she may fail her English, Maths, and Science exams.

Sakura reported that she found it difficult to take in and remember what the teachers were saying in lessons. Having previously been a conscientious pupil, Sakura had also started to avoid homework and often completed it in a panic at the last moment. She had become more withdrawn, rarely leaving her bedroom, and stopped attending basketball practice. Sakura had a close group of friends but there had been frequent arguments within the group throughout the last year. She found it difficult to get to sleep at night and, subsequently, struggled to get up in the morning. During the clinical interview, she became very upset and disclosed that she had recently been self-harming by superficially cutting her arms.

THEORY

Mental health and neuropsychological difficulties frequently co-occur and reciprocally influence one another. Consideration of mental health is an essential component of neuropsychological assessment. A holistic biopsychosocial neuropsychological formulation should encompass both the child or young person's cognitive profile *and* mental health presentation in order to best understand the presenting difficulties and to most appropriately apply intervention.

Consideration of the reciprocal relationship between mental health and neuropsychology is key at three levels, as described below.

Neurological Underpinnings of Mental Health Difficulties

Children and young people with chronic neurological disorders, particularly those with structural brain abnormalities, are at significantly greater risk of developing mental health problems than their peers. Epidemiological studies find rates of psychiatric disorder in this population as high as 35% to 50% with even higher rates in those with accompanying intellectual disability or structural brain abnormalities (Sillanpaa et al. 2016). The reasons for such high rates are likely multifactorial. The environmental consequences of having a chronic health condition (e.g. medication regimes, missed social developmental opportunities, and individual and family stress associated with managing the condition and its implications) can all have an understandable impact on mental wellbeing. However, rates of mental health difficulties in children with neurological conditions are significantly higher than in populations of children with other chronic health conditions, such as diabetes, who face similar environmental consequences (Davies, Heyman, and Goodman 2003). This finding supports the evidence that the disruption of cortical networks, for example by seizure activity or brain lesions, can have direct behavioural, emotional, and cognitive implications (O'Muircheartaigh and Richardson 2012). Mental health difficulties are more frequent in adolescents with epilepsy compared to adolescents with migraine, which strengthens the case of an independent association between mental health difficulties and seizures, over and above the associations between mental health and other neurological disorders (Wagner et al. 2014).

There is some evidence that structural or neurochemical changes may predispose individuals to both mental health presentations and epilepsy. Acute neurological events can also have a significant negative impact upon a child's mental health; children with acquired brain injury have significantly higher rates of anxiety and depression compared to neurotypical controls and many also present with clinically low self-concept (Hendry et al. 2020). Moreover, children with head trauma are at increased risk for developing post-traumatic stress disorder, which is also associated with several comorbid conditions including emotional disturbances, such as depression, and substance use disorders (Iljazi et al. 2020). Rates of mental health difficulties increase from childhood to adolescence in the general population but particularly in children with neurological disorder, which may reflect the impact of neurophysiological changes on mental health during puberty and an increase in psychosocial stressors during this life stage (Wagner et al. 2014).

The impact of neuroactive drugs on mental health and cognitive function must also be considered. The most commonly used medications prescribed by paediatric neurologists are ASMs, although children with neurological disorders may also be treated with a range of other medications such as stimulants, steroids, and analgesia; it is beyond the scope of this chapter to consider the impact of radiotherapy and chemotherapy for children with neuro-oncological presentations. ASMs aim to maximise seizure control, thereby reducing the risk of cognitive delay and improving quality of life, but may also induce or exacerbate cognitive or behavioural difficulties and drug interactions must be considered for those on more than one medication (Helmstaedter and Witt 2020). Sustained attention and processing speed are the cognitive domains most commonly impacted by ASMs (Helmstaedter and Witt 2020) and such difficulties will inevitably have a negative impact on academic performance and social functioning for children. ASMs can also affect mood; for example the use of ASMs has been linked to increased levels of suicidal ideation in adults with depression (Arana et al. 2010). Conversely, some ASMs are considered to act as a mood stabiliser so previously masked mental health difficulties may emerge if the medication is weaned.

Impact of Mental Health Disorders on Cognition

As with neurological disorders, the relationships between mental health and specific cognitive difficulties may be found at both the neurological and the environmental level. Mental health disorders can directly influence cognitive ability and also influence performance on psychometric assessment. Adolescents and young adults with depression have been found to have reduced cognitive capacity in the domains of episodic memory, working memory, executive functioning, and processing speed, but there is no consistent profile of impairment (Baune et al. 2014). Depression may result in a generally lowered cognitive profile, impairment within specific cognitive domains, or impairment on cognitively effortful tasks, in contrast to typical functioning on automatic tasks (Hammar and Årdal 2009). Similarly, low mood can result in lack of effort or motivation during cognitive assessment, which can undermine the validity of findings from neuropsychological assessment (see Chapter 23 on validity testing and ethical considerations).

The overlap between 'neurological' and 'psychiatric' disorders is increasingly apparent, with both cognitive and mental health difficulties recognised as symptoms of underlying 'brain dysfunction'. For example cognitive deficits, particularly in the domains of working memory, attention, and executive functioning, are key components of schizophrenia, possibly underpinned by disruption to cortical networks involving the dorsolateral prefrontal cortex (Barch and Ceaser 2012). Similarly, psychotic-type symptoms such as paranoia are characteristic early symptoms of anti-N-methyl-D-aspartate receptor encephalitis, whilst systemic lupus erythematosus can lead to bipolar-type symptoms (Najjar et al. 2013).

Sleep difficulties are also common in the context of both neurological disorders and mental health difficulties and can result in cognitive underperformance. Working memory, verbal recall, processing speed, and attention can be particularly impacted by sleep deprivation, functions that are key for successful classroom learning (Drummond and Brown 2001).

Impact of Cognitive Difficulties on Mental Health

Cognitive difficulties are common in children with epilepsy and other neurological disorders. Significant discrepancies between the expectations upon children and their ability to meet them can result in reduced self-esteem and subsequent associated mental health difficulties in children and young people.

An emerging literature has started to highlight the impact of specific learning disabilities on young peoples' mental health trajectories. For example children with nonverbal or reading disabilities have higher rates of anxiety and depression than typically developing peers (Mammarella et al. 2016). The impact of undiagnosed cognitive difficulties on mental health for children and young people may be even more significant; however, evidencing this via research is inherently challenging.

ASSESSMENT AND FORMULATION

Clinical assessment should be influenced by both the referral question and theoretical models associated with the neurological condition. Given the rates of mental health problems in children with neurological conditions, at a minimum, a screen for likely difficulties needs to be incorporated into any neuropsychological assessment. Standardised questionnaires are a simple and time-efficient method of screening, although questions about the reliability of standardised measures in those with co-occurring physical health conditions are raised. Specifically, there may be concerns that symptoms of the physical condition may overlap with items used to screen for mental health difficulties; for example tiredness could be a side effect of neurological dysfunction or a symptom of depression. A variety of different screening measures can be used clinically including the Child Behaviour Checklist (Achenbach 2014), the Strengths and Difficulties Questionnaire (Goodman 1999), the Revised Children's Anxiety and Depression Scale (Chorpita, Moffitt, and Gray 2005), and the Behavior Assessment System for Children, Third Edition (Reynolds and Kamphaus 2015). In addition, online comprehensive assessments such as the Development and Well-Being Assessment (Goodman et al. 2000) can offer a full screening prior to formal assessment. Canning and Kelleher (1994) reviewed the literature and found that whilst the Child Behaviour Checklist and Child Depression Inventory (Kovacs 1992) both had high specificity in this population, they had low sensitivity making them unreliable for screening purposes. The Strengths and Difficulties Questionnaire has been shown to be useful in both epilepsy and other chronic conditions with the proviso that multiple informants are used and that the total score rather than specific subscales are focused on (Reilly et al. 2014). For many measures there has been no specific research into this. As such, clinicians are advised to carefully read answers on screening questionnaires and use their clinical judgement in interpreting them rather than relying solely on cut-off scores.

Raised scores (or clinically judged red flags such as items related to suicidality) on screening measures, will need follow-up with a combination of clinical interview and standardised measures for more specific mental health problems. Much has been written on the assessment of mental health problems in young people. Separate interviews with the child/young person and parents are essential to obtain both perspectives on the child's functioning, as parent–child discrepancies are frequent, particularly in adolescence. In addition, mental health problems may be overlooked by families or schools as part of medical conditions rather than an independent concern. A good developmental history as well as a detailed picture of current functioning in social, emotional, and academic domains are essential.

Mental health difficulties can result in reduced engagement with the assessment process so must be considered and accommodated. Underperformance on testing can result either in data that is not usefully interpretable or in incorrect conclusions about a child's underlying cognitive abilities. Adjustments within the assessment process can help minimise the impact of mental health difficulties on performance, such as additional explanations about the purpose and potential positive impacts of the assessment to increase their motivation to engage. Children and young people with depressive or anxious symptoms may be distracted by negative rumination or the belief that they are 'bad' at a specific task. Scheduling the assessment for a time when the young person is most likely to be awake and alert is also important if their mental health disorder is associated with sleep impairment. For children and young people who present with clinical anxiety, good preparation about what to expect in addition to allowing a period of acclimatisation and 'settling in' to the assessment room is helpful.

Following the above principles, a cognitive assessment battery assessing intellectual functioning, episodic memory, attention, and executive functioning was administered. Sakura was found to have average range verbal and nonverbal reasoning and visual memory abilities, but her working memory, executive functioning, and attention scores fell in the low average range. Sakura's performances on subtests measuring psychomotor speed of processing fell in the low range. On verbal memory tests, Sakura recalled more information following a delay than she did immediately, with her immediate recall score falling in the impaired range and her delayed recall and recognition score in the borderline low range. A symptom validity test (Test of Memory Malingering; Tombaugh 1996) was administered as Sakura presented as ambivalent towards the assessment, but she passed all trials of the test.

Comprehensive neuropsychological formulations can inform evidence-based interventions that focus on the root of a child's difficulties, rather than responding to symptoms alone. The interaction between neurological disorder, cognitive dysfunction, psychopharmacology, systemic factors, and mental health difficulties is likely to be multifactorial with bidirectional interactions. For example Noeker et al. (2005) have highlighted many likely contributing components to mental health dysfunction in epilepsy. Comorbidities of neurological disorders, such as epilepsy, could perhaps be more usefully reconceptualised as a spectrum of symptoms of the condition, rather than being categorised as separate 'neurodevelopmental' and 'mental health difficulties' (Wagner et al. 2014), although the distinction persists in day-to-day clinical work.

The pattern of performance on neuropsychological assessment can provide useful evidence regarding the underlying causation of reported cognitive difficulties. For example the recall of greater volumes of information following a delay, compared to immediate recall, is inconsistent with organic amnesic difficulties, where the reverse would be expected but may reflect the impact of anxiety on performance. Inconsistencies between cognitive performances in different settings (i.e. a child may be able to complete maths tasks at home but struggle with the same task under exam conditions) can also point towards functional cognitive difficulties being underpinned by mental health, rather than organic, difficulties.

A negative cycle may develop for children and young people in which cognitive difficulties impact on attainment, which can increase anxiety and/or lower their self-esteem and mood, which subsequently reduces motivation and the ability to focus, leading to further academic difficulties (Fig. 19.1). Equally, neurological disorders may underpin both cognitive and mental health difficulties. Formulation around the likely cause and effect of difficulties is important to inform the level at which intervention is most likely to be helpful, particularly if resources are limited. Often it is initially difficult to identify the pattern of cause and effect, but response to treatment can help to clarify the picture over time. For example cognitive assessment could be repeated once symptoms of low mood or anxiety have been reduced via intervention to determine if findings of the initial cognitive assessment had been influenced by the child or young person's mental health.

Case Study – Sakura

In Sakura's case, an individual interview with her allowed disclosure of self-harm and hopelessness. Questions about biological factors such as sleep and appetite disruption in addition to parental report about withdrawal from family life and reduced participation in previously enjoyed activities highlighted depression. Use of the Strengths and Difficulties Questionnaire as well as the Revised Children's Anxiety and Depression Scale highlighted a high likelihood of mental health problems and specifically clinically significant depression symptoms. Using the International Classification of Diseases, 10th Revision/Diagnostic and Statistical Manual of Mental Disorders, Fifth Edition, Sakura met diagnostic criteria for a major depressive disorder. Knowledge of her specific symptoms informed the plan for cognitive assessment; specifically, the assessment was rescheduled to a time when she was less emotionally overwhelmed, breaks were offered when it was noted that negative rumination was impacting on her performance at assessment, and a performance validity test was administered to assess the likely validity of neuropsychological test findings.

For Sakura, many years of uncontrolled epilepsy and polypharmacy appeared to have resulted in cognitive compromise, affecting her attention and the efficiency with which she could process information. Whilst there was no evidence of a loss of skills over time, her rate of development in some cognitive domains had been slower than same-aged peers and unsuccessful trials of polypharmacy may have exacerbated the difficulties. Sakura's underlying neurological dysfunction is likely to have had a direct impact on her mental health, but environmental factors, such as the reduction of learning support as her seizures came under control and increasing awareness of the difference between her and her peers as she got older, are also likely to have been significant contributors. Sakura's previously undiagnosed cognitive difficulties, in conjunction with high expectations from her parents and teachers, had resulted in depressive and often self-critical thinking styles, which negatively impacted on her performances on tasks. This pattern was apparent in her performance on verbal memory tasks in which she performed better at delayed recall, when she perceived less pressure to remember everything, compared with immediate recall.

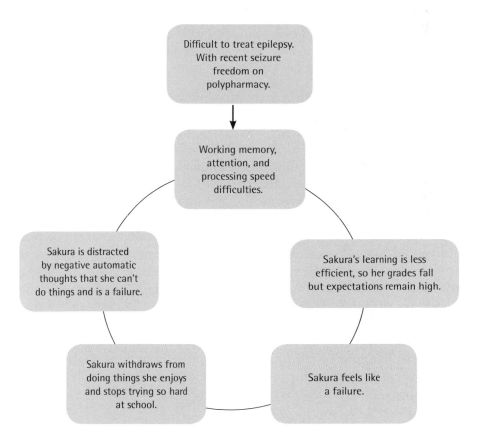

Figure 19.1 Psychological formulation of the 'vicious cycle' relationship between Sakura's neurological, cognitive, and mental health difficulties.

INTERVENTION AND MANAGEMENT

The neurodevelopmental and mental health comorbidities associated with neurological disorders can have a significant negative impact on quality of life, possibly even to a greater extent than the medical presentation themselves (Barch and Ceaser 2012; Wagner et al. 2014), so interventions to address them are essential. Close coworking between neuropsychologists, neurologists, clinical psychologists, psychiatrists, and educational psychologists is helpful to provide multifaceted interventions to improve quality of life for the child or young person (e.g. reviewing a child's ASM and seizure control concurrently to prescribing anxiolytic medication, provision of talking therapy, and the introduction of educational support for a child with epilepsy, high levels of anxiety, and school avoidance).

Despite the high rates of psychiatric disorders in children with neurological difficulties, evidence suggests that many of these go undetected or untreated, with, for example, one study showing that 60% of children with epilepsy who met criteria for a psychiatric disorder (on screening) never having had any contact with a mental health professional (Ott et al. 2003). Children with neurological conditions or other physical health problems are often excluded from randomised controlled trials of evidence-based interventions on the basis of comorbidity and there appears to be a belief amongst some clinicians that such interventions will not work for them.

Increasingly, research has established a number of evidence-based psychological interventions for mental health problems in children and adolescents. It is beyond the scope of this chapter to review these in detail here, but they have then been supported in various national guidelines for treatment. For example in the UK the National Institute of Clinical Excellence guidelines recommend cognitive behavioural therapy (CBT) for childhood social anxiety disorders, CBT for depression in adolescents (with interpersonal therapy, psychodynamic therapies, and family therapy as second-line treatment options), and parenting-based interventions for behavioural disorders in young children. Research on the application of evidence-based mental health treatment for children and adolescents with neurological conditions is, however, depressingly sparse. A number of small-scale studies and single case studies (primarily in children with epilepsy) provide some preliminary evidence that CBT is a safe and effective intervention for anxiety and depression in this group (e.g. Chorpita and Weisz 2009; Blocher et al. 2013), but there is much further work to do. Heyman et al. (2015) highlight that whilst evidence that standard treatments work for children and young people with neurological conditions is lacking, there is even less evidence that they do not work. In this situation the most parsimonious and ethical solution seems to be to offer those with neurological conditions the same evidenced-based treatments those without would receive.

The majority of studies investigating interventions targeting specific cognitive domains (e.g. working memory) for children with neurological disorders demonstrate short-term improvements on similar tasks but little long-term gain or generalisation to academic, behavioural, or social performance (Robinson et al. 2014). Cognitive interventions have the most impact for children who start with the highest level of impairment (Robinson et al. 2014). More systemic or skills-based interventions, such as reducing the working memory load in the classroom or providing training in the use of external memory aids help to locate the problem in the environment, and may therefore be more acceptable and accessible for those with comorbid mental health difficulties. Recently, innovations in the delivery of treatment have utilised teletherapy for delivery of intervention (Bennett et al. 2021a; Bennett et al. 2021b), which is an area with potential, but far more research is needed around uptake and successful delivery (see Chapter 24 for more detail on teleneuropsychology).

Case Study – Clinical Application

Feedback to Sakura and her family focussed on the interrelatedness of her depression, cognitive difficulties, and epilepsy. The context of her receiving less support following the resolution of her seizures was discussed and appropriate support recommended. Recommendations for increased counselling support at school, a reduced timetable, extra time in exams, and time limits on the time she spent on homework were discussed. Strategies to reduce the attentional and working memory demands on Sakura in the classroom were disseminated to her teachers; for example the use of a dictaphone, homework being set via an electronic learning platform, and having task instructions in front of her. An educational psychology review was recommended to translate the findings of the assessment into an Individual Education Plan and a targeted intervention to address gaps in her math abilities. Sakura was referred to her local child and adolescent mental health service with a recommendation that she be offered a CBT-based intervention for depression with an emphasis on behavioural activation; liaison with the mental health professional helped them to understand the formulation and to recognise that the primary mental health disorder was related to but not fully explained by the neurological disorder. Adjustment of delivery of the intervention to consider her attention, working memory, and processing speed difficulties was suggested. Possible adjustments included offering more sessions so less needed to be covered per session and involving parents and digital strategies to help Sakura recall content from the sessions. A self-help book, covering psychoeducation about depression, sleep hygiene, and behavioural activation was provided for Sakura and her parents whilst they waited for treatment.

Outcome

Following the assessment, Sakura and important people around her had a better understanding of her needs. The pressure that Sakura perceived to be upon her was reduced. Sakura dropped two subjects at school, which allowed her more time for homework and revision, and she was back on track to achieve passes in all exams. Sakura responded well to the CBT intervention. At 1-year follow-up, she was back to socialising and participating in extracurricular activities, she had stopped self-harming, and reported her mood was more stable. Both Sakura and her parents were positive about her future but were aware that the depression could return. However, this time, as part of a relapse management, they were aware of the process by which they could access support.

SUMMARY

Cases such as Sakura's demonstrate the often complex relationship between neurological, cognitive, and emotional difficulties. If a child or young person presents with neurological and cognitive difficulties, it is essential to consider potential comorbid mental health difficulties. Similarly, it is important to consider cognitive difficulties as a mediating factor if a child or young person presents with mental health difficulties in the context of neurological disorder. Failing to consider each of these components may undermine the success of any interventions. For example providing talking therapy for a child with depression and a neurological disorder may fail to make much of an impact if the child's specific learning difficulties, which make life difficult for them at school, are not also identified and addressed. Increasing recognition that mental health and cognitive difficulties are potentially intrinsic symptoms of neurological disorders will hopefully elevate the weight given to addressing these difficulties and reduce the unhelpful distinctions between psychiatric and neurological health. Consideration of the systemic influences on a child's difficulties is equally as important as environmental adjustments can significantly increase quality of life, particularly in the context of intractable neurological disorders.

Whilst there is limited evidence specifically identifying mental health interventions for children and young people with neurological difficulties, children and young people should not be automatically denied access to psychological or pharmacological interventions for mental health difficulties on the grounds of comorbid neurological difficulties. Reasonable adjustments should be made to make psychological interventions accessible for children and young people with specific cognitive difficulties, for example providing written summaries of sessions for those with memory difficulties or using fewer written materials for those with specific reading difficulties.

Mental health difficulties continue to be chronically underdetected in children with neurological disorders (Ott et al. 2003). This is an area that must continue to be highlighted with neurologists and service commissioners with the aim of moving towards a criterion standard of the provision of mental health screening programs in all neurology clinics, particularly for children and young people with epilepsy. Further research on the effectiveness of interventions for those with mental health difficulties is also urgently needed, and in the meantime ensuring those with neurological difficulties have equitable access to mental health services compared to their physically well counterparts is key.

REFERENCES

Arana A, Wentworth CE, Ayuso-Mateos JL, Arellano FM (2010) Suicide-related events in patients treated with antiepileptic drugs. *The New England Journal of Medicine* **363**: 542–551.

Barch DM, Ceaser A (2012) Cognition in schizophrenia: Core psychological and neural mechanisms. *Trends in Cognitive Science* **16**: 27–34.

Baune BT, Fuhr M, Air T, Hering C (2014) Neuropsychological functioning in adolescents and young adults with major depressive disorder – A review. *Psychiatry Research* **218**: 261–271.

Bennett S, Heyman I, Varadkar S, Coughtrey A, Walji F, Shafran R (2021a) Guided self-help teletherapy for behavioural difficulties in children with epilepsy. *J Clin Psychol Med Settings* **28**(3): 477-490. doi: 10.1007/s10880-021-09768-2.

Bennett SD, Heyman I, Coughtrey AE et al. (2021b) Telephone-guided self-help for mental health difficulties in neurological conditions: A randomised pilot trial. *Arch Dis Child* **106**(9): 862–867. doi: 10.1136/archdischild-2019-318577.

Blocher JB, Fujikawa M, Sung C, Jackson DC, Jones JE (2013) Computer-assisted cognitive behaviour therapy for children with epilepsy and anxiety: A pilot study. *Epilepsy & Behaviour* **26**: 70–76.

Canning EH, Kelleher K (1994) Performance of screening tools for mental health problems in chronically ill children. *Arch Pediatr Adolesc Med* **148**(3): 272–278.

Chorpita BF, Weisz JR (2009) *Modular Approach to Therapy for Children with Anxiety, Depression, Trauma or Conduct Problems (MATCH-ADTC)*. Satellite Beach, FL: PracticeWise LLC.

Davies S, Heyman I, Goodman R (2003) A population survey of mental health problems in children with epilepsy. *Developmental Medicine & Child Neurology* **45**: 292–295.

Drummond SPA, Brown GG (2001) The effects of total sleep deprivation on cerebral responses to cognitive performance. *Neuropsychopharmacology* **25**: s68–s73.

Hammar Å, Årdal G (2009) Cognitive functioning in major depression – a summary. *Frontiers in Human Neuroscience* **3**: 1–7.

Helmstaedter C, Witt J-A (2020) Anticonvulsant drugs and cognition. In: Riederer P, Laux G, Mulsant B, Le W, Nagatsu T, editors, *Neuropsychopharmacotherapy*. Cham: Springer. https://ezproxy-prd.bodleian.ox.ac.uk:2102/10.1007/978-3-319-56015-1_375-1.

Hendry K, Ownsworth T, Waters AM, Jackson M, Lloyd O (2020) Investigation of children and adolescents' mood and self-concept after acquired brain injury. *Child Neuropsychology* **26**: 1005–1025.

Heyman I, Skuse D, Goodman R et al. (2015) Brain disorders and psychopathology. In: Thapar A, Pine D, Leckman J et al., editors, *Rutter's Child Adolescent Psychiatry*. Chichester: Wiley, pp. 389–402.

Iljazi A, Ashina H, Al-Khazali H, Ashina M, Schytz H, Ashina S (2020) Post-traumatic stress disorder attributed to traumatic brain injury in children: A systematic review. *Brain Injury* **34**(7): 857–863.

Kovacs M (1992) *Children's Depression Inventory*. North Tonawanda, NY: Multi-Health Systems, Inc.

Mammarella IC, Ghisi M, Bomba M et al. (2016) Anxiety and depression in children with nonverbal learning disabilities, reading disabilities or typical development. *Journal of Learning Disabilities* **49**: 130–139.

Najjar S, Pearlman D, Alper K, Najjar A, Devinsky O (2013) Neuroinflammation and psychiatric illness. *Journal of Neuroinflammation* **10**: 43.

Noeker M, Haverkamp-Krois A, Haverkamp F (2005) Development of mental health dysfunction in childhood epilepsy. *Brain and Development* **27**(1): 5–16.

O'Muircheartaigh J, Richardson MP (2012) Epilepsy and the frontal lobes. *Cortex* **48**: 144–155.

Ott D, Siddarth P, Gurbani S et al. (2003) Behavioural disorders in paediatric epilepsy: Unmet psychiatric need. *Epilepsia* **44**(4): 591–597.

Reilly C, Atkinson P, Das KB et al. (2014) Screening for mental health disorders in active childhood epilepsy: Population-based data. *Epilepsy Research* **108**: 1917–1926.

Robinson KE, Kaizar E, Catroppa C, Godfrey C, Yeates KO (2014) Systematic review and meta-analysis of cognitive interventions for children with central nervous system disorders and neurodevelopmental disorders. *Journal of Paediatric Psychology* **39**: 846–865.

Sillanpaa M, Besag F, Aldenkamp A, Caplan R, Dunn D, Gobbi G (2016) Psychiatric and behaviour disorders in children with epilepsy (ILEA Task Force Report): Epidemiology of psychiatric/behavioural disorder in children with epilepsy. *Epileptic Disorders* **18**(1): S2–S7.

Wagner JL, Wilson DA, Smith G, Malek A, Selassie AW (2014) Neurodevelopmental and mental health comorbidities in children and adolescents with epilepsy and migraine: A response to identified research gaps. *Developmental Medicine & Child Neurology* **57**: 45–52.

CHAPTER 20

Intellectual Disability

Kyle Deane, Lindsay Katz, and Scott Hunter

Presenting Concern

Mary is a 7-year-old girl who was referred by her paediatric psychiatrist for a neuropsychological evaluation in light of her parents' increasing concerns regarding her sleep, self-injurious behaviours, academic performance, high activity level, and behavioural problems. Mary was born at term at a normal weight following an uncomplicated pregnancy and delivery. She was not exposed to drugs, alcohol, tobacco, or medications while in utero. Concerns were noted early on about dysmorphic facial features. A developmental screening test was completed when Mary was 19 months of age revealing delays in language, social, and motor development. A magnetic resonance imaging scan around the same time noted mild, diffuse prominence of subarachnoid spaces and mild prominence of the ventricular system. Finally, genetic testing completed when Mary was 2 years of age revealed a partial deletion of the short arm of chromosome 4, otherwise known as Wolf-Hirschhorn syndrome.

Mary continues to demonstrate developmental delays. She is unable to walk smoothly. She has a vocabulary of around 20 words but primarily uses gestures to communicate. Her parents believe that her receptive language is much better developed than her expressive language, based on their shared observations. She is able to consistently follow single-step directives. Mary has been in speech therapy, occupational therapy, and physical therapy addressing these concerns since 1 year of age.

Mary has some difficulty sleeping. She uses melatonin but still requires around an hour to fall asleep each night. Mary often wakes up in the middle of the night at random intervals. Her appetite is poor. Her parents also noted that she does not have a physical or facial reaction when tasting strong flavours such as trying sour candy or spicy food. Her teachers voiced some concern that Mary demonstrates occasional unusual ocular movements whilst also appearing briefly unresponsive. Mary exhibits some mild sensory sensitivities, including being upset by certain loud noises, such as a hair dryer. Mary does not show particular interest in playing with others, including her younger sister, and does not engage in reciprocal play. Nevertheless, she does seem to enjoy being around others.

Mary has received special education services with an Individualised Education Plan under the label 'Developmental Delay' since 3 years of age. Her teachers note that Mary can match and identify letters of the alphabet from a field of three. She can identify 25 sight words when paired with pictures. She is able to rote count and sequence numbers 1 through 10. Her teachers are currently attempting to teach her functional skills, including money and telling time.

The parents report that Mary's school has been contacting them about increasing outbursts where she hits her head and bites herself. They stated that Mary has bitten others on occasion at school as well. These outbursts typically follow a change in routine during the day and have been more frequent over the past 6 months. Parents also acknowledged that Mary's behaviour has become more challenging at home. Mary has been unable to self-regulate, greatly affecting her ability to focus and learn. Her teachers reported that she frequently needs redirection in order to stay on task. Her parents are seeking assistance in understanding how to best support Mary's developmental, behavioural, and educational needs.

THEORY

Defining Intelligence and Adaptive Functioning

Characteristics of intelligence include the ability to comprehend abstract ideas, recognise patterns, learn from experience, and engage in various forms of reasoning in order to achieve goals in a wide range of environments (Neisser et al. 1996). There is no clear consensus across or within fields about how to define or measure intelligence. Nonetheless, intelligence may be broadly characterised as an individual's ability to achieve goals in a wide range of environments.

Related to this construct, the concept of adaptive functioning refers to a collection of conceptual skills (e.g. expressive language, memory, and problem-solving), social skills (e.g. interpersonal communication, empathy, and social judgment), and practical skills (e.g. personal care, money management, recreation, school, and word task organisation) that are learned and performed by people in their daily lives (American Association on Intellectual and Developmental Disabilities 2010; American Psychiatric Association 2013). Adaptive behaviour can be understood as how an individual functions independently and meets personal and social responsibilities based on culture and age. In other words, this construct refers to competency in meeting one's needs and social demands (Sattler 2014). Adaptive behaviour is not independent of intelligence, and the two constructs are highly correlated (Harrison and Oakland 2015). That being said, whilst intelligence influences adaptive functioning, education, socialisation, and cultural experience also contribute to overall adaptive functioning (Sattler 2014).

Intellectual Disability

Intellectual disability, which has replaced the former term of 'mental retardation', describes conditions with onset during the developmental period characterised by deficits in intelligence and adaptive behaviour (World Health Organization 2003; American

Psychiatric Association 2013; Sattler 2014). To assess intelligence, modern-day intelligence tests are standardised on stratified samples designed to reflect current population in terms of sex, socioeconomic status, ethnicity, and educational attainment of the parent. A standard bell curve model, with a mean of 100 and a standard deviation of 15, is typically employed to determine IQ scores.

Guidelines from the American Association on Intellectual and Developmental Disabilities, the International Statistical Classification of Diseases and Related Health Problems, 10th Revision (World Health Organization 2003), and the Diagnostic and Statistical Manual of Mental Disorders, Fifth Edition (DSM-5; American Psychiatric Association 2013), have moved beyond assigning an IQ score to determine intellectual disability (the current International Classification of Diseases, 11th Edition, uses the label 'intellectual developmental disorder') and requires deficits in both intellectual and adaptive functioning originating in the developmental period. In fact, the IQ test was removed altogether from the diagnostic criteria of intellectual disability though the concept of IQ in the description of the disorder remains. In doing so, clinicians are encouraged to emphasise daily functioning over intellectual capacity and move away from arbitrary cut-offs based on IQ scores and standard deviations. Nonetheless, IQ testing is a critical component of a thorough neuropsychological evaluation. The DSM-5 allows further specification of mild, moderate, severe, or Profound based on level of conceptual, social, and practical skills (see Table 20.1). In addition to deficits

Table 20.1 Clinical characteristics for individuals of differing intellectual disability severity

Level of intellectual disability	Percentage of population with intellectual disability	Language development	Academic skills	Living skills and employment
Mild	~85%	Some delay; fluency by adolescence; minimal impairment	May acquire academic skills up to 6th grade level (~11 years of age)	May need supervision or guidance
Moderate	~10%	Functional language by adolescence	May acquire academic skills up to a 2nd grade level (~7 years of age)	Moderate supervision required
Severe	~3–4%	Limited	May become familiar with simple counting and alphabet	Close supervision required
Profound	~1–2%	May learn single words	None	Pervasive supervision required

Adapted from Janke and Jacola (2018). Based on American Psychiatric Association (2013) and World Health Organization (2003).

in adaptive functioning, multiple domains of intellectual abilities may be impacted, including visual spatial skills, language, executive functions, attention, memory, as well as emotional and behavioural regulation.

Neuroanatomy

Whilst it is difficult to determine neuroanatomical correlates of general intelligence, structural neuroimaging has identified a modest correlation between intelligence and brain volume across the lifespan (McDaniel 2005). In typically developing children, research has documented a relationship between changes in cortical thickness and scores on measures of intelligence (Shaw et al. 2006). Using functional magnetic resonance imaging Shaw and colleagues (2006) found that children of highest intelligence have superior levels of brain plasticity, characterised by a longer phase of increased cortical thickening, followed by equally intense cortical thinning during early adolescence.

Many nonidiopathic cases of intellectual disability (e.g. genetic syndromes) are associated with specific patterns of abnormal neuroanatomical development and activation patterns related to cognitive deficits (Kesler et al. 2011). Across intellectual disability syndromes, abnormalities in lateralisation and specialisation have been reported, ultimately leading to a lack of automaticity over time (Somers et al. 2015). In their review, Dierssen and Ramakers (2006) highlighted evidence for abnormal neuronal connectivity, including a suboptimal number of connections as well as an increased number of inappropriate neuronal connections, amongst individuals with intellectual disability.

Prevalence and Aetiology

Approximately 1% to 3% of the global population meets criteria for intellectual disability. A meta-analysis of 52 populated-based studies conducted between 1980 and 2009 found the overall average to fall at 1.04%; however, this may vary depending on region, socioeconomic status, and age (Maulik et al. 2011). Of note, studies conducted with children and adolescents had a higher prevalence rate compared to adults. A diagnosis of global developmental delay typically precedes a diagnosis of intellectual disability for children under the age of 5 years. This label is utilised to account for the lack of stability in IQ during this developmental period (Williams, 2010).

Males appear to be approximately 1.2 times more affected than females (Boyle et al. 2011). The most current estimated prevalence of intellectual disability falls at 1.48% for males and 0.9% for females (Zablotsky et al. 2017). These observed sex differences might be partially explained by sex-linked genetic causes of intellectual disability, particularly those that are X-linked, in addition to central nervous system differences (Durkin et al. 2007). While estimates vary, between 66% and 84% of individuals with intellectual disability fall in the mild range (Rojahn, Medeiros, and Farmer 2016). Individuals with moderate impairment make up 10% of the group, and 5% of individuals have moderate to profound impairments (Rojahn et al. 2016). Furthermore, individuals with intellectual disability are more likely to present with comorbid medical conditions and other health needs compared to children without intellectual disability, particularly those who fall in the moderate to profound range of intellectual impairment (Janke and Jacola 2018).

Idiopathic Intellectual Disability

A notable challenge in the field of intellectual disability is understanding and identifying aetiology, as 50% of cases are idiopathic (Mefford et al. 2012; Janke and Jacola 2018). Understanding the various aetiologies of intellectual disability is important for clinicians as it relates to developing impressions and providing recommendations. In idiopathic cases, there is often a family history of intellectual disability, suggestive of a genetic component in the development of intellectual disability. A disproportionate number of children with intellectual disability are from a low socioeconomic background, which may suggest an environmental impact as well (Janke and Jacola 2018). There is research suggesting that variance in IQ related to ethnicity may be attributed to socioeconomic disparities (Boyle et al. 2011).

Genetic Disorders

Of the other 50% of nonidiopathic cases of intellectual disability, about 25% to 50% of cases result from a genetic disorder, including chromosomal aberrations, single gene disorders, and genetic disorders of metabolism (Reichenberg 2016; Janke and Jacola 2018). These cases typically fall in the severe or profound range of functioning. Whilst over 1000 genetic causes of intellectual disability have been identified, notable specific genetic disorders associated with intellectual disability include Down syndrome, Fragile X syndrome, Angelman syndrome, Prader–Willi syndrome, Williams syndrome, 22q11 deletion syndrome, and others (see Table 20.2).

Prenatal and Early Childhood Factors

Prenatal exposure to substances also contributes to intellectual disability, with prenatal exposure to alcohol thought to be the most common nonhereditary cause of intellectual disability (see Chapter 16). Preterm birth, delivery complications, and maternal infection also contribute to intellectual disability prevalence, with the highest rates of intellectual disability among those born at less than 29 weeks gestation who are of low birthweight. Depending on the time of injury and exposure, childhood factors including exposure to environmental toxins and acquired brain injury contribute to the development of intellectual disability (Janke and Jacola 2018).

Table 20.2 Common syndromes and disorders associated with intellectual disability

Condition	Prevalence	Description
Down syndrome	1 in every 700 live births[a]	Additional copy of chromosome 21
Fragile X syndrome	1 in every 3600 live births[b]	Fragile mental retardation 1 gene (*FMR1*) becomes inactivated due to large number of repeats
Angelman syndrome	1 in every 24 000 live births[c]	Hemizygous microdeletion on chromosome 15 of maternal origin
Prader–Willi syndrome	1 in every 25 000 live births[d]	Hemizygous deletion on the paternal chromosome 15
Williams syndrome	1 in every 7500 live births[e]	Hemizygous microdeletion of at least 20 genes on chromosome 7q11.23
22q11 deletion syndrome	1 in every 4000 live births[f]	Microdeletion on chromosome 22q11
Autism spectrum disorder	1 in every 44 children at age 8 years[g]	Multiple genetic and environmental risk factors; majority of cases are idiopathic

[a]Parker et al. (2010). [b]Fernandez-Carvajal et al. (2009). [c]Mertz, Christensen, and Vogel (2013). [d]Butler (1990). [e]Strømme (2002). [f]Oskarsdóttir, Vujic, and Fasth (2004). [g]Maenner et al. (2021).

Common Comorbidities

Individuals with intellectual disability are vulnerable to many comorbid psychiatric conditions, including mood and behavioural disorders, psychotic disorders, and other neurodevelopmental disorders due to common genetic and environmental factors. Approximately one-third of individuals with intellectual disability meet criteria for another psychiatric condition and are three to four times more likely to meet criteria for a psychiatric condition compared to the general population (Harris 2014). Specifically, mood and anxiety disorders are often under- or misdiagnosed but appear to be more common in specific intellectual disability syndromes. Disruptive and conduct disorders are significantly more common among individuals with intellectual disability compared to the general population, with one study finding that 25% of individuals with intellectual disability met criteria for any conduct disorder, compared to 4.2% in the general population (Emerson 2003). The prevalence of psychotic disorders is generally similar; however, individuals with intellectual disability tend to have earlier onset and less favourable outcomes (Harris 2014).

Common neurodevelopmental disorders associated with intellectual disability are autism spectrum disorder (ASD) and attention-deficit/hyperactivity disorder. The majority of individuals with ASD fall in the broadly average range of intellectual functioning and present with a wide range of intellectual abilities (Ozonoff 2010); however, intellectual disability is present in approximately 35% of cases (Maenner et al. 2021). In contrast to intellectual disability prevalence in the general population, females with ASD are more likely to present with intellectual disability compared to males (Fombonne 2009; Loomes et al. 2017). Individuals with intellectual disability often present with symptoms consistent with a diagnosis of attention-deficit/hyperactivity disorder, including inattention and impulsivity (Huang and Ruedrich 2007; Deutsch et al. 2008), with some studies finding that children with intellectual disability are at increased risk for the diagnosis of attention-deficit/hyperactivity disorder (Neece et al. 2011), whilst other findings suggest that it may be similar overall but more prevalent in specific intellectual disability syndromes (Harris 2014).

ASSESSMENT AND FORMULATION

Neuropsychological assessment of intelligence may involve the examination of a child's discrete performance across a wide range of domains simultaneously, including visual spatial skills, language, executive functions, attention, memory, emotional/behavioural development, and general intellectual functioning. Whilst the clinical features of Wolf-Hirschhorn syndrome are described in the literature (see Zollino et al. 2008), it is a rare disorder and a neuropsychological profile has not been established. Thus, Mary's case required consideration of performance across all domains of functioning, as well as a comprehensive interview with her parents in order to obtain relevant medical, academic, and social history. We also reviewed pertinent medical and school records. In addition, Mary's parents and teacher completed standardised questionnaires to assess Mary's social-emotional, behavioural, adaptive, and executive functioning in daily life. Specifically, parents and teacher completed relevant forms of the Behavior Assessment System for Children, Third Edition (Reynolds and Kamphaus 2015), the Behavior Rating Inventory of Executive Functioning, Second Edition (Gioia et al. 2015), and the Scales of Independent Behavior, Revised (SIB-R) (Bruininks et al. 1996). The SIB-R covers 14 subscales, which are organised into four adaptive behaviour clusters, including Motor Skills, Personal Living Skills, Social Interaction and Communication Skills, and Community Living Skills. Parent and teacher ratings on the Adaptive Behavior Full Scale score from the SIB-R revealed Mary's independent functioning as falling in the severely impaired range consistent with her cognitive abilities. Overall, the scores were much lower than would be expected given Mary's age. Of note, behavioural observations were also closely documented given their importance to diagnosing an intellectual disability. Table 20.3 presents brief descriptions of frequently administered questionnaires used to assess adaptive functioning skills.

Typical clinical features outlined in cognitive-behavioural profiles of Wolf-Hirschhorn syndrome and other subtelomeric microdeletions reveal mild to profound intellectual disabilities with particularly limited speech and language skills (Zollino et al. 2008). Due to Mary's deficits in spoken language, a nonverbal measure of intelligence, the Leiter International Performance Scale, Third Edition (Roid et al. 2013), was administered to better assess Mary's overall cognitive abilities. While start points for item sets are based on chronological age on some instruments, such as the Leiter International

Table 20.3 Commonly used questionnaires to assess adaptive functioning

	Age range (y)	Description
Adaptive Behavior Assessment System, Third Edition (ABAS-III)	*Parent/Primary Caregiver Form:* 0–5 *Teacher/Daycare Provider Form:* 2–5 *Parent/Teacher Form:* 5–21 *Adult Form:* 16–89	Conceptual, social, and practical skills
Vineland Adaptive Behavior Scales, Third Edition (Vineland-3)	*Parent/Interview Form:* 0–90 *Teacher Form:* 3–21	Communication, daily living skills, socialisation, and motor skills
Scales of Independent Behavior, Revised (SIB-R)	3mo–80+	Motor, social/ communication, personal living, community living, and maladaptive indexes

Performance Scale, Third Edition, these can be altered based on the examiner's clinical judgement of the child's actual ability level. Overall, Mary demonstrated moderately impaired cognitive abilities (standard score=46, <1st percentile). Table 20.4 presents a brief description of other commonly administered measures to assess intellectual functioning. Again, while intellectual and developmental tests are integral facets of an intellectual disability evaluation, they may prove less useful than domain-specific neuropsychological tests for drawing inferences regarding brain function and range of competencies. Thus, other domains were assessed with Mary during this evaluation using the following additional instruments: Autism Diagnostic Observation Schedule, Second Edition (ADOS-2®) (Lord et al. 2012), the Beery-Buktenica Developmental Test of Visual Motor Integration, Sixth Edition (Beery et al. 2010), the Bracken Basic Concept Scale, Third Edition (Bracken 2006), the Expressive One-Word Picture Vocabulary Test, Fourth Edition (Martin and Brownell 2010), and the Peabody Picture Vocabulary Test, Fourth Edition (Dunn and Dunn 2007).

Given her difficulty with attention and social interaction, Mary struggled to engage in some assessment activities, which can be a common problem inherent in intellectual disability assessment. Due to this limitation, the results were interpreted with caution and used as a baseline rather than an estimate of optimal cognitive potential. Moreover, as with all testing involving intellectual disability, there are a number of differential diagnoses whose symptom presentation, such as social communication and behaviour deficits, may interfere with performance on neuropsychological measures. These include ASD, communication disorder, a specific learning disorder, and neurocognitive disorders, all of which were considered diagnostically. In terms of her developmental functioning, Mary demonstrated significant developmental delays across all areas of functioning with her cognitive functioning on testing falling between the 2 and 4-year-old level and her adaptive functioning in daily life as assessed by her teacher falling

Table 20.4 Commonly used measures to assess intellectual and developmental functioning

	Age range (y or y:mo)	Description
Wechsler Preschool and Primary Scales of Intelligence, Fourth Edition (WPPSI-IV)	2:6–7:7	Verbal comprehension, visual spatial, fluid reasoning, working memory, and processing speed
Wechsler Intelligence Scale for Children, Fifth Edition (WISC-V)	6:0–16:11	Verbal comprehension, visual spatial, fluid reasoning, working memory, and processing speed
Wechsler Adult Intelligence Scale, Fourth Edition (WAIS-IV)	16–90	Verbal comprehension, perceptual reasoning, working memory, and processing speed
British Ability Scales, Third Edition (BAS-3)	3–17	Verbal ability, nonverbal reasoning ability, and spatial ability
Differential Ability Scale, Second Edition (DAS-II)[a]	*Early Years:* 2:6–6:11 *School Age:* 7:0–17:11	Verbal, nonverbal, and spatial
Leiter International Performance Scale, Third Edition (Leiter-3)	3–75+	Nonverbal IQ, nonverbal attention, and nonverbal memory
Mullen Scales of Early Learning (MSEL)[a]	0–5:8	Visual reception, receptive language, expressive language, fine motor, and gross motor
Bayley Scales of Infant Development, Fourth Edition (Bayley-4)	0:1–3:6	Cognitive, language, motor, social-emotional, and adaptive behaviour
Stanford–Binet, Fifth Edition (SB-5)	2–85+	Fluid reasoning, knowledge, quantitative reasoning, visual spatial, and working memory

[a]Can be administered out of age range to calculate age equivalencies.

between the 1 and 4-year-old level. Based on her history and evaluation results, Mary met criteria for a diagnosis of Moderate Intellectual Disability (DSM-5 318.01). While the aetiology of Mary's neurocognitive profile is not entirely clear, it is likely that Mary's cognitive impairment is related not to another underlying diagnosis but rather to her medical history.

INTERVENTION AND MANAGEMENT

Overall, intellectual disability cannot be cured but is instead supported through a set of interventions and adaptations that are focused on promoting optimal outcomes. Often, the emphasis is on the acquisition of functional living skills as well as broader skills that will allow the most successful engagement with the broader social and vocational environments the individual engages with daily. There are a variety of evidenced-based services and treatments that families with children with intellectual disability can pursue to promote development.

Neuropsychological Intervention

The primary goal of neuropsychological intervention for this population is to identify specific recommendations for children across home, school, and community environments. Evaluations may have an inherent therapeutic effect as well (see Chapter 25). For example during feedback neuropsychologists can empower parents to seek services and provide psychoeducation and diagnostic clarification. For children with intellectual disability, much of the recommendations provided involve family-centred care and parent-focused interventions in addition to educational interventions. Mary's parents were encouraged to share the results of the evaluation with other providers as well as school teachers in order to organise support services. Ultimately, a significant role of the paediatric neuropsychologist in a multidisciplinary setting is to recognise the cognitive and adaptive level of the child at the point of assessment, focus on skill development across multiple domains, and seek to guide a community-oriented integrational approach to intervention designed to promote maximal independence.

Cognitive and Behavioural Interventions

Based on clinical and standardised observations of ability, it was recommended that Mary receive applied behaviour analysis (ABA) from a licensed provider in order to meet behaviour and social communication goals. ABA refers to a behavioural intervention based on learning theory principles including contingency management and identifying and altering antecedent conditions (Miltenberger 2012). The overall goal of ABA for those with intellectual disability is to decrease problem behaviour and increase desired behaviour whilst also teaching and reinforcing new skills (Storey and Miner 2011), which was deemed crucial to support a positive outcome for Mary. Additionally, it was suggested that ABA would help the family to develop appropriate expectations for Mary. We also recommended that she receive intensive school-based and private individual speech/language therapy if possible.

While cognitive behaviour therapy has been implemented with adults with intellectual disability (Hassiotis et al. 2013; Koslowski et al. 2016), there is a lack of randomised controlled trials using cognitive behaviour therapy to treat psychiatric illness among children with intellectual disability, despite the fact that these children are more likely to present with emotional and behavioural challenges compared to their typically developing peers (Oeseburg et al. 2010). There are, however, a number of pilot studies and case studies suggesting the effectiveness of the use of specific cognitive behaviour therapy-oriented approaches in conjunction with other behavioural interventions

(Hartley et al. 2015; Hronis et al. 2019). Addressing psychopathology with psychotherapy in this population with randomised controlled trials is an important future direction for research.

Pharmacological Interventions

Despite limited research to support their efficacy for individuals with intellectual disability, polypharmacy in this population is common, particularly among those with comorbid mental health diagnoses (McMahon, Hatton, and Bowring 2020). While it can be assumed that medications beneficial for the general population should apply to individuals with intellectual disability, unfortunately, this population is often excluded from clinical trials. Psychotropic medications are often prescribed to treat problem behaviours in this population. Atypical antipsychotics have research to support their use to treat problem behaviours in children and adults with intellectual disability (Matson and Neal 2009; Unwin and Deb 2011); however, other studies have found no benefit over placebo (Tyrer et al. 2009). Given the nature of the referral, which came from Mary's paediatric psychiatrist, we recommended that Mary's parents discuss pharmacological intervention with the inhouse psychiatrist in order to address Mary's activity level, behavioural difficulties, and self-injurious behaviours. We emphasised that medication will not address all of Mary's behavioural deficits but that it may decrease some of her behavioural issues, which would give her more opportunities to learn.

Other Interventions and Considerations

For individuals with language difficulties, improving functional communication is often an important treatment goal. Families may wish to adopt a Picture Exchange Communication System (PECS) where the child can use pictures to communicate wants and needs or other electronic augmentative and alternative communication devices (AACs). There is research to suggest that using PECS and augmentative and alternative communication devices can also assist in the development of spoken language (Almirall et al. 2016). Given Mary's extremely limited vocabulary and increased agitation in the face of frustration, we strongly encouraged the school and her parents to use PECS or an augmentative and alternative communication devices across environments to expand her ability to communicate. We also recommended the use of the communication system to be practised in her speech/language therapy as well as in the general classroom. It was also recommended that Mary carry a small PECS book at all times.

In keeping with the role of a neuropsychologist in a multidisciplinary setting as taking the lead role in coordinating comprehensive care, it was recommended that the family speak with their neurologist about obtaining an updated electroencephalogram to rule out the presence of absence seizures given the school's concern that Mary occasionally appears unresponsive whilst demonstrating unusual ocular movements as well as the elevated risk for seizures in children with intellectual disability syndromes (Kirch and Weller 2001). Importantly, transition to adulthood will also be an important point of intervention in Mary's future. Neuropsychologists within the multidisciplinary setting are in a unique position to identify strengths and challenges in order to promote successful transition. As she was only 7 years of age at the point of the evaluation, we discussed this process generally with the parents, briefly discussing and providing further resources on guardianship, employment, managing money, and independent living.

Outcome

One year following this evaluation, Mary came into the hospital for a follow-up neuropsychological evaluation that had been recommended by our team. Reports from Mary's parents, teacher, and speech therapist revealed that Mary had made significant progress in the area of functional communication. Parent feedback revealed that Mary's behaviours in the home had improved, which they attributed to improved communication using PECS as well as parent training with the assistance of ABA therapy. The parents had decided to attempt these behavioural interventions prior to starting psychotropic medication, to which the paediatric psychiatrist had agreed. They noted that self-injurious behaviours now occurred rarely. Continued monitoring by the multidisciplinary team, with the paediatric neuropsychologist taking a lead role in coordinating these efforts, will be important in order to monitor change as well as address any additional concerns that arise for Mary and her family.

SUMMARY

This case illustrates that issues surrounding the assessment of intellectual and adaptive functioning can be quite complex. Children and adolescents with intellectual disability require coordinated and comprehensive care within an integrated medical setting. Paediatric neuropsychologists are in a unique position to take a lead role in coordinating this team or may work as coleader with multiple allied health staff. As intellectual disability is heterogeneous in presentation and aetiology, a key role of paediatric neuropsychologists is to apply an understanding of neurocognitive disorders and syndrome-specific neuropsychological profiles to the comprehensive assessment of a child's strengths and challenges across multiple domains. The provision of recommendations for intervention in the context of the child's functioning across multiple domains can then be communicated to the family and other health providers. Importantly, these recommendations should be in the context of a parent/family-centred approach and should emphasise educational opportunities and integration with the community in order to maximise the child's independence and quality of life.

REFERENCES

American Association on Intellectual and Developmental Disabilities (2010) *Intellectual Disability: Definition, Classification, and Systems of Supports*, 11th edition. Washington, DC: AAIDD.

American Psychiatric Association (2013) *Diagnostic and Statistical Manual of Mental Disorder*, 5th edition. Arlington, VA: Author.

Almirall D, Distefano C, Chang Y et al. (2016) Longitudinal effects of adaptive interventions with a speech generating device in minimally verbal children with ASD. *Journal of Clinical Child and Adolescent Psychology* 45(4): 442–456.

Butler MG (1990) Prader-Willi syndrome: Current understanding of cause and diagnosis. *American Journal of Medical Genetics* 35(3): 319.

Boyle CA, Boulet S, Schieve LA et al. (2011) Trends in the prevalence of developmental disabilities in US children 1997–2008. *Pediatrics* 127(6): 1034–1042.

Deutsch C, Dube WV, McIlvane WJ (2008) Attention deficits, attention-deficit hyperactivity disorder, and intellectual disabilities. *Developmental Disabilities Research Reviews* 14(4): 285–292.

Dierssen M, Ramakers GJA (2006) Dendritic pathology in mental retardation: from molecular genetics to neurobiology. *Genes, Brain and Behavior* 5(2): 48–60. https://doi.org/10.1111/j.1601-183X.2006.00224.x.

Durkin MS, Schupf N, Stein ZA, Susser MW (2007) *Public Health and preventive Medicine*, 15th edition, Wallace R, editor. Stamford, CT: Appleton & Lange, pp. 1173–1184.

Emerson E (2003) Prevalence of psychiatric disorders in children and adolescents with and without intellectual disability. *Journal of Intellectual Disability Research* 47(1): 51–58.

Fernandez-Carvajal I, Walichiewicz P, Xiaosen X, Pan R, Hagerman P, Tassone F (2009) Screening for expanded alleles of the FMR1 gene in blood spots from newborn males in a Spanish population. *The Journal of Molecular Diagnostics* 11(4): 324–329.

Fombonne E (2009) Epidemiology of pervasive developmental disorders. *Pediatric Research* 65(6): 591–598.

Harris JC (2014) Intellectual disability (intellectual developmental disorder). In: Gabbard GO, editor, *Gabbard's Treatments of Psychiatric Disorders*. Arlington, VA: American Psychiatric Association, pp. 3–20.

Hassiotis A, Serfaty M, Azam K et al. (2013) Manualised individual cognitive behavioural therapy for mood disorders in people with mild to moderate intellectual disability: A feasibility randomised controlled trial. *Journal of Affective Disorders* 151: 186–195.

Hartley S, Esbensen A, Shalev R, Vincent L, Mihaila I, Bussanich P (2015) Cognitive behavioral therapy for depressed adults with mild intellectual disability: A pilot study. *Journal of Mental Health Research in Intellectual Disabilities* 8(2): 1–26.

Hronis A, Roberts R, Roberts L, Kneebone I (2019) Fearless me!: A feasibility case series of cognitive behavioral therapy for adolescents with intellectual disability. *Journal of Clinical Psychology* 75(6): 919–932. https://doi.org/10.1002/jclp.22741.

Huang H, Ruedrich S (2007) Recent advances in the diagnosis and treatment of attention-deficit-hyperactivity disorder in individuals with intellectual disability. *Mental Health Aspects of Developmental Disabilities* 10(4): 121–128.

Janke K, Jacola L (2018) Intellectual disability syndromes. In: Donders J, Hunter SJ, editors, *Neuropsychological Conditions Across the Lifespan*. New York, NY: Cambridge University Press, pp. 61–78.

Koslowski N, Klein K, Arnold K, Kosters M, Schutzwhol HJS, Puschner B (2016) Effectiveness of interventions for adults with mild to moderate intellectual disabilities and mental health problems: Systematic review and meta-analysis. *The British Journal of Psychiatry* 6: 469–474.

Kesler SR, Wilde E, Bruno JL, Bigler ED (2011) Neuroimaging and genetic disorders. In: Goldstein S, Reynolds CR, editors, *Handbook of Neurodevelopmental and Genetic Disorders in Children*. New York, NY: The Guilford Press, pp. 58–63.

Kirch R, Weller E (2001) Do cognitive normal children with epilepsy have a higher rate of injury than their nonepileptic peers? *Journal of Child Neurology* 16: 100–104.

Loomes R, Hull L, Mandy WPL (2017) What is the male-to-female ratio in autism spectrum disorder? A systematic review and meta-analysis. *Journal of the American Academy of Child & Adolescent Psychiatry* 56(6): 466–474.

Maenner MJ, Shaw KA, Bakian AV et al. (2021) Prevalence and characteristics of autism spectrum disorder among children aged 8 years – autism and developmental disabilities monitoring network, 11 Sites, United States, 2018. *MMWR Surveillance Summaries* 70(SS-11): 1–16. doi: http://dx.doi.org/10.15585/mmwr.ss7011a1.

Matson JL, Neal D (2009) Psychotropic medication use for challenging behaviors in persons with intellectual disabilities: An overview. *Research in Developmental Disabilities* 30: 572–586.

Maulik PK, Mascarenhas MN, Mathers CD, Dua T, Saxena S (2011) Prevalence of intellectual disability: A meta-analysis of population-based studies. *Research in Developmental Disabilities* 32(2): 419–436. doi: 10.1016/j.ridd.2010.12.018.

McDaniel MA (2005) Big-brained people are smarter: A meta-analysis of the relationship between in vivo brain volume and intelligence. *Intelligence* 33: 337–346.

McMahon M, Hatton C, Bowring DL (2020) Polypharmacy and psychotropic polypharmacy in adults with intellectual disability: A cross-sectional total population study. *Journal of Intellectual Disability Research* 64(11): 834–851. https://doi.org/10.1111/jir.12775.

Mefford HC, Batshaw ML, Hoffman EP (2012) Genomics, intellectual disability, and autism. *The New England Journal of Medicine* 366(8): 733–743. https://doi.org/10.1056/NEJMra1114194.

Mertz LG, Christensen R, Vogel I et al. (2013) Angelman syndrome in Denmark. Birth incidence, genetic findings, and age at diagnosis. *American Journal of Medical Genetics* 161(9): 2197–2203.

Miltenberger RG (2012) *Behavior Modification: Principles and Procedures*. Belmont, CA: Wadsworth Cengage Learning.

Neece C, Baker B, Blacher J, Crnic KA (2011) Attention-deficit/hyperactivity disorder among children with and without intellectual disability: An examination across time. *Journal of Intellectual Disability Research* 55(7): 623–635.

Neisser U, Boodoo G, Bouchard TJ et al. (1996) Intelligence: Knowns and unknowns. *American Psychologist* 51: 77–101.

Oeseburg B, Jansen D, Groothoff J, Dijkstra G, Reijneveld S (2010) Emotional and behavioural problems in adolescents with intellectual disability with and without chronic diseases. *Journal of Intellectual Disability Research* 54(1): 81–89.

Oskarsdóttir S, Vujic M, Fasth A (2004) Incidence and prevalence of the 22q11 deletion syndrome: A population-based study in Western Sweden. *Archives of Disease in Childhood* **89**(2): 148–151.

Ozonoff S (2010) Autism spectrum disorders. In: Yeates K, Ris D, Taylor HG, Pennington B, editors, *Pediatric Neuropsychology: Research, Theory and Practice*, 2nd edition. New York, NY: Guilford Press, pp. 418–446.

Parker SE, Mai CT, Canfield MA et al. (2010) Updated National Birth Prevalence estimates for selected birth defects in the United States, 2004–2006. *Birth Defects Research* **88**(12): 1008–1016.

Reichenberg A, Cederlöf M, McMillan A et al. (2016) Discontinuity in the genetic and environmental causes of the intellectual disability spectrum. *Proceedings of the National Academy of Sciences – PNAS* **113**(4): 1098–1103. https://doi.org/10.1073/pnas.1508093112.

Rojahn J, Medeiros K, Farmer CA (2016) Intellectual and developmental disabilities. In: Norcross JC, VandenBos GR, Freedheim DK, Pole N, editors, *APA Handbook of Clinical Psychology: Psychopathology and Health*. Washington, DC: American Psychological Association, pp. 335–351.

Sattler JM (2014) *Foundations of Behavioral, Social, and Clinical Assessment of Children*. La Mesa, CA: Jerome M. Sattler, Publisher Inc.

Shaw P, Greenstein D, Lerch J et al. (2006) Intellectual ability and cortical development in children and adolescents. *Nature* **440**: 676–679.

Somers M, Shields L, Boks M, Kahn R, Sommer I (2015) Cognitive benefits of right-handedness: A meta-analysis. *Neuroscience and Biobehavioral Reviews* **51**: 48–63.

Storey K, Miner C (2011) *Systematic Instruction of Functional Skills for Students and Adults With Disabilities*. Springfield, IL: Charles C. Thomas Publisher.

Strømme P, Bjømstad P, Ramstad K (2002) Prevalence estimation of Williams Syndrome. *Journal of Child Neurology* **17**(4): 269–271.

Tyrer P, Oliver-Africano PC, Ahmed Z et al. (2008) Risperidone, haloperidol, and placebo in the treatment of aggressive challenging behaviour in patients with intellectual disability: A randomised controlled trial. *The Lancet (British Edition)* **371**(9606): 57–63. https://doi.org/10.1016/S0140-6736(08)60072-0.

Unwin G, Deb S (2011) Efficacy of atypical antipsychotic medication in the management of behaviour problems in children with intellectual disabilities and borderline intelligence: A systematic review. *Research in Developmental Disabilities* **32**: 2121–2133. http://dx.doi.org/10.1016/j.ridd.2011.07.031.

Williams J (2010) Global developmental delay – globally helpful? *Developmental Medicine & Child Neurology* **52**(3): 227.

Wingate M, Kirby RS (2014) Prevalence of autism spectrum disorder among children aged 8 years – autism and developmental disabilities monitoring network, 11 sites, United States, 2010. *Morbidity and Mortality Weekly Report. Surveillance Summaries (Washington, DC: 2002)* **63**(2): 1–21.

World Health Organization (2003) *The ICD-10 Classification of Mental and Behavioural Disorders: Clinical Descriptions and Diagnostic Guidelines*, 10th rev., 2nd edition. Geneva: World Health Organization.

Zablotsky B, Black LI, Blumberg SJ (2017) *Estimated Prevalence of Children With Diagnosed Developmental Disabilities in the United States, 2014–2016. NCHS Data Brief, no 291.* Hyattsville, MD: National Center for Health Statistics.

Zollino M, Murdolo M, Marangi G et al. (2008) On the nosology and pathogenesis of Wolf–Hirschhorn syndrome: Genotype–phenotype correlation analysis of 80 patients and literature review. *American Journal of Genetics* **148**: 257–269.

CHAPTER 21

Speech, Motor Impairments, and Physical Limitations

Seth A Warschausky

Presenting Concern

At the initial assessment, Sarah was an 8-year-old born preterm at 27 weeks' gestation and diagnosed with spastic bilateral cerebral palsy (Gross Motor Function Classification System level V; Palisano et al. 1997). Sarah utilised a manual wheelchair with assistance. She could not manipulate objects and was severely limited in her ability to perform simple actions such as pointing (Manual Ability Classification System level IV; Eliasson et al. 2006). Sarah needed total assistance for activities of daily living. She was not able to direct her care. She demonstrated anarthria (loss of speech due to motor impairment) and used eye movements to indicate yes/no. She responded to humour. Initially, she did not have an augmentative and alternative communication (AAC) device. She did not initiate communication with peers, though she appeared to be interested in their activities. Her communication was largely restricted to interactions that were initiated and facilitated by her parent.

Sarah was in a special education program. She had not had standardised testing; thus, there was limited information regarding her potential to develop academic skill. She appeared to have difficulties with attention. Sarah's mother was seeking basic information regarding Sarah's cognitive capabilities and the school wanted basic information regarding learning potential, including reading.

In the initial session to develop an assessment strategy, Sarah demonstrated some accurate eye gaze. She appeared able to make dichotomous choices with some vocalising to indicate 'yes'. She attempted items from the Columbia Mental Maturity Scale (Reuter and Mintz 1970) using eye gaze. She could make some distinctions between different shapes and demonstrated some abstract reasoning. Sarah was able to participate in an evaluation for a maximum of an hour and a half with breaks to address fatigue and motivation. She did not endorse reports of pain nor did her mother observe expressions of pain or discomfort.

THEORY

Children who receive special education services often have significant impairments in speech/articulation and/or dexterity that can preclude participation in traditional psychological and educational assessments (National Longitudinal Transition Study-2 2008). Approximately 28% of all children who receive special education services have difficulty speaking and 5.3% have difficulty with dexterity. Thus, there is a terrible irony in the assumed prerequisite ability to speak and manipulate objects inherent in the development of traditional neuropsychological assessment instruments. The inaccessibility of test instruments has hindered our understanding of the cognitive risks and needs associated with specific neurodevelopmental conditions, including cerebral palsy, the most common cause of childhood physical disability. For example there is limited information about processing speed and phonological processing in this population. Other neurodevelopmental conditions include attention-deficit/hyperactivity disorder and autism spectrum disorder. Deficits in these areas have significant implications for educational accommodations and interventions. Accessible testing is also needed to monitor the cognitive side effects of pharmacological and other medical interventions, as well as access to clinical trials that require cognitive assessment. The focus of this chapter is primarily regarding children who experience speech, motor, and physical limitations on the more severe end of the spectrum.

There have been efforts to create modified test procedures that are accessible to children with multiple impairments. Strategies have included converting response options to a forced-choice format (Sabbadini et al. 2002), using assistive technologies such as pressure switches and a wireless head-controlled mouse for response (Warschausky et al. 2012), eye-gaze interfaces (Poletti et al. 2017), event-related brain potentials (Byrne, Dywan, and Connolly 1995), and brain-computer interface (Alcaide-Aguirre et al. 2017). The problem is that modifying standardised procedures to make them accessible changes the psychometric properties of tests, including construct validity. *Construct irrelevance*, or the extent to which scores reflect extraneous factors, can be inherent in measurements from tests that are not accessible to the participant (Magasi et al. 2017; Magasi, Harniss, and Heinemann 2018).

The Standards for Psychological and Educational Testing in the US (American Educational Research Association et al. 2014) identify modifications in stimulus and response formats, time constraints, and test selection. These standards were developed to ensure fairness and accuracy in administration and interpretation. Hill-Briggs et al. (2007) described common accommodations for physical impairments that include adjusting time limits and avoiding timed tests, use of relatively motor-free instruments, use of adaptive equipment/assistive technologies for response, limited and multiple assessment sessions, and accessible seating and tables. The standards for testing individuals with specific impairments recommend piloting test modifications prior to clinical use and providing test validity and normative data regarding standard modification recommendations. In discussing the development of accessible computer-assisted testing in particular, Magasi et al. delineate a six-step process for accessible test development, with an endpoint description of reasonable accommodation guidelines as an essential component of instrument development (Magasi et al. 2018).

Psychometrics and Validation

There is longstanding recognition of the potential of computerised neuropsychological assessment instruments, with detailed discussions of benefits and challenges to a computerised approach. In some of the most prominent discussions of computerised assessment, however, there has been a surprising paucity of comment on the potential accessibility for people with disabilities. The American Academy of Clinical Neuropsychology/National Academy of Neuropsychology joint statement made no mention of this potential advantage (Bauer et al. 2012). Similarly, prominent papers in flagship neuropsychology journals did not discuss these potential applications (Miller and Barr 2017; Parsons, McMahan, and Kane 2018).

Recently, in the course of studying the accessibility of the National Institutes of Health (NIH) Toolbox Cognition Battery computerised tests (Gershon et al. 2013), Magasi et al. (2017) noted that when testing individuals who had sustained brain or spinal cord injury, almost a quarter required accommodations for test access, particularly for motor-response demands. Yet, more than half the examiners when implementing accommodations breached Reasonable Accommodations Guidelines such that results could not be interpreted. However, there have been promising efforts to create motor-free composites scores from the NIH Toolbox Cognition Battery for individuals who have impairments in upper extremity functioning (Carlozzi et al. 2017).

Assistive Technology and Cognitive Load

As clinicians and researchers consider the use of computerised assessment including the use of AAC and assistive technologies to make assessment instruments more accessible, a paradox arises in the mental workload inherent in various technological approaches to item presentation and response. Mental workload has been defined as 'the level of attentional resources required to meet both objective and subjective performance criteria, which may be mediated by task demands, external support, and past experience' (Young and Stanton 2005, p. 1). Importantly, technological modifications for accessibility can result in both overload such as overly complex perceptual demands or higher working memory demands, as well as underload – a somewhat vague term that implies inadequate stimulation. There is some evidence from AAC research that direct selection is less cognitively demanding than responding with a pressure switch to scanning of response options (Wagner and Jackson 2006). However, there is a lack of information regarding mental workload effects of modifications for accessibility on test performance and Warschausky et al. (2012) comparing the Peabody Picture Vocabulary Test, Third Edition (PPVT-III) (Dunn and Dunn 1997) performance with a head mouse to a scanning/pressure switch procedure did not find test performance differences in children who had cerebral palsy.

ASSESSMENT AND FORMULATION

A basic assessment approach for children with physical and other impairments is summarised in Figure 21.1.

Review of Literature on Adapted Assessment

There is a paucity of psychometric studies of instruments that were adapted for accessibility in accordance with the approach recommended in the Standards for Psychological and Educational Testing. In one of the few studies to date, initial findings provided preliminary evidence that the modification of existing quadrant forced-choice response instruments (using pressure switch or head mouse access) did not result in significant change in scores or evidence of validity (Warschausky et al. 2012). However, similar modified access to the Raven's Coloured Progressive Matrices (Raven, Raven, and Court 1998), a test that includes a stimulus image separated from response options, was not fully successful. An attempt to modify a phonemic awareness task from verbal response to forced-choice format computer access resulted in significantly higher

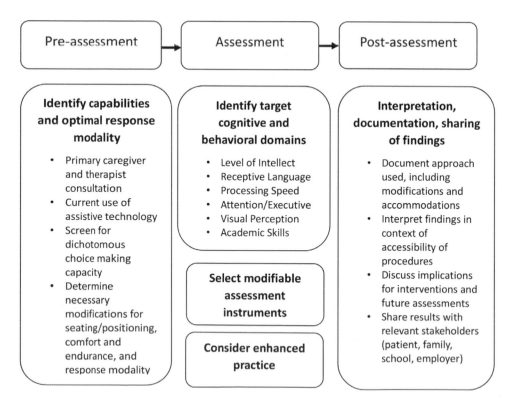

Figure 21.1 Basic approach to neuropsychological assessment of children with physical and other impairments.

scores compared with scores on the standard version. Thus, there was evidence that modifying quadrant forced-choice instruments for accessible responding via assistive technologies did not appear to alter the psychometric properties of the instruments in children with or without cerebral palsy. However, changing the standard response modality (from production to forced choice) or having a separate stimulus image did alter the construct validity.

Little or No Overt Volitional Response: Eye-Gaze and Brain-Computer Interfaces

To more accurately assess cognition in people with severe speech and motor impairments, clinicians and researchers have used assistive technologies such as touch pads, switches, and eye trackers. With the exception of eye-gaze technologies, these assistive technologies also require significant speech or motor input, so cognitive assessments remain inaccessible to those with the most severe impairments. Eye-gaze testing strategies have been used with low-technology materials and more recently using eye-gaze computer interface technologies (Desideri et al. 2016; Poletti et al. 2017) with promising results. Yet, even eye-gaze strategies require oculomotor capabilities.

A potentially promising and largely motor-free approach could be to use brain activity to register the individual's response to test items. There have been promising efforts to conduct event-related potential-based cognitive testing using standardised tests with minimal modifications of test items (Perego et al. 2011). That said, to date the evidence supports using eye-gaze computer interface over brain computer interface (BCI) strategies when the person is capable of the former (Pasqualotto et al. 2015). As BCIs continue to develop, there is an emerging literature on ethical implications of and guidance for their use, including mental privacy issues and ethics for research that promotes the well-being of and includes the perspectives of participants, does not overstate the value of BCIs, and recognises the social and societal implications among others (Pham et al. 2018).

Prerequisites for Testing: Basic Choice-Making Capabilities

A commonly encountered difficulty in developing an accessible approach to testing cognition in children with the most severe speech and motor impairments is establishing the extent to which they have basic choice-making capabilities. Typically, choice-making is defined and assessed as the expression of personal preference that would not in and of itself be a sufficient level of choice-making to participate in testing. There is a paucity of objective, systematic approaches to conceptualisation and assessment of choice-making abilities. Van Tubbergen et al. (2008) have described a progression of capabilities and skills involved in choice-making, a framework for understanding the abilities that constitute the foundation for these skills and behaviours, and a preliminary screening strategy. This progression of skills ranges from basic orienting, to indications of preference, to directed responses, and finally abstraction responses. Participation in standardised testing would require a demonstration of at least directed response capabilities. There is a paradox inherent in identifying these prerequisite skills in those who do not have overt volitional responses, including the need for BCI-facilitated assessment of choice-making.

Selected Domain-Specific Considerations

The reader is referred to the NIH Common Data Elements for cerebral palsy for a compilation of current recommended instruments for neuropsychological research with this population, including descriptions of accessibility for individuals with motor and speech impairments. Many of the instruments are validated for use in clinical assessments.

RECEPTIVE LANGUAGE WITH NO SPEECH RESPONSE DEMANDS

Receptive language has served as a proxy for level of intellect, with some caveats. There are a number of tests that assess receptive vocabulary by utilising forced-choice format responding, typically in a quadrant array. The PPVT has been identified as the most frequently used test in this regard (Geytenbeek et al. 2010), although the British Picture Vocabulary Scale, Third Edition (Dunn et al. 2009), is likely to be utilised in the UK. The limited psychometric studies of utilising other access strategies with quadrant forced-choice format response options provide some support for robust measurement agreement (Kurmanaviciute and Stadskleiv 2017).

VISUOSPATIAL AND PERCEPTUAL REASONING

There is a paucity of effort to study motor-free and speech-free assessment of perceptual reasoning and visuospatial functions. The Raven's Progressive Matrices tests, although utilising forced-choice and nonverbal response formats, have been recognised as largely loading on g-factor intelligence. Raven's tests were designed to be administered with flexible response options; however, there have been a few efforts to examine the feasibility and psychometric effects of accommodated responses. Findings have been mixed, suggesting greater measurement agreement when using finger or eye pointing than when using scanning/pressure switch technologies or a head mouse in typically developing individuals (Warschausky et al. 2012; Kurmanaviciute and Stadskleiv 2017; Poletti et al. 2017). Preliminary work has supported the potential utility of adapting the Kaufman Brief Intelligence Test, Second Edition, Matrices subtest (Kaufman and Kaufman 2004) for eye-tracking administration (Desideri et al. 2016). There are a number of tests including Motor-Free Visual Perception Test, Fourth Edition (Colarusso and Hammill 2015) and the Developmental Test of Visual Perception, Third Edition (Hammill, Pearson, and Voress 2014), designed to specifically assess visual perception utilising potentially motor-free response options; however, there are limited studies of the validity and measurement agreement using modified response formats (Brown and Peres 2018).

Processing Speed

Information processing speed is a particularly important domain given its sensitivity to change in neurological status and contribution to a number of higher-level cognitive processes. Slowed processing speed is one of the most robust neuropsychological sequelae of traumatic brain injury and a wide range of neurological diseases (Marco et al. 2012; Shultz et al. 2016). Processing speed increases through childhood and is associated with increased working memory capacity (Fry and Hale 2000).

Processing speed tests such as the Symbol Digit Modalities Test (Smith 1991) that can be conducted with verbal rather than motor responses potentially reduce speeded motor demands, although oromotor speed is still involved. Carlozzi et al. (2017) utilised the Symbol Digit Modalities Test in creating a motor-free composite for the NIH Toolbox Cognition Battery and demonstrated the utility of this test for people with spinal cord injury and/or traumatic brain injury. Technological solutions to the motor confound problem have included promising efforts to develop accessible inspection time tests of processing speed that minimise speeded response demands by varying stimulus presentation time on a computer screen, with untimed and accessible response to a dichotomous choice prompt (Shank et al. 2010; Kaufman, Donders, and Warschausky 2014). There also have been promising efforts to develop eye-tracking versions of the Trail Making Test (Reitan 1955) as well as the D2 (Brickencamp and Zillmer 1998), as tests of processing speed and sustained attention (Hicks et al. 2013; Keller et al. 2015).

Executive Functions: Working Memory

Assessment of working memory typically focuses on auditory and visuospatial working memory functions. The Digit Span subtest from the Wechsler scales, the most common clinical test of auditory working memory, is accessible to those with physical impairments, if speech is comprehensible. As more complex working memory tests that involve receptive language demands, the Token Test (De Renzi and Vignolo 1962) and the Developmental Neuropsychological Assessment, Second Edition (NEPSY-II) Comprehension of Instructions test (Korkman, Kirk, and Kemp 2007) require a motor response. Visuospatial working memory tests such as the Wechsler Picture Span subtest and Corsi Block-Tapping Test (Corsi 1972) typically require a physical response. For those with combined physical and speech impairments, there have been efforts to develop accessible formats including an eye-tracking version of a Digits Sequencing Task (Poletti et al. 2018). A cautionary note is that historically in the typically developing population articulation rate was identified as a strong correlate of working memory; subsequently, in children with cerebral palsy, it was shown that oral speech rate was not a strong correlate, with findings suggesting that covert rehearsal rates were the important correlate (White et al. 1994).

Case Study – Assessment

Three further sessions were required to complete the assessment with Sarah. In the first session, she attempted to use a simple switching device to participate in a modified PPVT-III administration. Her attention and motivation were limited. There appeared to be discomfort with her positioning in the wheelchair, and she was more comfortable in a standard chair. The switching device was not of immediate benefit. She understood cause and effect and was able to hit the switch to activate a computer-generated response. Sarah gave correct responses to items in her age item set but an accurate ceiling was not obtained. An initial attempt to administer a quadrant forced-choice academic achievement test utilising a similar procedure was not successful, again, at least in part, tied to attention and motivation. It was clear that an accurate assessment was only possible over multiple evaluation sessions trying different types of modifications of test materials and communicative devices. At that point, the plan was to have Sarah undergo a re-evaluation in the AAC/assistive technologies lab.

Subsequent to the AAC/assistive technologies assessment, Sarah's AAC specialist worked with Sarah using a head mouse to move a cursor and make choices from images scanned and presented on a computer screen. In preparation for the assessment, the AAC specialist was able to help in identifying optimal presentation formats. For example she had attempted presentations using quadrants versus horizontal arrays. She had found greater accuracy in pictures presented in a horizontal array, but quadrant presentation appeared sufficiently accurate for assessment using the standard formats.

During the second assessment session, Sarah used a head mouse and made choices from images presented on a laptop screen. She performed at a higher level when a slow cursor was used and pictures were sufficiently separated so that choices could be indicated in part by the trajectory of the movement as well as ability to hold the cursor in a quadrant for approximately 3 seconds. When quadrant stimuli were presented in a modified three-choice format, she was able to respond quite quickly and accurately to initial items. The Raven's Coloured Progressive Matrices was administered in a modified four-choice format and Sarah was able to demonstrate some accurate completion and matching, but there were indications of visuospatial and perceptual impairments that included selecting choices with orientation and configuration errors. There continued to be some concern with the ways in which her headrest was permitting optimal head movement. In particular, Sarah had difficulty with types of vertical movement. If it were possible to dampen some of the extraneous movement, it appeared that this would have been helpful.

The use of assistive technologies allowed Sarah to more consistently demonstrate her capabilities. Apart from evaluating the best format and examining her skills with a head mouse, Sarah was able to complete the PPVT-III. She continued to exhibit some inconsistency making it difficult to establish an accurate basal but her ceiling was established. It was clear that the PPVT-III was capturing vocabulary in a number of instances; for example when testing the limits with words such as 'tortoise' or 'huge', Sarah was able to accurately select pictures corresponding to more familiar terms, i.e. 'turtle' and 'big'. On the other hand, there were visuoperceptual difficulties noted that were similar to what had been observed with the Raven's Coloured Progressive Matrices, including difficulty distinguishing similar shapes.

During the third assessment session, the positioning issues again were noted with difficulty getting optimal movement in the vertical axis. Sarah had significant difficulty moving the cursor to the top or bottom choices at times. Again, visuoperceptual difficulties were noted. Sarah was able to do precise matching with very simple patterns and had clear difficulty when attempting to match more complex patterns. She did not demonstrate right/left intrapersonal orientation. Portions of a quadrant forced-choice academic achievement test were administered using the standard quadrant presentation. Reading recognition subtest items were administered and Sarah could easily match words. She also demonstrated basic sound-symbol association. When asked to find words beginning with 'the same sound' she tended to choose words where the ending letter matched the sound. This may be associated with some of the difficulty with orientation of figures previously described. In mathematics, Sarah was inconsistent in demonstrating basic computational skills, although reportedly she had done well with this in other settings.

Outcome

In summary, the results suggested a significant discrepancy between relative strength in receptive language and greater impairments in visuoperceptual and visuospatial functions. Receptive vocabulary fell between 2 and 3 standard deviations below peers. Levels of adaptive behaviour in aspects of communication and social functioning fell 2 to 3 standard deviations below peers, as well. Sarah's profile was consistent with a mild intellectual disability. Sarah was learning some basic academic skills and it was anticipated that she would make greater progress in the academic domains, given how recently she had been introduced to assistive technologies.

Recommendations:

✓ There was progress in Sarah's seating and positioning, although discomfort and mild pain were noted in some instances. It was advised to assess and address discomfort and pain prior to and during Sarah's activities. Her head movement was not optimal yet for use of the type of head mouse utilised in the assessment. In addition to addressing freedom of movement, Sarah was referred to occupational and physical therapy to develop techniques to dampen her extraneous movement.

✓ Regarding assistive technologies, Sarah was most successful when using a laptop that could be easily repositioned.

✓ There was a significant strength with verbal compared with nonverbal skills for Sarah. Use of verbal mediation strategies or verbal explanations were recommended with minimisation of visuoperceptual demands in instructional materials.

✓ The reported level of intellect was given as an estimate. It was noted that Sarah had only recently accessed the types of technology utilised in the evaluation. It will be important to return to questions of skill development and capabilities in the future to monitor progress and gain a review of her abilities.

✓ Findings supported the importance of emphasising academic skill development in educational programming. At that point, it was not clear if there was relative difficulty in the development of written language versus mathematics, although the profile would predict relative strength in the former versus the latter.

✓ Fatigue greatly affected Sarah's performance. Sarah took breaks approximately every 20 to 25 minutes and this will need to be considered in future evaluations as well as academic programming.

✓ Plan follow-up assessment when AAC training is completed and consistent AAC use is observed.

SUMMARY

There are significant health disparities associated with the inaccessible nature of standardised neuropsychological test instruments that include barriers to refined educational planning, barriers to monitoring iatrogenic and medical treatment effects, and barriers to participation in clinical trials.

Prior to developing an accessible testing strategy, it is essential to establish dichotomous choice-making capabilities at a minimum, and this may involve collaborating with clinicians such as speech-language pathologists. In developing an accessible testing strategy, the cognitive load of alternative response formats must be considered. When communicating findings, it is important to fully document test modifications and accessibility strategies, and to carefully consider the validity and limitations of testing in interpretation of the data and final conclusions. Models of neuropsychological functions such as working memory do not necessarily fully apply to those with multiple impairments.

There is a compelling need for further study of the psychometrics of accessible test procedures in children with disabilities, including children who have impairments and capabilities similar to those of Sarah in the case study. There is significant complexity, however, to this research endeavour. Assistive technologies access needs to be tailored to each individual child's optimal sensorimotor capabilities, raising a number of issues. First, it is conceivable that assistive technologies access methods differ in cognitive load (Mizuko and Esser 1991; Wagner and Jackson 2006; Dropik and Reichle 2008). If indeed there are such differences, there is the potential for a mismatch between what is optimal for physical accessibility versus cognitive capabilities. Future efforts to standardise adaptations are likely to include collaboration with test publishers to comply with copyright laws as well as professional standards regarding test security. There are neuropsychological domains including processing speed in which test accessibility will require the development of new instruments rather than modification of traditional measures. Finally, for those with the most severe physical and speech impairments, there is a critical need to develop assessment strategies that identify choice-making capabilities.

REFERENCES

Alcaide-Aguirre RE, Warschausky SA, Brown D, Aref A, Huggins JE (2017) Asynchronous brain-computer interface for cognitive assessment in people with cerebral palsy. *Journal of Neural Engineering* 14(6): 066001. doi: 10.1088/1741-2552/aa7fc4.

American Educational Research Association, American Psychological Association, National Council on Measurement in Education, Joint Committee on Standards for Educational and Psychological Testing (US) (2014). *Standards for Educational and Psychological Testing*. Washington, DC: American Educational Research Association.

Bauer RM, Iverson GL, Cernich AN, Binder LM, Ruff RM, Naugle RI (2012) Computerized neuropsychological assessment devices: Joint position paper of the American Academy of Clinical Neuropsychology and the National Academy of Neuropsychology. *Archives of Clinical Neuropsychology* 27(3): 362–373. doi: 10.1093/arclin/acs027.

Brown T, Peres L (2018) A critical review of the Motor-Free Visual Perception Test – fourth edition (MVPT-4). *Journal of Occupational Therapy Schools and Early Intervention* 11(2): 229–244. doi: 10.1080/19411243.2018.1432441.

Byrne JM, Dywan CA, Connolly JF (1995) An innovative method to assess the receptive vocabulary of children with cerebral palsy using event-related brain potentials. *J Clin Exp Neuropsychol* **17**(1): 9–19. doi: 10.1080/13803399508406576.

Carlozzi NE, Goodnight S, Umlauf A et al. (2017) Motor-free composites from the National Institutes of Health Toolbox Cognition Battery (NIHTB-CB) for people with disabilities. *Rehabilitation Psychology* **62**(4): 464–473. doi: 10.1037/rep0000185.

Desideri L, Tarabelloni G, Nanni I, Malavasi M, Nori R, Bonifacci P (2016) An eye-controlled version of the Kaufman Brief Intelligence Test 2 (KBIT-2) to assess cognitive functioning. *Computers in Human Behavior* **63**: 502–508. doi: 10.1016/j.chb.2016.05.077.

Dropik PL, Reichle J (2008) Comparison of accuracy and efficiency of directed scanning and group-item scanning for augmentative communication selection techniques with typically developing preschoolers. *American Journal of Speech-Language Pathology* **17**(1): 35–47. Available at: https://www.learntechlib.org/p/107983/ [Accessed 24 October 2021].

Eliasson AC, Krumlinde-Sundholm L, Rosblad B et al. (2006) The Manual Ability Classification System (MACS) for children with cerebral palsy: Scale development and evidence of validity and reliability. *Developmental Medicine and Child Neurology* **48**(7): 549–554.

Fry A, Hale S (2000) Relationships among processing speed, working memory and fluid intelligence in children. *Biological Psychology* **54**: 1–34.

Gershon RC, Wagster MV, Hendrie HC, Fox NA, Cook KF, Nowinski CJ (2013) NIH Toolbox for assessment of neurological and behavioral function. *Neurology* **80**(11 Suppl 3): S2–S6.

Geytenbeek J, Harlaar L, Stam M et al. (2010) Utility of language comprehension tests for unintelligible or non-speaking children with cerebral palsy: A systematic review. *Developmental Medicine and Child Neurology* **52**(12): 1098–1098. doi: 10.1111/j.1469-8749.2010.03833.x.

Hicks SL, Sharma R, Khan AN et al. (2013) An eye-tracking version of the trail-making test. *Plos One* **8**(12): e84061. doi: UNSP e8406110.1371/journal.pone.0084061.

Hill-Briggs F, Dial JG, Morere DA, Joyce A (2007) Neuropsychological assessment of persons with physical disability, visual impairment or blindness, and hearing impairment or deafness. *Archives of Clinical Neuropsychology* **22**(3): 389–404. doi: 10.1016/j.acn.2007.01.013.

Kaufman JN, Donders J, Warschausky S (2014) A comparison of visual inspection time measures in children with cerebral palsy. *Rehabilitation Psychology* **59**(2): 147–154. doi: 10.1037/a0036019.

Keller J, Gorges M, Horn HT et al. (2015) Eye-tracking controlled cognitive function tests in patients with amyotrophic lateral sclerosis: A controlled proof-of-principle study. *Journal of Neurology* **262**(8): 1918–1926. doi: 10.1007/s00415-015-7795-3.

Kurmanaviciute R, Stadskleiv K (2017) Assessment of verbal comprehension and non-verbal reasoning when standard response mode is challenging: A comparison of different response modes and an exploration of their clinical usefulness. *Cogent Psychology* **4**. doi: 10.1080/23311908.2016.1275416.

Magasi S, Harniss M, Heinemann AW (2018) Interdisciplinary approach to the development of accessible computer-administered measurement instruments. *Archives of Physical Medicine and Rehabilitation* **99**(1): 204–210. doi: 10.1016/j.apmr.2017.06.036.

Magasi S, Harniss M, Tulsky DS, Cohen ML, Heaton RK, Heinemann AW (2017) Test accommodations for individuals with neurological conditions completing the NIH Toolbox-Cognition Battery: An evaluation of frequency and appropriateness. *Rehabil Psychol* **62**(4): 455–463. doi: 10.1037/rep0000191.

Marco EJ, Harrell KM, Brown WS et al. (2012) Processing speed delays contribute to executive function deficits in individuals with agenesis of the corpus callosum. *Journal of the International Neuropsychological Society: JINS* **18**(3): 521–529. https://doi.org/10.1017/S1355617712000045.

Miller JB, Barr WB (2017) The technology crisis in neuropsychology. *Archives of Clinical Neuropsychology* **32**(5): 541–554. doi: 10.1093/arclin/acx050.

Mizuko M, Esser J (1991) The effect of direct selection and circular scanning on visual sequential recall. *Journal of Speech & Hearing Research* **34**(1): 43–48. https://doi.org/10.1044/jshr.3401.43.

National Longitudinal Transition Study-2 (2008) Retrieved from http://www.nlts2.org/.

Palisano R, Rosenbaum P, Walter S, Russell D, Wood E, Galuppi B (1997) Development and reliability of a system to classify gross motor function in children with cerebral palsy. *Dev Med Child Neurol* **39**(4): 214–223.

Parsons TD, McMahan T, Kane R (2018) Practice parameters facilitating adoption of advanced technologies for enhancing neuropsychological assessment paradigms. *Clinical Neuropsychologist* **32**(1): 16–41. doi: 10.1080/13854046.2017.1337932.

Pasqualotto E, Matuz T, Federici S et al. (2015) Usability and workload of access technology for people with severe motor impairment: A comparison of brain-computer interfacing and eye tracking. *Neurorehabilitation and Neural Repair* **29**(10): 950–957. doi: 10.1177/1545968315575611.

Perego P, Turconi AC, Andreoni G et al. (2011) Cognitive ability assessment by brain-computer interface validation of a new assessment method for cognitive abilities. *Journal of Neuroscience Methods* **201**(1): 239–250. doi: 10.1016/j.jneumeth.2011.06.025.

Pham M, Goering S, Sample M, Huggins JE, Klein E (2018) Asilomar survey: Research perspectives on ethical principles and guidelines for BCI research. *Brain-Computer Interfaces* **5**(4): 97–111.

Poletti B, Carelli L, Faini A et al. (2018) The Arrows and Colors Cognitive Test (ACCT): A new verbal-motor free cognitive measure for executive functions in ALS. *Plos One* **13**(8). doi: 10.1371/journal.pone.0200953.

Poletti B, Carelli L, Solca F et al. (2017). An eye-tracking controlled neuropsychological battery for cognitive assessment in neurological diseases. *Neurological Sciences* **38**(4): 595–603. doi: 10.1007/s10072-016-2807-3.

Sabbadini M, Bombardi P, Carlesimo GA, Rosato V, Pierro MM (2002) Evaluation of communicative and functional abilities in Wolf-Hirshhorn syndrome. *J Intellect Disabil Res* **46**(Pt 7): 575–582.

Shank LK, Kaufman J, Leffard S, Warschausky S (2010) Inspection time and attention-deficit/hyperactivity disorder symptoms in children with cerebral palsy. *Rehabil Psychol* **55**(2): 188–193. doi: 10.1037/a0019601.

Shultz EL, Hoskinson KR, Keim MC et al. (2016) Adaptive functioning following pediatric traumatic brain injury: Relationship to executive function and processing speed. *Neuropsychology* **30**(7): 830–840. https://doi.org/10.1037/neu0000288.

Van Tubbergen M, Warschausky S, Birnholz J, Baker S (2008) Choice beyond preference: Conceptualization and assessment of choice-making skills in children with significant impairments. *Rehabilitation Psychology* **53**(1): 93–100. doi: 10.1037/0090-5550.53.1.93.

Wagner BT, Jackson HM (2006) Developmental memory capacity resources of typical children retrieving picture communication symbols using direct selection and visual linear scanning with fixed communication displays. *Journal of Speech Language and Hearing Research* **49**(1): 113–126. doi: 10.1044/1092-4388(2006/009).

Warschausky S, Van Tubbergen M, Asbell S, Kaufman J, Ayyangar R, Donders J (2012) Modified test administration using assistive technology: Preliminary psychometric findings. *Assessment* **19**(4): 472–479. doi: 10.1177/1073191111402458.

White DA, Craft S, Hale S, Park TS (1994) Working memory and articulation rate in children with spastic diplegic cerebral palsy. *Neuropsychology* **8**(2): 180–186.

Young MS, Stanton NA (2005) Mental workload. In: Stanton NA, Hedge A, Brookhuis K, Salas E, Hendrick HW, editors, *Handbook of Human Factors and Ergonomics Methods*. London: Taylor & Francis.

PART 3

Factors Influencing Assessment and Feedback

CHAPTER 22

Culture

Daniel Stark

Presenting Concern

Samuel is a 14-year-old boy who was born in Ecuador where he spent the first 11 years of his life. He was born at term in the local community hospital with no concerns for his early social, motor, or language development. Samuel's parents separated when he was a few months old. Samuel attended a Spanish-speaking school characterised by large class sizes where he learned to read and write at approximately the same time as his peers, although maths was reported as a challenge. Samuel was described as highly active and a 'troublemaker' by his teachers.

At the age of 9 years, Samuel's mother moved to Portugal to pursue work opportunities whilst Samuel and his older sister remained in Ecuador in the care of their grandparents. Samuel experienced his first seizure around this time, although it was not identified as such and was instead considered a reaction to his mother's absence. Samuel experienced successive episodes of eye deviations, motor 'jerks', and changes in behaviour and laughter. These progressed until he experienced a generalised seizure at the age of 10 years. There is a paucity of medical information available from Ecuador, although his mother reports that no electroencephalogram was performed, and he was diagnosed with epilepsy and started on medication as a result. At the age of 11 years, Samuel and his sister moved to the UK to live with his mother.

In the UK, Samuel's epilepsy was identified as juvenile myoclonic epilepsy and he began sodium valproate. Samuel enrolled in the local secondary school and began learning English. He was provided with relatively little support in and adjusting to the academic curriculum and in learning English. Whilst his sister adjusted well to life in the UK, a range of concerns was noted with Samuel. His neurology team had noted difficulties with conversational English. These difficulties did not appear to be resolved with an interpreter, who queried his understanding and described him as 'immature'. The majority of media that Samuel consumed was from Ecuador. Samuel was reported to have several friends, although he rarely saw them out of school hours. Finally, there were queries about Samuel's academic progress, with views of his level of ability and progress being mixed, although the cause of this could not be fully determined. A referral was made to evaluate Samuel's neuropsychological profile given the presence of the juvenile myoclonic epilepsy in the context of a young person who had made a significant transition from one language/cultural environment to another.

THEORY

Background

Neuropsychologists are often asked to assess children from a diverse range of cultural, linguistic, and and educational backgrounds, often in the context of varying clinical presentations. The assessment of a child using standardised, norm-referenced instruments that differ from the child's cultural and language background can pose substantial challenges during a neuropsychological evaluation. Challenges posed by such referrals are increasing in clinical practice with the last 50 years having seen an exponential rise in international migration and globalisation. As a result, there have been substantial shifts in the demographic makeup of many countries, characterised by increasing rates of cultural and linguistic diversity (e.g. Coleman 2008). Whilst clinical neuropsychologists have a clear ethical and professional responsibility to undertake clinical evaluations within this context, there is a paucity of research to guide the process of culturally informed evaluations, particularly within paediatric populations.

In their broadest sense, cultural and language factors represent an array of heterogeneous environmental variables. Modern accounts of brain development emphasise the interplay of environmental and genetic factors in determining structural and functional specialisation in the developing brain (e.g. Interactive Specialisation Theory; Johnson 2011). Within this context, many cognitive abilities (e.g. memory) are recognised as universal. However, repeated participation and exposure to one's cultural environment has been proposed to mould brain structure and function through neuroplastic processes. There is now accumulating evidence for differences between cultural groups using diverse methodologies such as magnetic resonance imaging, event related potential, and functional magnetic resonance imaging (Kitayama and Uskul 2011). These include motor function and visual perceptual abilities (e.g. colour perception and spatial reasoning; Ardila 2017). Differences in the activation of the frontoparietal attention network, for example, have been found between those from East Asian and Western cultures, varying with self-reported ratings of cultural identity (Hedden et al. 2008).

Bias in Culturally Informed Neuropsychological Assessments

Cultural factors can also affect the way an individual performs during neuropsychological assessment. Poorer test performance has consistently been demonstrated amongst individuals from non-Western cultures on Western instruments (e.g. Shuttleworth-Edwards et al. 2004), and individuals from Western cultures demonstrating poorer performance on non-Western assessments (e.g. The Panga Munthu Test). These findings would suggest there is a substantial degree of 'bias' on neuropsychological instruments with individuals from different cultural backgrounds. Bias of this kind is considered to impact neuropsychological assessments at multiple points, which are summarised in Table 22.1 (for further information, see Van de Vijver and Tanzer 2004; Fernández and Abe 2018).

Table 22.1 Summary of potential sources of bias in cross-cultural neuropsychological assessments

Factor affecting assessment	Definition	Example
Construct bias	The construct being assessed is not equivalent across cultural groups	Intelligence and 'intelligent behaviour' are recognised as a culturally defined construct and may be viewed differently by different cultures
Instrument or item bias	Items on assessments have different meanings or occur with different frequency across cultural groups. It can also include the omission of items that are key to the target culture	An item that assesses knowledge common to one culture but less frequent to another. For example 'Name a prime minister of the UK in the Second World War' or the use of Roman alphabet stimuli on a continuous performance task with a child with a non-Germanic first language
Administration bias	Difficulties/differences in factors affecting the administration of an instrument. This is typically language and communication differences between the clinician and child	The child's language abilities are insufficient to understand and complete tasks adequately, or cultural norm violations on behalf of the clinician

It is also important to recognise that clinical neuropsychology is a culturally embedded practice that relies on culturally based assumptions and values. This is further compounded by findings that, in contrast to many cognitive domains, constructs such as intelligence are not universal. Instead, intelligence is a culturally defined concept, which has been demonstrated to differ from culture to culture. Bias can also operate through the individual's familiarity with the text materials; instruments are likely to contain stimuli that are culturally or linguistically specific, and not common to other cultures. Administration bias can also be substantial, with language and communication issues having a significant impact on the child's ability to understand what is expected of them in the assessment. Other sources of bias may be less evident. For example in the USA, one adult study demonstrated how a range of interacting factors could influence test performance. These included differences in the ethnic background between an assessor and the examinee, manipulating the degree of 'threat' posed in the assessment (e.g. instructions that emphasise 'relax and try your best' vs 'tests that emphasise comparing performance with that of others'), as well as the examinee's perceived degree of discrimination faced on a day-to-day basis (Thames et al. 2013). Differential effects have been demonstrated across different domains of cognitive function.

Approaches to Cultural Differences in Neuropsychological Assessment

Different approaches to the difficulties encountered in cross-cultural assessments have been proposed. Historically, the use of 'culture fair' or 'culture free' instruments has been proposed, which typically require minimal verbal instructions or expression for completion (e.g. Rey Complex Figure Test). However, cultural influences on test performance extends beyond that of language with empirical data now demonstrating substantial cultural differences on non-verbal and visual-spatial tasks (see Rosselli and Ardila 2003 for a review).

There have been a number of solutions attempted by test developers. These have typically included efforts to match the normative data to the census data of the country in question, through inclusion of data from different racial/ethnic groups. However, such approaches do not allow the clinician to account for the precise combination of demographic, cultural, and linguistic factors that impact an individual's neuropsychological function. An alternative approach is renorming of assessment instruments, which is often unfeasible given the large number of cultures and languages present in many societies. Such approaches are controversial and criticisms can be broadly divided into the following arguments:

1. Race and ethnicity have tenuous scientific meaning and are more commonly based upon sociopolitical considerations (Collins 2004).
2. May promote the use of 'race-based norms' (Gasquoine 2009).
3. Race and ethnicity have no cause–effect relationship on cognitive development and instead serve as a proxy for the underlying cultural, language, and educational factors of interest (Manly 2006).
4. There is substantial risk of misunderstanding and stigmatisation as well as potentially denying individuals services available to the rest of the population (Manly and Echemendia 2007).

ASSESSMENT AND FORMULATION

Preparation

One consistent factor when preparing for cross-cultural assessments is the need to develop a 'cultural knowledge base' appropriate to the child and family in question. This will assist in providing a context for the selection and interpretation of assessment data. This starts at the point of referral, where information regarding the child's cultural background and language abilities can be gathered. It will also allow for information on other factors that have influenced the child's cognitive development to be collected such as sociopolitical variables and educational background. Some authors have argued for the need for clinicians to be self-reflective and evaluate their own beliefs and cultural identities when working with individuals from different cultural backgrounds, a concept termed 'cultural humility' (Yeager and Bauer-Wu 2013).

It is also important to determine whether an interpreter is required for the evaluation and for which components. It is beyond the scope of this chapter to discuss the complexities arising from this issue, and there are professional guidelines available (e.g. British Psychological Society 2017). However, there is substantial recognition that such approaches can invalidate assessment data and many authors have argued the practice to be unethical. As such, the use of interpreters should only be considered when there are no other options and the child would otherwise be denied clinical services. The literature guiding working with interpreters in paediatric neuropsychology is extremely sparse. Therefore a pragmatic approach is advised that includes preparation of the interpreter ahead of time around expectations of the format of the assessment, preparation of any reasonable adaptations of the material, and discussion with the child and carer involved.

Interview

In addition to a standard clinical interview related to the child's clinical condition (e.g. epilepsy in the case of Samuel), it is important to adapt the interview to consider cultural differences in communication style and possible lack of familiarity with the concepts involved in a neuropsychological evaluation.

The assessment of a child's level of acculturation and linguistic capability is a fundamental component of the interview. Acculturation has been well investigated in health care research and has been proposed as an attempt to operationalise the degree of cultural and linguistic variability at the individual level so that this can be incorporated into the assessment. Higher degrees of acculturation serve as a proxy for the individual more closely resembling the normative group of the neuropsychological test in question and are thereby less susceptive to the degree of bias in the evaluation. Higher degrees of acculturation have been associated with higher test scores on a range of standardised assessments, including both language and nonlanguage-based measures (e.g. Manly et al. 2004). However, acculturation has also been found to be domain specific. For example findings of greater language acculturation have been associated with greater performance on language measures but not on measures of attentional control (Tan and Burgess 2020). This is an important factor prior to selection and administration of a test battery as well as when interpreting the results.

Consistent with modern models of acculturation, it is important to recognise a number of factors, which include: (1) that acculturation is domain specific and (2) that acculturation is not a linear process and individuals can retain one culture as well as adopting another within each domain. Crucially, in child settings, it is also important to emphasise that a child's level of acculturation will likely differ from that of other family members. There are a range of measures designed to assess levels of acculturation such as the

Stephenson Multigroup Acculturation Scale (Stephenson 2000; see Matsudaira 2006 for a review). Questions such as those in Table 22.2 can assist in attempting to operationalise the child and family's separate levels of acculturation to the culture in which the assessment is to be undertaken. Following this, three broad options have been suggested. The first decision is whether the child should be referred to someone with

Table 22.2 Example questions to assess the child and family's degrees of acculturation

Practical aspects of relocation
When did the child and family move?
Under what circumstances was the move?
Have there been any other moves of this kind?
What were the means of support following the move? Community integration?
How welcomed have they felt?
What are the socioeconomic variables in home country? Income, education, etc.
What are the socioeconomic variables in host country?
What is the access to health care and usage in home country like?

Language
How well does the child speak the language of the host country?
How well does the child speak English?
What language(s) were they exposed to in the early developmental period?
What language(s) have they been educated in?
Have there been any substantial language transitions? If so, at what age?

Education
Which countries have they received education in? What languages were classes in?
What language were they taught to read and write in? Did they achieve this at the same time as their peers?
What is the educational system/expectations of the relevant schools?
What was the 'quality' of their education? Questions as to class sizes, availability of resources in school, rigour of teaching, subjects taught etc., are likely to be useful in this area.
How was the child performing educationally before any big transitions?

Culture
How knowledgeable is the child about the history, traditions, and practices of their country of origin?
How knowledgeable is the child about the history and culture of their current country?
What is their relationship with the culture of origin and the dominant culture?
Who does the child socialise with? Do they have friends from other cultural backgrounds?
What is the exposure like to television, movies, and radio? Which culture?
What social media are they active on and with whom?
What are the family's expectations for the child?

greater familiarity with the child's cultural and language background. Other proposed options include employing a 'behavioural neuropsychological approach', in which no standardised assessments are used and clinical impressions are made based upon the individual's day-to-day functioning. This is likely to be extremely complex, particularly in the context of a developmental framework. In addition, it has been criticised for being highly subjective. The final approach, which is employed most commonly, is undertaking a standardised assessment whilst attempting to minimise cultural and linguistic factors in the selection and interpretation of instruments.

Test Selection and Interpretation

A number of strategies have been advocated for reducing the impact of culture on assessment instruments. Some authors (e.g. Nell 1999) advocate extended 'practice periods' with guided learning on easier items to ensure that the child in question has a better understanding of the expectations of the task. Other authors have suggested that a strong emphasis is placed on qualitative information, such as the child's response style, or encouraging the child to 'think aloud' so that their strategy can be more easily identified. Modifications to test stimuli or instructions have also been advocated. These include eliminating words and concepts that are specific to a particular language or cultural group or modification of administration instructions or stimuli. For example children with little exposure to a particular form of currency will struggle on questions asking them to state the value of particular numbers of coins. Alternatively, whilst the Stroop Color-Word Test is typically taken as a task of executive function, if individuals have limited exposure to reading in the language of administration, it ceases to function as it was intended as a result of material bias. In each assessment of this kind, the clinician must balance potential compromises to the reliability and validity of the instrument against the degree of bias in the assessment.

INTERVENTION AND MANAGEMENT

Intervention and management recommendations are a central feature of a neuropsychological evaluation, with the overarching aim to promote the child's cognitive, behavioural, emotional, social, and academic outcomes. However, these same tenets hold true when working with children and families from differing cultural backgrounds. 'Culture' is not an avenue for intervention in and of itself, although interventions for the child's clinical condition have the potential to be divisive and contentious if cultural variables are not taken into account.

Report and Feedback

Feedback of findings and the neuropsychological formulation is a central feature of the assessment process (see Chapter 25 on Feedback). In addition to traditional aspects of the report (e.g. reasons for referral, developmental history, and details of the assessment/formulation) a number of differences are likely required. These have been termed 'making the implicit explicit' (Fujii 2017). The aim of this is to highlight the role of cultural factors that had the potential to impact upon the evaluation and the means taken to minimise these. It is anticipated that these are likely to include descriptions of the languages used in the assessment, the role and impact of an interpreter, and modifications made to the test materials and the justification for doing so. Given that cultural factors will vary depending on the child and family's specific cultural background, language, and levels of acculturation, these details will differ from report to report. The clinician will also need to consider whether to include an interpreter in the feedback and whether to provide a translated copy of the report for the family.

Working With Different Belief Systems

When undertaking culturally informed neuropsychological assessments, there is a requirement for a high degree of ability to understand and work effectively with children and families from varying cultural backgrounds. Clinicians are typically advised to research this and seek adequate supervision before undertaking an assessment. This is a highly complex area in which multiple factors have the potential to interact and 'trade off' with one another.

There are well-documented cultural differences in health beliefs, including more collectivistic perspectives (i.e. common in countries such as China, Japan, and Brazil) or the role of religious beliefs in a child's difficulties (Armstrong and Swartzman 2001). As part of this process, it is important to recognise that paediatric neuropsychology is itself a cultural practice. Practitioners will have their own worldviews, attitudes, and beliefs, particularly around the clinical conditions, which they treat. However, these are not necessarily shared by children and families, particularly amongst those at greater cultural distance. As such, there is a need to work within a neuropsychological framework but also to engage with the belief systems of the child and family in question. For example Ismail et al. (2005) reported that amongst South Asian individuals with epilepsy in the UK, over half endorsed views that epilepsy was the will of god or as punishment for sins in a past life. A diverse network of traditional healers was also reported, providing a parallel system of health care. This was often undertaken with recognition that Western treatments had failed to arrive at a 'cure'. Similarly, amongst individuals with epilepsy in Ecuador, lower levels of education and information provided relative to epilepsy have been found to be associated with higher levels of perceived discrimination (Luna et al. 2017).

One well-established concept that is particularly important when considering recommendations or intervention is that of ethnocentrism. This can be defined as the act of judging another culture based upon the values and beliefs of one's own culture and has been associated with patient alienation, poorer clinical outcomes, and faulty clinical decision-making (Capell, Dean, and Veenstra 2008). Multiple models for culturally competent clinical practice have been proposed. Common factors amongst models include aspects of knowledge (e.g. of culture in health care delivery), attitudes (e.g. respecting variation in cultural norms), and clinical skills (e.g. eliciting patient's explanatory model of illness) (Saha, Beach, and Cooper 2008) in clinical practice. These can form a useful framework from which a joint formulation or model of the child's difficulties can be constructed. This has been identified as a powerful tool in enhancing clinical outcomes and a variety of methods have been proposed in the literature. These include discussing the child and family's understanding of the causes of illness, the timeline of events, the consequences of the illness, including impact on day-to-day life, their interactions with health care services and healers, patterns of distress, and the degree of control they have as well as their beliefs around the prospect for a 'cure' (see Dinos et al. 2017 for further information).

Outcome

Samuel and his mother attended the assessment together and the interview was facilitated by an interpreter. Samuel was assessed in English given his 3 years of education in English with his level of acculturation incorporated in the assessment. He was able to converse in English but favoured Spanish when at home. However, his metalinguistic abilities (e.g. inferencing) in English were unclear. Both Samuel and his family maintained a strong sense of identity with Ecuador, particularly when outside of school. There was evidence of both assimilative and separative acculturation styles in different contexts.

Overall, Samuel's broader cognitive abilities were estimated to be below the level for his age group, including on measures that were anticipated to be less susceptible to cultural and language factors in this case (e.g. Beery-Buktenica Visual-Motor Integration Test, Beery, Buktenica, and Beery 2010; Wechsler Intelligence Scale for Children, Fifth Edition visual-spatial and fluid-reasoning subtests, Wechsler 2016). This was not unexpected given the context of the epilepsy. Samuel's performance on measures of English language was lower, although it was unclear whether low-language based scores represented difficulties with language or was a combination of learning English as an additional language combined with reduced exposure due to the family's acculturative strategy. It was recognised that to delineate this would require further assessment in Spanish.

Other low scores (e.g. Conners' Continuous Performance Test, Third Edition, Conners 2014, and executive function measures) were thought to reflect inherent weaknesses with Samuel's attention and executive functions abilities, particularly on measures with minimal language demands with less bias in test materials. This was consistent with standardised parental report measures of day-to-day executive function and was a likely consequence of juvenile myoclonic epilepsy on Samuel's development. Samuel's academic knowledge and abilities were well below the level expected, with a range of clinically significant discrepancies in his profile. This suggestion of broad-based 'impairment' in Samuel's academic ability was hypothesised to reflect poorer 'quality' relative to Western standards of education, combined with inherent difficulties with Samuel's ability to access English language teaching.

In addition to a series of psycho-education sessions on epilepsy for Samuel and his family, recommendations included environmental interventions for the vulnerabilities in his average cognitive profile, assessment for possible attention-deficit/hyperactivity disorder and support in school given his status as an English as an Additional Language student in combination with his academic 'under-achievement'.

SUMMARY

Cultural and linguistic factors are recognised to exert a powerful but poorly understood influence on neuropsychological evaluations, particularly when employing standardised, norm-referenced instruments. Culture has a profound effect on the development and expression of universal, core cognitive abilities, with differences evident on language-based assessments, as well as non-language measures. This is further compounded given that neuropsychological assessment takes place within a cultural context, with its own culturally informed views of what constitutes many constructs such as 'intelligence'. In addition, multiple sources of bias have been identified in the assessment, particularly for individuals from non-Western cultures. These include lack of familiarity with stimuli in the test materials, different response styles as well as variables influencing administration (e.g. language and stereotype threat). This poses substantial challenges to paediatric neuropsychologists when undertaking assessments with individuals from different cultural groups or those who are at the intersection of different cultures. At present, there are no assessments that address these issues in child populations.

In addition to factors related to the administration and interpretation of standardised assessments during neuropsychological assessment, it is also important to be aware of broader cultural issues relating to the reasons for the referral. Children and families will have their own understanding on the aetiology and treatment of the presenting clinical condition and differences in such illness beliefs will be contingent upon a diverse range of factors. In addition, it is also important to be mindful of culturally specific presentations of psychological distress. These have been well documented at the intersection of multiple cultural groups. For example 'ataque de nervios' has been described as a presentation of psychological distress thought to be specific to Hispanic/Latin cultural groups (e.g. Yusim et al. 2009). Similarly, 'thinking too much' has been studied across multiple geographic areas and recognised as representing different forms of psychological distress that vary both within and across cultures (Kaiser et al. 2015).

Clinicians therefore not only have to adjust existing neuropsychological assessments and incorporate cultural factors into the interpretation of assessments and their formulations but also consider culturally specific presentations of the child and family's emotional well-being and psychological distress. Taking account of language factors and competence, level of acculturation, and the child's educational history provides a useful framework to reduce confounding cultural effects when assessing a young person's neuropsychological function.

REFERENCES

Ardila A (2017) Culture and cognitive testing. In: Ardila A, editor, *Historical Development of Human Cognition: A Cultural-Historical Neuropsychological Perspective* (Vol. 3). Singapore: Springer, pp. 135–139.

Armstrong TL, Swartzman LC (2001) Cross-cultural differences in illness models and expectations for the health care provider-client/patient interaction. *Handbook of Cultural Health Psychology*. San Diego: Elsevier, pp. 63–84.

British Psychological Society (2017) *Working with Interpreters: Guidelines for Psychologists*. Leicester, UK: British Psychological Society.

Capell J, Dean E, Veenstra G (2008) The relationship between cultural competence and ethnocentrism of health care professionals. *Journal of Transcultural Nursing* 19(2): 121–125.

Coleman D (2008) The demographic effects of international migration in Europe. *Oxford Review of Economic Policy* 24(3): 453.

Collins FS (2004) What we do and don't know about 'race', 'ethnicity', genetics and health at the dawn of the genome era. *Nature Genetics* 36(11 Suppl): S13–15. doi: ng1436 [pii] 10.1038/ng1436.

Dinos S, Ascoli M, Owiti J, Bhui K (2017) Assessing explanatory models and health beliefs: An essential but overlooked competency for clinicians. *BJPsych Advances* 23(2): 106–114. doi: 10.1192/apt.bp.114.013680.

Fernández AL, Abe J (2018) Bias in cross-cultural neuropsychological testing: Problems and possible solutions. *Culture and Brain* 6(1): 1–35.

Fujii D (2017) *Conducting a Culturally Informed Neuropsychological Evaluation*. Washington DC: American Psychological Association.

Gasquoine PG (2009) Race-norming of neuropsychological tests. *Neuropsychology Review* 19(2): 250–262. doi: 10.1007/s11065-009-9090-5.

Hedden T, Ketay S, Aron A, Markus HR, Gabrieli JD (2008) Cultural influences on neural substrates of attentional control. *Psychological Science* 19(1): 12–17. doi: 10.1111/j.1467-9280.2008.02038.x.

Ismail H, Wright J, Rhodes P, Small N (2005) Religious beliefs about causes and treatment of epilepsy. *British Journal of General Practice* 55(510): 26–31.

Johnson MH (2011) Interactive specialization: A domain-general framework for human functional brain development? *Developmental Cognitive Neuroscience* 1(1): 7–21. doi: 10.1016/j.dcn.2010.07.003.

Kaiser BN, Haroz EE, Kohrt BA, Bolton PA, Bass JK, Hinton DE (2015) 'Thinking too much': A systematic review of a common idiom of distress. *Social Science & Medicine* 147: 170–183. doi: 10.1016/j.socscimed.2015.10.044.

Kitayama S, Uskul AK (2011) Culture, mind, and the brain: Current evidence and future directions. *Annual Review of Psychology* 62: 419–449. doi: 10.1146/annurev-psych-120709-145357.

Luna J, Nizard M, Becker D et al. (2017) Epilepsy-associated levels of perceived stigma, their associations with treatment, and related factors: A cross-sectional study in urban and rural areas in Ecuador. *Epilepsy & Behavior* 68: 71–77. doi: 10.1016/j.yebeh.2016.12.026.

Manly JJ (2006) Deconstructing race and ethnicity: Implications for measurement of health outcomes. *Medical Care* 44(11 Suppl 3): S10–16. doi: 10.1097/01.mlr.0000245427.22788.be 00005650-200611001-00005 [pii].

Manly JJ, Byrd DA, Touradji P, Stern Y (2004) Acculturation, reading level, and neuropsychological test performance among African American elders. *Applied Neuropsychology* 11(1): 37–46. doi: 10.1207/s15324826an1101_5.

Manly JJ, Echemendia RJ (2007) Race-specific norms: Using the model of hypertension to understand issues of race, culture, and education in neuropsychology. *Archives of Clinical Neuropsychology* 22(3): 319–325. doi: S0887-6177(07)00013-3 [pii] 10.1016/j.acn.2007.01.006.

Matsudaira T (2006) Measures of psychological acculturation: A review. *Transcult Psychiatry* **43**(3): 462–487. doi: 10.1177/1363461506066989.

Nell V (1999) *Cross-Cultural Neuropsychological Assessment: Theory and Practice*. New York: Psychology Press.

Rosselli M, Ardila A (2003) The impact of culture and education on non-verbal neuropsychological measurements: A critical review. *Brain and Cognition* **52**(3): 326–333. doi: S0278262603001702 [pii].

Saha S, Beach MC, Cooper LA (2008) Patient centeredness, cultural competence and healthcare quality. *Journal of the National Medical Association* **100**(11): 1275–1285.

Stephenson M (2000) Development and validation of the Stephenson Multigroup Acculturation Scale (SMAS). *Psychological Assessment* **12**(1): 77–88.

Shuttleworth-Edwards AB, Kemp RD, Rust AL, Muirhead JG, Hartman NP, Radloff SE (2004) Cross-cultural effects on IQ test performance: A review and preliminary normative indications on WAIS-III test performance. *Journal of Clinical and Experimental Neuropsychology* **26**(7): 903–920. doi: 10.1080/13803390490510824.

Tan YW, Burgess GH (2020) Multidimensional effects of acculturation at the construct or index level of seven broad neuropsychological skills. *Culture and Brain* **8**: 27–451–19.

Thames AD, Hinkin CH, Byrd DA et al. (2013) Effects of stereotype threat, perceived discrimination, and examiner race on neuropsychological performance: Simple as black and white? *Journal of the International Neuropsychological Society* **19**(5): 583–593. doi: 10.1017/S1355617713000076.

Van de Vijver F, Tanzer NK (2004) Bias and equivalence in cross-cultural assessment: An overview. *Revue Européenne de Psychologie Appliquée/European Review of Applied Psychology* **54**(2): 119–135.

Yeager KA, Bauer-Wu S (2013) Cultural humility: Essential foundation for clinical researchers. *Applied Nursing Research* **26**(4): 251–256. doi: 10.1016/j.apnr.2013.06.008.

Yusim A, Anbarasan D, Hall B, Goetz R, Neugebauer R, Ruiz P (2009) Somatic and cognitive domains of depression in an underserved region of Ecuador: Some cultural considerations. *World Psychiatry* **8**(3): 178–180. doi: 10.1002/j.2051-5545.2009.tb00247.x.

CHAPTER 23

Validity Testing in Paediatric Neuropsychology

Brian L Brooks and William MacAllister

Presenting Concern

Jane is a right-handed girl who was born at term subsequent to an unremarkable pregnancy. She was the fourth of five children in this sibship. Developmental milestones were reported to have all been achieved on time based on family report. Though she was described as having 'mild dyslexia' when younger, she went on to perform quite well academically, earning mostly As and Bs throughout her schooling. Despite her strong academic history, she was described as an anxious and perfectionistic child. She was involved in multiple competitive sports.

Jane sustained a concussion at age 14 years when she collided head-to-head with another player in field hockey, subsequently falling and then striking her forehead on the ground. Emergency department records note that, although there was no clear loss of consciousness, she was unable to remember the event but was aware that she was attended to by her coach, walked to the first aid office, and was brought to the emergency department via ambulance. Medical records from the emergency department visit documented that she complained of dizziness, forehead pain, and neck pain. Cervical X-rays were completed and read by the radiologist as unremarkable. She returned to the emergency department 1 week later with new complaints starting that day that included vomiting, headache, vertigo, photophobia, poor sleep, and difficulties walking independently. Due to her concerns with walking, Jane refused to ambulate on her own, and she began using a wheelchair. Cognitive complaints included difficulty processing conversations, trouble remembering personal details, and difficulty reading. Mood was also labile, but she did not appear distressed by her presentation. Treatment for headache was initiated in the emergency department which provided temporary relief. A brain computerised tomography scan was completed at that time and was interpreted by the neuroradiologist as unremarkable. Jane returned to the emergency department again at about 3 weeks postinjury with similar complaints of vomiting, headache, vertigo, photophobia, poor sleep, and difficulties walking independently. At the second emergency department visit, a referral to the outpatient brain injury program was generated.

Jane was seen 1 month postinjury by the nurse practitioner in the tertiary care hospital's brain injury outpatient clinic. Headaches, poor sleep, emotional disruption, cognitive problems (now including the progression to a complete inability to read), absence from school, and persistent difficulties with walking were documented. A somewhat limited physical examination was reported as normal. She was advised to begin returning to school, was prescribed an antiemetic for nausea, and was provided with suggestions for sleep (sleep hygiene and melatonin). Referrals for physical therapy, neuropsychology, and a brain magnetic resonance imaging scan were all generated to begin investigating and treating the presenting complaints. A consultation with a neurologist was also requested.

Jane was referred for a neuropsychological evaluation given her cognitive complaints, mood changes, and medically unexplained symptoms. She was seen 1.5 months postinjury. On clinical interview, Jane was a good historian and eloquently recounted her concerns. She presented with several atypical and unlikely symptoms given her injury, including an inability to report her birthday, changes in reading ability due to 'words appearing scrambled and having to figure out the sounds of letters', and ambulation problems. Notably, she did not seem distressed about being in a wheelchair but was distressed about not being at school and was concerned about being able to attend a sporting event in 2 weeks.

THEORY

Lagging behind the adult neuropsychology literature base, validity testing in paediatric evaluations has only recently garnered attention in the last decade. Performance validity tests (PVTs) are included in neuropsychological assessments to provide tangible measurement of task engagement, response bias (i.e. a tendency to answer inaccurately or falsely), and intentional underperformance, and, as such, facilitate the neuropsychologist's ability to objectively judge the accuracy of test results. PVTs are not administered or interpreted in isolation. They are used in conjunction with other methods to determine validity, including but not limited to: behavioural observations, consistency with medical history, consistency with known effects of a disease, and symptom validity scales on questionnaires (e.g. designed to detect if someone is completing a rating scale inconsistently or randomly, if someone is reporting an excessive level of problems and presenting themselves too negatively, if someone is under-reporting common concerns and presenting themselves too favourably).

The observed lag in paediatric-focused literature for validity testing may translate into lower levels of use of these types of measures in clinical practice. Although a recent survey of neuropsychologists across North America who specifically evaluate children and adolescents suggested that 92% of clinicians report using at least one PVT in all neuropsychological assessments (Brooks, Ploetz, and Kirkwood 2016), subsequent investigation calls these results into question and suggests that fewer than 6% of paediatric clinicians routinely use these measures in clinical settings (MacAllister, Vasserman, and Armstrong 2019). PVT use remains quite controversial in paediatric neuropsychology, although we assert that this should not be the case. Many believe that those routinely using PVTs are motivated to 'catch liars'; this is a misguided assumption arising from a false belief that scoring below established cut-offs on validity tests can only be equated to malingering (Baker and Kirkwood 2015). Instead, the raison d'être of PVTs is to help a clinician determine and ensure accuracy of test results within the context of all available information, directly leading to accurate diagnostic conclusions and appropriate treatment recommendations (Slick and Sherman 2012; Sherman 2015). It is worth highlighting that PVT use in all assessments (i.e. regardless of whether they are conducted for clinical or legal purposes) is consistent with recommendations from major professional organisations (e.g. the American Academy of Clinical Neuropsychology, National Academy of Neuropsychology; see Bush et al. 2005; Heilbronner et al. 2009) and is also consistent with ethical guidelines to ensure clinical decisions are based on the most accurate data possible (MacAllister and Vasserman 2015).

Ethics codes and practice standards vary by region, most include guidelines regarding the appropriate use of psychological tests and the interpretation thereof. For example in our region, the College of Alberta Psychologists Practice Guideline regarding the Control and Use of Tests by Psychologists notes that psychologists should 'uphold the highest standards of accuracy' when administering (and, by extension, interpreting) test results (College of Alberta Psychologists 2013). The American Psychological Association has the clearest codified and referenced ethics code regarding test usage and interpretation (American Psychological Association 2002). For example standards 9.01c and 9.06 of the American Psychological Association ethics code note that psychologists 'provide opinions on the psychological characteristics of individuals *only after they have conducted an examination of an individual adequate to support their statements or conclusions*' (p. 1071, emphasis added) and that, in interpreting the results of assessments, psychologists must consider 'the purpose of the assessment as well as the *various test factors*', which include factors that may '*reduce the accuracy*' of test interpretation (p. 1072, emphasis added). Without an objective assessment of an individual's engagement in the testing process using PVTs, the results of objective cognitive testing should be considered tentative. In fact, in the presence of PVT performance below established cut-off scores, these measures are the single most important factor in appropriate diagnosis and treatment planning. For example Sherman (2015) and Slick and Sherman (2012) provide critical analyses of differential diagnoses associated with noncredible performances that are necessary for said planning, with some reasons being firmly rooted in psychological distress (e.g. see Baker and Kirkwood 2015).

All of this begs the question of why have paediatric neuropsychologists been slow to routinely adopt PVTs in their assessments? Reimbursement issues (i.e. in the USA), low base rates of invalidity, longstanding practice habits, and time constraints for assessment likely factor in for many; to some extent, this has reflected the fact that validation of PVTs in young populations has been slow. Clinician knowledge of appropriate tools has been hampered. However, the last decade or so has shown an explosion of research validating the use of both embedded and freestanding PVTs for young populations. Considerable effort has been dedicated towards validating those PVTs originally developed for use in adults to be used in younger populations (i.e. a downward translation of measures), but there has also been recent movement towards developing both standalone PVTs (Kirkwood et al. 2014; Sherman and Brooks 2015b; Brooks and Sherman 2018; Brooks et al. 2019a) and embedded PVTs (Sherman and Brooks 2015a; Brooks et al. 2018; Brooks et al. 2019b) that are designed a priori specifically for use in paediatric populations.

The lag in routine validity test use for paediatric assessments may also lie in misperceptions of the purpose of these measures and an underappreciation for the reasons why invalid data could be obtained. A common misperception is that these tests are only necessary when a patient is involved in litigation or when the clinician feels their role is to catch someone feigning test results. Prior survey studies from the UK (e.g. McCarter et al. 2009), western European countries (e.g. Dandachi-FitzGerald, Ponds, and Merten 2013), and North America (e.g. Sharland and Gfeller 2007) have supported this misperception that PVTs are less important for clinical work than forensic work. This approach fails to appreciate that young people are very capable of underperforming on testing, even in the absence of a litigious situation.

Validity tests help facilitate a clinical decision about whether or not obtained results are meaningful, which is essential regardless of the reason why an assessment is being conducted. As noted previously, PVTs are one component within a comprehensive decision-making process that are used to determine validity of obtained results. Key differences between PVTs and other methods, such as behavioural observations, inconsistencies in presentation over time, and differences between known disease and patient presentation, are that PVTs are rooted in evidence, are continually subjected to research scrutiny, and they are objective measures with tangible scores to interpret (instead of an opinion that may be more easily swayed by bias or may be subject to a lack of sensitivity at detecting subtle underperforming). The objective nature of PVTs is key to keeping one's clinical judgment consistent over time and minimising drift that can creep into even the most seasoned clinician's opinion. In addition, routinely giving validity tests to all patients helps establish and maintain clinical acumen about how easily these measures are passed by even those with frank neurological disease (MacAllister et al. 2009; Brooks, Sherman, and Krol 2012; Carone 2014; Ploetz et al. 2016; Brooks et al. 2019b; MacAllister et al. 2020). The 'why' someone obtains a score below established cut-offs on any PVT is the sine qua non of clinical decision-making. An automatic label of 'faking' or 'malingering' without consideration of all the factors is not only premature, it can be detrimental to clinical rapport, and it can miss an important direction for patient care (Baker and Kirkwood 2015).

ASSESSMENT AND FORMULATION

In considering the validity of neuropsychological test findings, the skilled neuropsychologist should employ several strategies. First and foremost, at the outset of the evaluation, the clinician should be familiar with the presenting complaints/diagnoses, such that a mismatch between expected findings and observed test data can be judged. For example those performing epilepsy evaluations in a tertiary care setting servicing medically refractory epilepsy may anticipate significant cognitive impairments. In contrast, outcomes in mild traumatic brain injury (i.e. concussion) are generally favourable, with resolution of physical and cognitive symptoms generally occurring within a few days to weeks for the vast majority (Barlow et al. 2010; Zemek et al. 2016) and evidence suggesting long-term acquired cognitive deficits are unlikely (e.g. see a systematic review of meta-analyses by Karr, Areshenkoff, and Garcia-Barrera 2014). In cases of concussion with prolonged symptom recovery, however, obtaining scores below established cut-offs for PVTs is far more common (e.g. Kirkwood et al. 2014).

All neuropsychologists pay close attention to behavioural observations during examinations and there are several red flags that may lead one to conclude that test data are invalid; the obvious include outright task refusal, extreme oppositionality, dramatic exaggeration of symptomatology, and/or playfulness, with the latter more commonly seen in preschool aged children. Other behaviours that may render test results invalid include not paying attention, misunderstanding test instructions, or physical limitations that may not be readily known to the examiner (e.g. being colour blind, having poor hearing, requiring prescription glasses). Although we certainly advocate for careful observation of test-taking behaviours, it has become clear that, except in the most egregious of cases (e.g. blatant refusal to answer), behavioural observations alone cannot be relied on to determine data validity. For example Kirkwood and colleagues (Kirkwood and Kirk 2010; Kirkwood et al. 2010) have shown that children and adolescents can successfully feign neuropsychological deficits, even in cases where secondary gain is not obvious.

The most empirically supported method for determining test validity is the use of formal PVTs that have validity evidence for use in children and adolescents. This term, PVT, warrants some further clarification at this point. The term PVT should be distinguished from symptom validity tests (SVTs); while PVTs refer to performance-based tasks (either standalone or embedded within a cognitive test) that assess feigning or exaggeration of cognitive deficits, SVTs generally refer to questionnaire items that point to exaggeration of reported symptoms. It is generally recommended that neuropsychological evaluations include both PVTs to detect invalid objective test performance and SVTs to detect exaggerated subjective symptom reporting.

A review of available and validated tools is outside the scope of this chapter, but we refer the interested reader to resources such as Kirkwood's text *Validity Testing in Child and Adolescent Assessment: Evaluating Exaggeration, Feigning, and Noncredible Effort* (Kirkwood 2015) as well as reviews by Emhoff, Lynch, and McCaffrey (2018) and Kirk et al. (2020; in particular, Tables 2 and 3). We wish to note that freestanding validity measures (i.e. measures specifically designed as standalone validity measures) typically boast stronger psychometric properties than embedded indices (i.e. interpretation of aspects of bona fide cognitive tasks that may suggest poor task engagement). In short, there is currently a small but useful arsenal of PVTs validated for use in children and adolescents undergoing neuropsychological evaluations.

INTERVENTION AND MANAGEMENT

In considering the case of Jane, there are several important factors to consider regarding the validity of her presentation from the perspective of consistency with known effects from a diagnosis (e.g. concussion or mild traumatic brain injury). First and foremost, the injury characteristics are minimal, with no clear loss of consciousness at the time of injury, an absence of prolonged dense posttraumatic amnesia, and unremarkable neuroimaging. In short, a complete recovery would be expected from this single, uncomplicated, mild concussion. Even if the literature suggests that a significant minority will have lingering symptoms beyond the 2 months when she was evaluated by neuropsychologists, the literature would also support that the trajectory would be positive over time, not worsening with onset of new significant neurological problems well after the injury. This should lead the astute clinician to consider other factors in explaining her symptom presentation, which is in part keeping with the early requisitions for a brain magnetic resonance imaging scan, neuropsychological evaluation, and neurology consultation to rule out potential occult processes.

Jane came to the neuropsychology appointment in a wheelchair, reporting that whilst she is physically capable of walking, she has a difficult time doing so given balance problems and her legs 'not moving quickly.' She clarified that 'I have to tell my legs what to do' and stated 'I can walk, but I'm slow.' She was also fearful that she would fall if she stood up and walked, but, interestingly, she was not psychologically distressed by being in a wheelchair. Profound fatigue was also reported, with her mother commenting that Jane will experience extreme fatigue by only taking a few steps and will reportedly 'pass out'. Other somatic symptoms included daily vomiting, headaches that 'never go away', and poor sleep. With respect to cognitive symptoms, she reported difficulty focusing, with no improvement in concentration seen since injury. Curiously, her mother did not observe any concentration challenges when Jane was completing a recent art project. With respect to anxiety, she expressed concerns about falling behind in school and her grades suffering.

Embedded within this history are also several red flags for symptom exaggeration; although symptoms of nausea, vomiting, and dizziness immediately postinjury are certainly common, again, the emergence of new symptoms weeks later is unexpected, especially in light of normal neuroimaging. It is also noteworthy that the reported daily vomiting was never witnessed by another person, including her mother. Further, the development of an inability to walk and deficits in autobiographical memory are inconsistent with concussion and are rarely medically probable (e.g. delirium), raising significant concerns regarding the viability of the claims. Moreover, our clinical experience is that even the most neurologically impacted children do not forget something as personal and important as their own birthday. Further, behaviourally, there were several inconsistencies within her own presentation that were noted (e.g. awkward pencil grip then followed by normal pencil grip; being slow to respond on some tests and then so rapid on other tests that it was hard to keep up with her responses; negative learning curves where repetition of information led to much lower performance). Essentially, the first step of determining validity of presentation is consistency of a clinical presentation with known diagnosis, which was not met with Jane. Even if all validity measures are passed by a patient with this clinical history, the current presentation is not consistent with concussion and differential diagnoses must rise to the surface rapidly.

On formal testing, objective test results were quite uneven, and certainly not consistent with what may be expected with head injury. For example her verbal learning and memory were measured to be well above her same-age peers, falling at the 95th percentile. This level of considerable strength in memory clearly bolstered the clinical opinion that her obtained scores below established cut-offs on the PVTs were true positives; her performances on the Test of Memory Malingering (Tombaugh 1996), the Memory Validity Profile (Sherman and Brooks 2015b), and the Medical Symptom Validity Test (Green 2004) were all well below established cut-offs, and not far above random guessing/statistical chance. It is improbable to have superior skills on formal memory testing but perform so grossly below established levels on simple validity tests.

Outcome

A neuropsychological evaluation of Jane was conducted, which included about 2 hours of objective testing and completion of standardised questionnaires. The testing included measures of attention, learning, memory, psychomotor processing speed, executive functioning, several standalone PVTs, embedded PVTs, and SVTs (this is a standard battery regardless of specific complaints). Every PVT in this battery was below acceptable cut-off scores and several SVTs suggested improbable symptom reporting. Interestingly, as noted previously, she scored below established cut-offs on PVTs but had superior abilities on other measures. The neuropsychological evaluation report concluded that her objective test results 'are not valid and should not be interpreted as being a meaningful representation of her abilities' given multiple flagged PVTs and SVTs.

It was further noted that her 'presentation and complaints are *not consistent* with concussion'. With the progressive ruling out of neurological explanations for her presentation, the presentation suggested psychological aetiologies instead, including queries of anxiety with somatisation and/or factitious disorder.

Treatment recommendations were discussed with the team, with intensive psychotherapy being considered one of the most important interventions. Jane was seen for psychotherapy by one of the hospital psychologists; given the nature of her presentation and the level of functional disability, she was engaged in daily therapy. The psychologist focused effort on education of concussion symptoms and recovery, challenging false beliefs about returning to sport and school that appeared to be driven by her anxiety, increasing behavioural activation, and teaching strategies for improving sleep at night. She was also concomitantly seen for an urgent psychiatric evaluation to help determine medical treatment, with a somatic symptom disorder being diagnosed and Jane being prescribed fluoxetine. An urgent brain magnetic resonance imaging scan was also completed during this time, which was read as normal by the neuroradiologist. Although physical therapy was part of her treatment programming, this mainly targeted the physical deconditioning that occurred secondary to her wheelchair usage; importantly, had symptoms been taken at face value, physical therapy would have been the main focus of treatment, but deemed of limited utility given the psychological underpinning of her presentation. Plans for continued school reintegration were also discussed.

At a psychiatry follow-up after a few weeks, Jane reported that 'everything is better' and commented that 1 week ago, she 'just woke up and everything was over', further clarifying that she was able to walk, was no longer dizzy, and nausea and vomiting subsided. She felt that she no longer needed psychotherapy but did agree to continue taking the fluoxetine Jane continued her integration back to full-time school and care was returned to her primary care physician.

SUMMARY

The present case highlights a few key points. Most notably, detection of invalid test engagement was critical for accurate diagnosis. Specifically, had PVTs not been appropriately employed, the neuropsychologist may have erroneously concluded that there were longstanding cognitive deficits secondary to her concussion. Not only would this conclusion have been grossly out of keeping with our current knowledge about concussion outcomes, but it would have led to inappropriate treatment recommendations and further costly investigations. That is had cognitive impairment (and physical impairments) been taken at face value, treatment recommendations would have included intensive cognitive rehabilitation and physical therapy, and further recommendations would have been necessary to determine the neurological basis of her acquired deficits. Given the psychiatric nature of her presentation, these treatments would have not only been unhelpful, but also placed undue burden on health care practitioners and the health care system at large. More importantly, however, the unintentional iatrogenesis stemming from the inappropriate medicalisation of her psychiatric symptoms would have further prolonged her recovery, violating the central tenet of most ethics codes: *Do no harm*.

It should be acknowledged that Jane's overall presentation was somewhat of a caricature of what is more commonly seen in clinical practice; although this was an actual case seen by one of the chapter authors, the overdramatised symptom presentation and implausible physical and cognitive complaints would likely be misattributed to the concussion by only the most naïve clinician. The vast majority of children and adolescents with performance on validity tests below established cut-offs are far more subtle and less detectable in casual observation. Still, there are cases where insufficient performance on validity tests are seen in very 'high stakes' neuropsychological evaluations. Aside from concussion evaluations where there is a known high rate of PVT scores falling below established cut-offs, PVTs are critical in any child or teen evaluation being conducted in a situation where potential gain is at hand (e.g. academic accommodations, access to stimulant medications, reduction of external pressures, etc.). Perhaps most dramatically, one of the authors has seen unexpected validity concerns in medical cases, most notably in a young teen undergoing a presurgical epilepsy evaluation. Failure to detect invalid results in this case could have led to a devastating surgical outcome. Specifically, this patient may have been deemed to be at low risk for cognitive decline with surgery, and the surgeon may have been less conservative in the resection, leading to a loss of cognitive skill falsely deemed already impaired.

To summarise, validity testing is a critical element of paediatric neuropsychological evaluation. Although, in years past, there was a dearth of PVTs validated for use in child evaluations, this is no longer the case; several PVTs developed for use with adults have shown utility in younger populations and there are now instruments developed specifically for children. Not only is the routine use of validity testing consistent with guidelines from professional organisations but also professional ethics; validity testing helps the clinician to ensure the accuracy of our test data in the pursuit of accurate diagnostic conclusions and appropriate treatment planning.

REFERENCES

American Psychological Association, Ethics Committee (2002) Ethical principles of psychologists and code of conduct. *American Psychologist* **57**(12): 1060–1073.

Baker DA, Kirkwood MW (2015) Motivations behind noncredible presentations: Why children feign and how to make this determination. In: Kirkwood MW, editor, *Validity Testing in Child and Adolescent Assessment: Evaluating Exaggeration, Feigning, and Noncredible Effort*. New York: The Guilford Press, pp. 125–144.

Barlow KM, Crawford S, Stevenson A, Sandhu SS, Belanger F, Dewey D (2010) Epidemiology of postconcussion syndrome in pediatric mild traumatic brain injury. *Pediatrics* **126**(2): e374–381.

Brooks BL, Fay-McClymont TB, MacAllister WS, Vasserman M, Sherman EMS (2019a) A new kid on the block: The Memory Validity Profile (MVP) in children with neurological conditions. *Child Neuropsychol* **25**(4): 561–572.

Brooks BL, MacAllister WS, Fay-McClymont TB, Vasserman M, Sherman EMS (2019b) Derivation of new embedded performance validity indicators for the Child and Adolescent Memory Profile (ChAMP) Objects subtest in youth with mild traumatic brain injury. *Arch Clin Neuropsychol* **34**(4): 531–538.

Brooks BL, Ploetz DM, Kirkwood MW (2016) A survey of neuropsychologists' use of validity tests with children and adolescents. *Child Neuropsychology* **22**(8): 1001–1020.

Brooks BL, Sherman EM, Krol AL (2012) Utility of TOMM Trial 1 as an indicator of effort in children and adolescents. *Archives of Clinical Neuropsychology* **27**(1): 23–29.

Brooks BL, Sherman EMS (2018) Using the Memory Validity Profile (MVP) to detect invalid performance in youth with mild traumatic brain injury. *Appl Neuropsychol Child* **8**(4): 319–325.

Brooks BL, Plourde V, MacAllister WS, Sherman EMS (2018) Detecting invalid performance in youth with traumatic brain injury using the Child and Adolescent Memory Profile (ChAMP) lists subtest. *Journal of Pediatric Neuropsychology* **4**(3–4): 105–112.

Bush SS, Ruff RM, Troster AI, Barth JT, Koffler SP, Pliskin NH (2005) Symptom validity assessment: Practice issues and medical necessity NAN policy & planning committee. *Archives of Clinical Neuropsychology* **20**(4): 419–426.

Carone DA (2014) Young child with severe brain volume loss easily passes the Word Memory Test and Medical Symptom Validity Test: Implications for mild TBI. *The Clinical Neuropsychologist* 28(1): 146–162.

College of Alberta Psychologists (2013) Control and use of tests by psychologists. Available at: https://www.cap.ab.ca/Portals/0/pdfs/ControlAndUseOfTests.pdf [Accessed January 2022].

Dandachi-FitzGerald B, Ponds RWHM, Merten T (2013) Symptom validity and neuropsychological assessment: A survey of practices and beliefs of neuropsychologists in six European countries. *Archives of Clinical Neuropsychology* 28: 771–783.

Emhoff SM, Lynch JK, McCaffrey RJ (2018) Performance and symptom validity testing in pediatric assessment: A review of the literature. *Dev Neuropsychol* 43(8): 671–707.

Heilbronner RL, Sweet JJ, Morgan JE, Larrabee GJ, Millis SR (2009) American Academy of Clinical Neuropsychology Consensus Conference Statement on the neuropsychological assessment of effort, response bias, and malingering. *The Clinical Neuropsychologist* 23(7): 1093–1129.

Karr JE, Areshenkoff CN, Garcia-Barrera MA (2014) The neuropsychological outcomes of concussion: A systematic review of meta-analyses on the cognitive sequelae of mild traumatic brain injury. *Neuropsychology* 28(3): 321–336.

Kirk JW, Baker DA, Kirk JJ, MacAllister WS (2020) A review of performance and symptom validity testing with pediatric populations. *Applied Neuropsychology: Child* 9(4): 292–306. doi: 10.1080/21622965.2020.1750118.

Kirkwood MW, editor (2015) *Validity Testing in Child and Adolescent Assessment: Evaluating Exaggeration, Feigning, and Noncredible Effort.* New York: The Guilford Press.

Kirkwood MW, Connery AK, Kirk JW, Baker DA (2014) Detecting performance invalidity in children: Not quite as easy as A, B, C, 1, 2, 3 but automatized sequences appears promising. *Child Neuropsychology* 20(2): 245–252.

Kirkwood MW, Kirk JW (2010) The base rate of suboptimal effort in a pediatric mild TBI sample: Performance on the Medical Symptom Validity Test. *The Clinical Neuropsychologist* 24(5): 860–872.

Kirkwood MW, Kirk JW, Blaha RZ, Wilson P (2010) Noncredible effort during pediatric neuropsychological exam: A case series and literature review. *Child Neuropsychology* 16: 604–618.

Kirkwood MW, Peterson RL, Connery AK, Baker DA, Grubenhoff JA (2014) Postconcussive symptom exaggeration after pediatric mild traumatic brain injury. *Pediatrics* 133(4): 643–650.

MacAllister WS, Désiré N, Vasserman M, Dalrymple J, Salinas L, Brooks BL (2020) The use of the MSVT in children and adolescents with epilepsy. *Applied Neuropsychology: Child* 9(4): 323–328. doi: 10.1080/21622965.2020.1750127.

MacAllister WS, Nakhutina L, Bender HA, Karantzoulis S, Carlson C (2009) Assessing effort during neuropsychological evaluation with the TOMM in children and adolescents with epilepsy. *Child Neuropsychology* 15(6): 521–531.

MacAllister WS, Vasserman M (2015) Ethical considerations in pediatric validity testing. In: Kirkwood MW, editor, *Validity Testing in Child and Adolescent Assessment: Evaluating Exaggeration, Feigning, and Noncredible Effort.* New York: The Guilford Press, pp. 164–184.

MacAllister WS, Vasserman M, Armstrong K (2019) Are we documenting performance validity testing in pediatric neuropsychological assessments? A brief report. *Child Neuropsychology* 25(8): 1035–1042.

McCarter RJ, Walton NH, Brooks ND, Powell GE (2009) Effort testing in contemporary UK neuropsychological practice. *The Clinical Neuropsychologist,* 23: 1050–1066.

Ploetz D, Mazur-Mosiewicz A, Kirkwood MW, Sherman EMS, Brooks BL (2016) Performance on the Test of Memory Malingering in children with neurological conditions. *Child Neuropsychology,* **22**(2): 133–142.

Sharland MJ, Gfeller JD (2007) A survey of neurologists' beliefs and practices with respect to the assessment of effort. *Archives of Clinical Neuropsychology* **22**: 213–223.

Sherman EMS (2015) Terminology and diagnostic concepts. In Kirkwood MW, editor, *Validity Testing in Child and Adolescent Assessment: Evaluating Exaggeration, Feigning, and Noncredible Effort* New York: The Guilford Press, pp. 22–41.

Slick DJ, Sherman EMS (2012) Differential diagnosis of malingering and related clinical presentations. In: Sherman EMS, Brooks BL, editors, *Pediatric Forensic Neuropsychology*. New York: Oxford University Press, pp. 113–135.

Zemek R, Barrowman N, Freedman SB, Gravel J, Gagnon I, McGahern C (2016) Clinical risk score for persistent postconcussion symptoms among children with acute concussion in the ED. *JAMA* **315**(10): 1014–1025.

CHAPTER 24

Paediatric Teleneuropsychology

Elizabeth Roberts, Rosie Brett, and Tara Murphy

Presenting Concern

Kate is an 11-year-old girl of White British heritage who lives at home with her mother, father, and older sister. There is no family history of neurological or neurodevelopmental disorders. Kate met her developmental milestones until age 3 years when she presented with balance problems. She was taken to hospital and diagnosed with an anaplastic astrocytoma (a rare malignant brain tumour) of the left frontal lobe. She underwent neurosurgery to remove the tumour, which resulted in focal epilepsy. Kate's seizures became increasingly debilitating over time and a brief educational psychology assessment showed considerable cognitive challenges.

At age 10 years, Kate had approximately 12 seizures a day. Several antiseizure medications were trialled with unsuccessful results. At 11 years, Kate underwent a left hemispherotomy that led to a loss of functional skills (difficulties walking, using her left arm, and with self-care activities). In order to optimise her skills, Kate entered a 4-month period of inpatient neurorehabilitation. Kate's language skills were weak (similar to her level presurgery). She was able to understand basic conversations with adults and could produce sentences with a maximum of six words. She had difficulty with higher-level aspects of language (i.e. inference, sequencing, and reasoning).

Around the time of the assessment, the UK went into lockdown as the result of the COVID-19 pandemic, and, therefore, the neuropsychological assessment was completed remotely.

THEORY

Teleneuropsychology is the use of video-teleconferencing (VTC) techniques to administer neuropsychological services without face-to-face contact (Munro Cullum et al. 2014). This may include teleassessment, where neuropsychological assessments are carried out using VTC or telerehabilitation, defined as a course of therapy carried out via VTC remotely (Parmanto and Saptano 2009; McCue and Munro Cullum 2013).

The practical application of using teleneuropsychology involves a high level of technology, use of screens, a reliable internet connection, and well-developed clinical skills. The need for this novel approach to carrying out neuropsychological work has been driven by many factors such as work with geographically remote communities and the high demands of travel to specialist centres. Most recently, it came to the forefront of many neuropsychologists' practice due to the COVID-19 pandemic. Up until this point, the vast majority of the literature and practice had been focused on adult neuropsychology and, given the constraints that the pandemic has placed on paediatric practice, this area is likely to grow rapidly in the coming years.

This chapter seeks to give an overview of the current literature, highlighting benefits and limitations, ethical considerations, and practical considerations. We will draw on best-practice guidelines provided by professional bodies to date alongside the existing paediatric literature. Our aim is to highlight limitations and make recommendations based on the information currently available, which primarily focuses on teleassessment.

Models of Delivery

Stolwyk (2020) identifies three models of teleneuropsychology from the paediatric literature. These vary based on the location of both the clinician and client and can be chosen based on the patients' needs, ability to travel for sessions, and the intended test requirements. These models of teleneuropsychology have the potential to facilitate greater access to telerehabilitation for a wider patient population.

Remote – Patient and Clinician in Separate Hospitals/Clinics

Several studies have utilised the remote model. Hodge et al. (2019) assessed 33 children aged 8 to 12 years, with specific learning disorder in reading. Ten of the children had a co-occurring diagnosis of attention-deficit/hyperactivity disorder. A remote psychologist administered the Wechsler Intelligence Scale for Children, Fifth Edition (Wechsler 2014) whilst the participant was at the centre accompanied by a local centre psychologist. Assessment was delivered via Coviu (2020), a video communication facility that uses peer-to-peer communication with encryption, synchronised image viewing, remotely visible click-markers for pointing at images, and cameras to share activities that involve physical manipulatives (e.g. blocks). Webcams and speakers were used with touchscreens and standard personal computers.

The remote method yielded comparable results to the face-to-face method. Correlation analyses showed high associations between the testing methodologies. Subtests that required less clinical interpretation and judgement were most highly correlated. Feedback was elicited from the parents and Centre psychologists. The majority (84%) of Centre psychologists endorsed that the child's performance was not affected by mode of assessment.

Of the responses that indicated the child's performance was affected, two reported that it had a positive impact on the child (e.g. improved their attention and engagement with the assessment), whilst one reported it had a negative impact (i.e. the child was less animated in the telehealth assessment compared with face-to-face). Local psychologists reported the majority of sessions to have 'good' audio quality. Psychologists' satisfaction with video quality was slightly lower. All parents reported being 'comfortable' throughout the telehealth administration, and many reported support for teleneuropsychology as a means to improve accessibility of specialist assessment services for children in remote geographical locations.

Waite et al. (2010) and Sutherland et al. (2019) report on data using the Clinical Evaluation of Language Fundamentals, Fourth Edition, Australian adaptation (Semel, Wiig, and Secord 2003) in children. Waite et al. assessed 25 children aged 5 to 9 years, previously diagnosed or suspected of having language impairment, whereas Sutherland assessed 13 children with autism aged 9 to 12 years. An online or face-to-face speech-language pathologist carried out testing. Permission to reproduce stimulus materials in a digitised format was obtained from the test publisher (Harcourt Assessment Inc.). Two speech-language pathologist simultaneously rated each participant. The participant's computer monitor was an analogue capacitive touchscreen that enabled recording of the participant's responses to stimuli displayed on the screen. No significant differences were found between face-to-face and online evaluation. The kappa and weighted kappa analyses revealed very good agreement between the online and face-to-face ratings for the individual item scores on all subtests.

Another early pilot study by Stain et al. (2011) included 11 adolescents and young adults with early psychosis. The adult tests and inventories reported in Table 24.1 were administered. The mode of assessment was alternated with half of the sample undergoing the VTC first and half undergoing the face-to-face assessment first. There was a strong correlation between modes of assessment for most instruments. Results indicated that in general the mean difference between face-to-face and VTC modes of assessment was close to zero with significant bias only evident for general cognitive functioning (Wechsler Test of Adult Reading; Wechsler 2001), where VTC produced higher ratings than face-to-face assessments. No comment was made on control of practice effects. Feedback from the participants indicated strong acceptability of VTC in a high-risk psychiatric population of young adults.

WITHIN CLINIC – PATIENT AND CLINICIAN IN ADJACENT ROOMS

A pilot study by Ragbeer et al. (2016) included three males with juvenile Batten disease, and one nonaffected brother of an affected child. With the examiner in one room, and the participants and a graduate student in another, remote neuropsychological assessment via one of two methods was carried out.

Table 24.1 Measures that have been compared video-teleconferencing versus face-to-face

No difference	Difference
Wechsler Intelligence Scale for Children, Fifth Edition – Full Scale (Wechsler 2014)	Wide Range Assessment of Memory and Learning, Second Edition – Verbal Fluency subtest (Sheslow and Adams 2003)
Wechsler Intelligence Scale for Children, Fourth Edition – Similarities, Vocabulary, Information, Digit Span subtests (Wechsler 2003)	
Controlled Oral Word Association Test (Benton, Hamsher, and Sivan 1983)	Wechsler Test of Adult Reading (Wechsler 2001)
Wechsler Memory Scale – Logical Memory subtest (Wechsler 1987)	
Social and Occupational Functioning Assessment Scale (Rybarczyk 2011)	
Brief Psychiatric Rating Scale (Overall and Gorham 1962)	
Clinical Evaluation of Language Fundamentals, Fourth and Fifth Editions – Concepts and Following Directions, Word Structure, Recalling Sentences, and Formulated Sentences subtests (Semel, Wiig, and Secord 2003; Wiig, Semel, and Secord 2013)	
California Verbal Learning Test-Children's Version (CVLT-C)/ California Verbal Learning Test, Second Edition (CVLT-II)	
Delis-Kaplan Executive Function System (D-KEFS)	
Beery-Buktenica Developmental Test of Visual Motor Integration, Sixth Edition (VMI-6)	

The two methods involved either:

- Method 1: Remote expert assessment with in-person technical assistance. The investigator remotely administered tests, whilst a (graduate) student sat with the child in an adjacent room and provided technical assistance. Redirection provided by the student (such as verbatim clarification) was prompted by the examiner.

- Method 2: In-person assessment with remote expert guidance. Testing was administered directly by a student seated in the same room as the child. An examiner watched the evaluation remotely and gave prompts (e.g. time allowances for verbal responses) to the student.

Selective verbal subtests from the Wechsler Intelligence Scale for Children, Fourth Edition (Wechsler 2003) and the Wide Range Assessment of Memory and Learning, Second Edition (Sheslow and Adams 2003) alongside the Verbal Fluency test were administered. The percentage agreement values were generally good for the tests; interscorer agreement between the examiners ranged from 78% to 100%. Agreement was highest when only data were included from children with the condition, albeit a very small cohort from which to draw conclusions.

Home – Patient at Home and Clinician in Clinic/Home

A recent study by Harder and colleagues (2020) assessed 53 children (aged 10–17 years) with paediatric demyelinating disorders from the USA. Each child was seen twice to complete a brief neuropsychological battery; one face-to-face and one with a remote home-based VTC. Tests included: California Verbal Learning Test-Children's Version/ California Verbal Learning Test, Second Edition; Vocabulary and Digit Span subtests from the Wechsler Intelligence Scale for Children, Fifth Edition/Wechsler Adult Intelligence Scale, Fourth Edition; Beery-Buktenica Developmental Test of Visual Motor Integration, Sixth Edition; selective subtests from the Delis-Kaplan Executive Function System, and the Woodcock-Johnson, Third Edition Tests of Achievement. The order of the assessments was counterbalanced and participants were assessed in a room alone in English or Spanish. Testing materials were sent in a sealed envelope prior to the assessment with permission from the publishers.

No significant differences in results were obtained in the face-to-face or remote sessions, and there was no significant change in performance across sessions. Satisfaction ratings from the majority (>85%) of children and caregivers supported VTC and most involved did not have a preference of face-to-face over VTC delivery of assessment. Technological problems were found in 21% (despite purposefully using a low bandwidth application) and environmental distractions occurred in 47% of VTC sessions and yet did not appear to impact the results. Notably, almost a quarter of participants did not have access to the required technology and had to borrow a device and a significant number of children (26 from 95) were lost to follow-up.

Test Selection

Based primarily on the adult literature (e.g. Brearly et al. 2017), certain tests require little modification for use in teleneuropsychology. Verbally mediated tasks such as Digit Span, Verbal Fluency, and List Learning (e.g. California Verbal Learning Test), appear unaffected by the use of VTC methods (Brearly et al. 2017). Premorbid ability and attention tests (e.g. Oral Symbol Digit Modalities Test; Smith 1991) as well as learning and memory tests (e.g. Rey Complex Figure Test Delay) and executive functioning tests (e.g. Letter Fluency, Wechsler Adult Intelligence Scale, Fourth Edition similarities) have been found to elicit highly consistent performance conditions with stroke survivors (Chapman et al. 2021).

Neuropsychologists have argued that not all tests are appropriate for teleassessment. For example there is the concern that teleassessment methods can limit opportunities for examiners to observe behaviour due to quality of camera angles or picture as well as due to problems with strength of internet connection (Brearly et al. 2017). This can lead to the presentation of test stimulus falling below the required standards (Parsons 2016). The evidence base may need to be expanded on for some tests before their use via VTC. For example the Boston Naming Test (Kaplan, Goodglass, and Weintraub 1983) has been found to have mixed feasibility results, and there has been a push for motor-dependent tasks to be investigated further. In the meantime, validated face-to-face administration of motor-free assessments might be useful (Piovesana et al. 2019).

Brearly et al. (2017) conducted a systematic review and meta-analysis of the adult literature, with the purpose of investigating the effect of VTC on adult neurocognitive tests. The findings from this study are useful in helping to guide test selection. Brearly et al. (2017) divided the tests used within these studies into two categories: synchronous (single-trial and timed tests) and nonsynchronous (untimed tests). They hypothesised that issues with VTC, such as poor quality of transmission or lost internet connection, would be more likely to impact tests that are synchronous, due to them being timed and allowing for no repetition.

Overall, no significant differences were found between VTC and face-to-face test scores, with VTC test scores falling around 1/33rd of a standard deviation less than face-to-face scores. With nonsynchronous tests (including visuoconstructional tasks such as Figure Recall from the Repeatable Battery for the Assessment of Neuropsychological Status, Randolph et al. 1998), however, there was a significant difference, with VTC test scores around 1/10th of a standard deviation lower than face-to-face administration. Data from the synchronous tests were too heterogeneous to be grouped together, so were investigated at the test level. Subtests including Digit Span, Phonemic Fluency, Category Fluency, and List Learning all produced comparable results to face-to-face testing when carried out using VTC. There was greater variability in the effect of VTC on synchronous tasks that required the manipulation of physical objects (e.g. Mini Mental State Examination, Second Edition, Folstein et al. 2010; and Clock-Drawing Test, Agrell and Dehlin 1998), which impeded interpretation as to the effect of VTC on such tasks.

The six paediatric studies reviewed at the beginning of the chapter (Waite et al. 2010; Stain et al. 2011; Ragbeer et al. 2016; Hodge et al. 2019; Sutherland et al. 2019; Harder et al. 2020) also provide findings to help guide test selection between VTC and face-to-face scores, as per Table 24.1.

ASSESSMENT AND FORMULATION

A neurocognitive assessment was requested as part of Kate's neurorehabilitation program in order to understand the impact of the hemispherotomy on her cognition and to inform transition back to school. Kate's early discharge from the neurorehabilitation setting due to the COVID-19 pandemic meant that the neuropsychological assessment was completed remotely. It was felt that this would be feasible as Kate was familiar with technology and able to talk with people using video call platforms. Her attention

Table 24.2 Kate's scores on the assessment battery

Assessment	Score
Completed in person	
Wechsler Intelligence Scale for Children, Fifth Edition Full Scale IQ	<0.1st percentile
Completed via video-teleconferencing	
Children's Memory Scale: Verbal Immediate Memory	1st percentile
Children's Memory Scale: Verbal Delayed Memory	0.4th percentile
Completed with mother via video-teleconferencing	
Adaptive Behavior Assessment System, Third Edition: General Adaptive Composite	0.5th percentile
Behavior Rating Inventory of Executive Functioning, Second Edition: General Executive Composite	99th percentile (clinically elevated)
Strengths and Difficulties Questionnaire: Total Difficulties Score	20 (very high)

was also such that it was felt she would be able to sit through a testing session if short breaks were provided throughout.

The psychologist had a brief session with Kate's mother to set up the technology and room ahead of the assessment. Kate's mother set the technology up in a quiet bedroom in their house, where she felt she would not get distracted. An iPad was used with an inbuilt camera, whilst the psychologist at home used a laptop with an inbuilt camera. The Microsoft Teams platform was used. Kate's mother sat close by throughout the assessment for technological support. However, she was prepared on the importance of not helping Kate with the test items, so that her performance reflected her ability accurately.

A battery of assessments including the Wechsler Intelligence Scale for Children, Fifth Edition (Wechsler 2014) and Children's Memory Scale (Stories and Word Pairs subtests; Cohen 1997) were administered. These were administered using the Q-Global platform, a web-based system that allows you to administer assessments via screen-share. Record forms that Kate required had been sent to her mother in advance and she had them ready, alongside a pencil, on the day. Kate engaged well with the remote assessment; she maintained attention for approximately 40 minutes at a time, at which point she was offered a 15-minute break. The entire testing session lasted approximately 2.5 hours. Kate was able to switch between tasks, either looking at stimuli on her screen or listening to verbally presented information. The use of VTC seemed to act as an incentive as Kate commented that it was 'fun' to use an iPad and to see the assessor 'through a screen'. However, as there are a lack of equivalence studies validating the use of teleconferencing software and screen-sharing delivery of neuropsychological batteries with children, the assessor was mindful of this within her formulation, as well as being transparent about the method of delivery within the assessment report. In addition, a reduced battery of assessments was completed.

In order to gain further understanding of Kate's skills, parent questionnaires were completed (Adaptive Behavior Assessment System, Third Edition, ABAS-III, Harrison and Oakland 2015; Strengths and Difficulties Questionnaires, SDQ, Goodman 1999; Behavior Rating Inventory of Executive Functioning, Second Edition, BRIEF-2, Gioia et al. 2015). The questionnaires were also completed via VTC, with both Kate's mother and the assessor based at home. It was felt that doing this via VTC rather than the typical self-report would yield more detailed and valid results. The results of the assessment were as follows:

Kate's scores across the assessment indicate global difficulties in cognition and learning. The lack of selective impact on language skills for Kate indicates that language functions developed in an atypical way due to her brain tumour, epilepsy, and treatments.

Use of the remote method enabled completion of the assessment, and Kate and her mother engaged well with the process. Kate's performance on the current assessment was in line with parental report, behaviour observations, and her previous presentation. Low scores on the assessment delivered were therefore predicted. This would suggest that the VTC assessment produced reliable results.

Practical Implications

Although studies support the feasibility of teleneuropsychology methods, teleassessment requires careful consideration at each stage. Additionally, using this mode of delivery with children may require additional preparation to that in adults. Due to the unprecedented level of interest in the use of teleneuropsychology amidst the COVID-19 pandemic, a number of guidelines have been put forward from professional bodies around teleneuropsychology (Association of Educational Psychologists 2020; British Psychological Society Division of Clinical Psychology 2020; British Psychological Society Division of Neuropsychology 2020b). Table 24.3 provides a summary of the key points emanating from these guidelines.

INTERVENTION AND MANAGEMENT

Whilst the majority of this chapter has focussed on teleassessment, due to there being a more extensive evidence base in this area, there is an emerging evidence base with regards to telerehabilitation. Corti et al. (2019) carried out a systematic review of 32 technology-based telerehabilitation programs that aimed to address cognitive and behaviour issues for children with acquired brain injury. In order to calculate effect sizes, meta-analysis was carried out on a subset of these studies (14), which utilised control group designs. With regards to cognition, this analysis suggests that telerehabilitation

Table 24.3 Practical considerations around paediatric assessment using video-teleconferencing

Consideration	Prior to assessment	During assessment	After assessment
Validity and reliability	**Suitability** Is video-teleconferencing appropriate for the child's chronological age and developmental level? Check that the assessments required are available for remote delivery (e.g. are they available through the Q-Global platform). Check that there is agreement on the licence from the publishers to send materials	**Threats to validity** Note any factors that may impact testing (e.g. interruptions/distractions in home environment, internet quality issues, technology problems etc.)	**Formulation and Reporting** Be mindful of the lack of equivalence studies validating the use of teleconferencing software and screen-sharing delivery within formulation and be transparent about the method of delivery within the assessment report
Hypotheses	**What hypotheses am I trying to test?** Can these hypotheses be tested adequately via remote means? If not, what are the alternative options, e.g. offer an in-person appointment when possible, gather information through other means, such as parent/teacher report etc.?	**Triangulate performance** Are the results consistent with other sources of information, e.g. self-report, parent/teacher report, and observation?	**Feedback session to family** Do the family agree with your formulation? Are the findings from the current assessment consistent with their view of the child? What implications do the findings have for what the young person needs going forward, e.g. compensations at school?
Preparing session participant	**Briefing** Has the parent/local supporter been adequately briefed on their role? Clearly explain the appropriate level of involvement in the participation to avoid them interjecting inappropriately	**During the assessment** Ensure that adequate breaks are built into the assessment. Plan these where possible to ensure they do not invalidate the assessment (e.g. causing there to be too long a delay between memory subtests)	**Feedback session** Discuss who will be present for the feedback session. Discuss ahead of time how to share screens or to share resources for this session

(Continued)

Table 24.3 Continued

Consideration	Prior to assessment	During assessment	After assessment
Technology	**Setting up assessment** Complete a pre-assessment video call with the young person's parent or guardian ahead of the assessment to test the technology. Ensure that they have a good internet connection and that the screen on the device they are using is of an adequate size for the young person to clearly see the stimuli	**Technology concerns during assessment** Examiners should familiarise themselves with technological problems and have established a contingency plan ahead of formal testing. Discuss with the parent and young person in advance what you will do in different situations, e.g. if the internet connection cuts out	**Feedback session to family** At the beginning of the feedback session, ensure that there is a good quality connection and agree what will happen if the connection fails
Test materials	**Preparation** Have all of the relevant materials been sent to the child and are they present for the examiner? Ensure that neither party has to leave the testing rooms to retrieve materials	**Using materials** Use the supporter to pass the child the relevant materials they need during the assessment and to clear away those not in use to avoid distraction	**Return of materials** Ensure that any testing materials are returned and supply a reply-paid envelope to encourage this
Location	**Environment** Consider potential distractions and ways to eliminate disturbances in order to ensure the patient's privacy	**Testing** Review the child's location with the camera at the beginning of testing. Ask the supporter to make any change to this as needed	**Location of feedback session** Ensure that those at the feedback session have access to a private space where they will not be disturbed or interrupted
Testing	**Practice and prepare** Examiners should practise beforehand the most appropriate and best validated tests with a colleague	**Engagement** Try to make the testing as similar to face-to-face testing as possible. Be patient with responses. Dress professionally and wear a name badge with a plain background visible	**Ending the testing session** Where possible, end the session with the support psychologist or parent present so that the next stage can be explained and any questions asked

(Continued)

Consideration	Prior to assessment	During assessment	After assessment
Ethical considerations	**Consent/assent** Ensure you seek informed consent from both guardian and child which specifies that telecontact is agreed to. Document this consent. It must be explained that it is prohibited for the family to record the testing session in any way	**Opting out** Ensure that both the child and parent are aware that they can 'opt out' of the testing session at any point, if they no longer want to continue	**Ending the feedback session** Check in with the family as to how they are feeling emotionally and direct them to sources of emotional support, as needed

programs were effective in targeting specific cognitive domains (e.g. executive functioning, working memory) but had limited generalised effects. With regards to behaviour, meta-analysis yielded a small to moderate effect size, suggesting that telerehabilitation programs were effective at improving behaviour.

Wade et al. (2020) adapted problem-solving (adapted from Nezu et al. 2006) and parenting (I-InTERACT, Internet-based Interacting Together Everyday, Recovery after Childhood TBI) training packages for delivery via telerehabilitation. They report findings from 14 clinical trials, which included in excess of 800 children and their families. The children represented in these trials had a range of diagnoses, including traumatic brain injury, epilepsy, brain tumours, congenital heart disease, and perinatal stroke. Their findings support the feasibility, acceptability, and efficacy of both problem-solving and parenting interventions. With regards to the efficacy of problem-solving telerehabilitation, a meta-analysis indicated that it leads to reduction in behavioural problems and parental distress, whilst improving family functioning. Their findings also support the efficacy of a telerehabilitation parenting intervention in reducing behavioural problems and increasing positive parenting practices.

Case Study – Kate

Within the current case study, the range of interventions that could be offered to Kate and her family to support her rehabilitation were also limited due to her being located remotely. However, a pragmatic approach was taken, and it was felt that psychoeducation was one such intervention that would lend itself well to this method of delivery. It was hypothesised that psychoeducation would support Kate's parents to improve their knowledge about their daughter's brain injury, build skills, and reduce stress (Brown et al. 2013).

Prior to the psychoeducation starting, the psychologist spoke with Kate's parents via VTC. The purpose of this meeting was to ascertain the parental goals for the intervention. Kate's parents said that they would like to learn more about Kate's brain tumour and the impact of her brain tumour resection and epilepsy on her development. They also wanted to think about Kate's strengths and needs alongside what this could mean for the future.

The psychologist prepared a slide presentation based on Kate's parents' goals. The psychoeducation was completed in two 60-minute sessions. During the first 40 minutes of each session the neuropsychologist delivered the presentation using the screen-sharing option so that everyone could view the material simultaneously. An administration assistant at the neurorehabilitation setting printed hard copies of the slides and the clinical report and posted these to the parents ahead of the sessions.

Throughout the presentation the psychologist regularly checked in with the parents to ascertain their understanding of the information. This seemed even more necessary than usual, as delivering the intervention via VTC limited the opportunities to observe parents' nonverbal communication. During the final 20 minutes of each session, parents were given space to ask questions and share their thoughts and feelings about the information.

On reflection, this intervention could have gone further by using the 'whiteboard' function of VTC to cocreate psychoeducation resources with Kate and her family.

Ethical Considerations

Ethical considerations across many domains are key with teleneuropsychology as this is a novel modality that has limited empirical testing to guide clinical delivery. The recommendations used below relate primarily to the remote and within clinic models. Considerations for the home model are far more extensive and beyond the scope of this chapter. Furthermore, these considerations will need to be expanded. For example in the USA, practice regulations can vary from state to state, and so psychologists must obtain licensure in each state they will be working in and inform patients of this (Grosch, Gottlieb, and Munro Cullum 2011).

Security

Only secure platforms that conform to ethical and data security guidelines should be used. At the time of writing this chapter many existing platforms were under validation. It may be helpful to draw on advice from insurance companies as to coverage for indemnity. For clinicians and researchers, it will be prudent to check with local guidelines and management procedures that your practice complies with regulations about storing and transmitting data.

Consent/Assent

The child and family should be aware of how information recorded might be used and stored. The British Psychological Society guidelines suggest that the child or young person should consent to using VTC before every session and that if the child is under 16 years, parental consent and child assent is needed (British Psychological Society Division of Clinical Psychology 2020; British Psychological Society Division of Neuropsychology 2020a). Specific consent may be needed for material recorded through audio or video in accordance with data protection guidance.

CONFIDENTIALITY

As with traditional delivery of neuropsychological assessment and intervention, the confidentiality of the information is important. The location of testing should be considered in terms of privacy, whether this is at a remote clinic or the patient's home. Many of the caveats with traditional assessment apply, such as avoiding interruptions to the testing room. The opportunities for breaches of information (with limited control over who might be present in a remote testing room), how information may be relayed back to the examiner, and how recordings might be used are increased with VTC.

Confidentiality of testing material should be carefully considered. There are guidelines from publishers regarding which materials can be shared with patients beyond the face-to-face setting and revisions and clarification were made to guidelines during the COVID-19 pandemic. The clinician should make sure there is no material visible to the patient that could breach data governance guidelines (British Psychological Society Division of Neuropsychology 2020a).

ACCESS

Although there has been increased access to internet connectivity and technological devices, recent research (Harder et al. 2020) shows that there is a significant proportion of health service users in high-income countries who will not automatically have access to the technological devices needed for VTC. This consideration must be made when funding the development of VTC in the provision of services.

Outcome
Kate's parents were asked to feed back how they had found the remote assessment and intervention. They reported that they had found it very useful and that they now felt better able to advocate for Kate. Moreover, they said that they were happy that VTC was an option, as it allowed the assessment and intervention to take place when it otherwise might not have. They also felt it worked particularly well for the delivery of psychoeducation. Kate's parents requested that the psychoeducation materials be shared with Kate's school, which was scheduled for remote delivery at a planned school training day.

SUMMARY

The use of teleneuropsychology has the potential to increase the availability of paediatric neuropsychology services to children of all ages and their families. Evidence is currently limited for teleneuropsychology in paediatric populations. The studies to date include small sample sizes, most commonly of populations with specific, often rare conditions, and are carried out in limited cultures and countries (Parsons and Kane 2018). Most research has focused on teleassessment as opposed to telerehabilitation, so we know less about how traditional rehabilitation would be received, although online intervention shows promise (Wade et al. 2018). Given the worldwide impact of the COVID-19 pandemic on neuropsychology and clinical paediatric team practice, teleneuropsychology is likely to grow for both assessment and intervention in the coming years.

There is evidence from the literature base, with regards to the feasibility and acceptability of teleneuropsychology. Teleassessment has been used with children from 5 years of age and has been found to produce comparable results to face-to-face assessment, particularly with regards to verbally mediated tasks. Telerehabilitation has been used effectively to improve cognition, behaviour, and positive parenting practices (Corti et al. 2019; Wade et al. 2020). However, it should be noted that most of the existing studies have utilised within clinic testing or remote testing, leaving a lack of studies assessing feasibility of the home testing model. It is possible that differences between these settings could lead to differences in feasibility, acceptability, reliability, and validity so studies exploring this are imperative. The current evidence base for feasibility of using VTC methods needs to grow, drawing on a wider participant population, and measurement of diverse cognitive domains.

There are also many practical considerations to consider when practising teleneuropsychology. First and foremost, the practitioner needs to consider whether remote methods are suitable and feasible for their client. If the young person is not at the cognitive or developmental level to engage with VTC, then this method will not be possible. Even if they do have the skills required, consideration then needs to be given as to whether they have access to the necessary technology, including an adequately sized screen and a good internet connection, as well as someone to support them in setting up the assessment, if required, and access to a quiet and distraction-free environment to complete the assessment in. Consideration also needs to be given as to whether the hypotheses that need to be tested can be done so via remote means, i.e. is there an assessment that has been adapted for remote delivery that assesses that domain? Practitioners also need to be transparent about their methods for delivery when reporting on results and should pay careful consideration to whether their findings triangulate as well as highlighting any potential implications that this method of delivery may have had on the results.

Finally, a significant obstacle in the way of acceptance of teleneuropsychology has been the reluctance of many teams to adopt this method of working. Rabin and colleagues found that it is not so much the patients that have reservations about remote working practices but the clinicians. When asked about their attitudes towards this delivery method, concerns were identified about costs, test accuracy, data security, and feasibility of assessment with specific clinical populations (Rabin et al. 2016). Gicas and colleagues (2020) reported on a survey carried out in 2020 that sought to identify barriers and opportunities to remote clinical psychology training in Canadian psychologists. The majority of respondents ($n=164$) reported an openness to working remotely with barriers around clinic closures, onsite training restrictions, and inadequate resources raised. In addition, concerns with test validity and health and safety concerns were mooted and counterbalanced by an appetite for future teaching, training, and supervision online. It may be that if future training is delivered remotely, practice in this manner may be more accessible. There may be limitations to this method of practice (which should be considered on a case-by-case basis), but it holds great promise for the future as internet connectivity improves worldwide and future research informs practice.

REFERENCES

American Psychiatric Association (2000) *Diagnostic and Statistical Manual of Mental Disorders*, 4th edition. Washington, DC: American Psychiatric Association.

Association of Educational Psychologists (2020) *Working remotely with children, young people and their families: Staying safe, maintaining data security, upholding professional standards and using technology*. [pdf] Available at: www.aep.org.uk [Accessed 22 May 2020].

British Psychological Society Division of Clinical Psychology (2020) *Considerations for psychologists working with children and young people using online video platforms*. [pdf] Available at: https://www.bps.org.uk/sites/www.bps.org.uk/files/Member%20Networks/Divisions/DCP/Considerations%20for%20psychologists%20working%20with%20children%20and%20young%20people%20using%20online%20video%20platforms.pdf [Accessed 22 May 2020].

British Psychological Society Division of Neuropsychology (2020a) *Neuropsychology in the current context*. [pdf] Available at: https://www.slideshare.net/secret/6suu8fs9tx1jYn [Accessed 22 May 2020].

British Psychological Society Division of Neuropsychology (2020b) *Division of Neuropsychology Professional Standards Units Guidelines to colleagues on the use of tele-neuropsychology*. [pdf] Available at: https://www.bps.org.uk/sites/www.bps.org.uk/files/Member%20Networks/Divisions/DoN/DON%20guidelines%20on%20the%20use%20of%20tele-neuropsychology%20%28April%202020%29.pdf [Accessed 22 May 2020].

Brearly TW, Shura RD, Martindale SL et al. (2017) Neuropsychological test administration by videoconference: A systematic review and meta-analysis. *Neuropsychology Review* 27: 174–186: doi: 10.1007/s11065-017-9349-1.

Brown FL, Whittingham K, Boyd B, Sofronoff K (2013) A systematic review of parenting interventions for traumatic brain injury: Child and parent outcomes. *The Journal of Head Trauma Rehabilitation* 28: 349–360. doi: 10.1097/HTR.0b013e318245fed5.

Chapman JE, Gardner B, Ponsford J, Cadilhac DA, Stolwyk RJ (2021) Comparing performance across in-person and video conference-based administrations of common neuropsychological measures in community-based survivors of stroke. *Journal of the International Neuropsychological Society* 27(7): 697–710.

Corti C, Oldrati V, Oprandi MC et al. (2019) Remote technology-based training programs for children with acquired brain injury: A systematic review and a meta-analytic exploration. *Behavioural Neurology* 1–31. doi: 10.1155/2019/1346987.

Coviu (2020) *About Coviu*, Coviu, viewed 30 June 2020, https://www.coviu.com/en-au/about [Accessed 4 July 2020].

Gicas KM, Paterson TSE, Narvaez Linares NF, Loken Thornton WJ (2020) Clinical psychological assessment training issues in the COVID-19 era: A survey of the state of the field and considerations for moving forward. *Canadian Psychology/Psychologie Canadienne* 62(1): 44–55. Advance online publication. http://dx.doi.org/10.1037/cap0000258.

Grosch MC, Gottlieb MC, Munro Cullum C (2011) Initial practice recommendations for teleneuropsychology. *The Clinical Neuropsychologist* 25: 1119–1133. doi: 10.1080/13854046.2011.609840.

Harder L, Hernandez A, Hague C et al. (2020) Home-based pediatric teleneuropsychology: A validation study. *Archives of Clinical Neuropsychology* 35(8): 1266–1275. https://doi.org/10.1093/arclin/acaa070.

Hodge MA, Sutherland R, Jeng K et al. (2019) Agreement between telehealth and face-to-face assessment of intellectual ability in children with specific learning disorder. *Journal of Telemedicine and Telecare* 25: 431–437. doi: 10.1177/1357633X18776095.

McCue M, Munro Cullum C (2013) Telerehabilitation and teleneuropsychology: Emerging practices. In: Noggle CA, Dean RS, Barisa MT, editors, *Neuropsychological Rehabilitation*. Cham: Springer, pp. 327–340.

Munro Cullum C, Hynan LS, Grosch M, Parikh M, Weiner MF (2014) Teleneuropsychology: Evidence for video teleconference-based neuropsychological assessment. *Journal of the International Neuropsychological Society* 20: 1028–1033. doi: 10.1017/S1355617714000873.

Nezu AM, Maguth Nezu C, D'Zurilla TJ (2006) *Solving Life's Problems: A 5-Step Guide to Enhanced Well-Being*. New York: Springer Publishing Company, LLC.

Parmanto B, Saptono A (2009) Telerehabilitation: State-of-the-art from an informatics perspective. *International Journal of Telerehabilitation* 1: 73–84. doi: 10.5195/ijt.2009.6015.

Parsons TD (2016) Telemedicine, mobile, and internet-based neurocognitive assessment. In: Parsons TD, editor, *Clinical Neuropsychology and Technology*. Cham: Springer, pp. 99–111.

Parsons TD, Kane R (2018) Technologically enhanced neuropsychological assessment – Review and update. In: Koffler S, Mahone EM, Marcopulos BA, Johnson-Greene DE, Smith G, editors, *Neuropsychology: Science and Practice*. New York: Oxford University Press, pp. 59–92.

Piovesana AM, Harrison JL, Ducat JJ (2019) The development of a motor-free short-form of the Wechsler Intelligence Scale for Children – Fifth Edition. *Assessment* 26(8): 1564–1572. doi: 10.1177/1073191117748741. Epub 2017 Dec 28. PMID: 29284274.

Rabin LA, Paolillo E, Barr WB (2016) Stability in test-usage practices of clinical neuropsychologists in the United States and Canada over a 10-year period: A follow-up survey of INS and NAN members. *Archives of Clinical Neuropsychology* 31: 206–230. doi: 10.1093/arclin/acw007.

Ragbeer SN, Augustine EF, Mink JW, Thatcher AR, Vierhile AE, Adams HR (2016) Remote assessment of cognitive function in juvenile neuronal ceroid lipofuscinosis (Batten disease). *Journal of Child Neurology* 31: 481–487. doi: 10.1177/0883073815600863.

Rybarczyk (2011) Social and Occupational Functioning Assessment Scale (SOFAS). In: Kreutzer JS, DeLuca J, Caplan B, editors, *Encyclopedia of Clinical Neuropsychology*. New York: Springer, pp. 2313–2313.

Semel E, Wiig E, Secord W (2003) *Clinical Evaluation of Language Fundamentals*, 4th edition. San Antonio, TX: The Psychological Corporation.

Stain HJ, Payne K, Thienel R, Michie P, Carr V, Kelly B (2011) The feasibility of videoconferencing for neuropsychological assessments of rural youth experiencing early psychosis. *Journal of Telemedicine and Telecare* 17(6): 328–331. https://doi.org/10.1258/jtt.2011.101015.

Stolwyk R, Hammers D, Harder L, Munro Cullum C (2020, April 2) Teleneuropsychology in response to COVID-19: Practical guidelines to balancing validity concerns with clinical need [Webinar]. The International Neuropsychology Society. https://www.the-ins.org/files/webinars/20200402_covid19/INS_COVID19_Webinar-20200402.pdf.

Sutherland R, Trembath D, Hodge MA, Rose V, Roberts J (2019) Telehealth and autism: Are telehealth language assessments reliable and feasible for children with autism? *Int J Lang Commun Disord* 54(2): 281–291. doi: 10.1111/1460-6984.12440. Epub 2018 Nov 22. PMID: 30565791.

Wade SL, Narad ME, Shultz EL et al. (2018) Technology-assisted rehabilitation interventions following pediatric brain injury. *Journal of Neurosurgical Sciences* 62:187–202. doi: 10.23736/S0390-5616.17.04277-1.

Wade SL, Gies LM, Fisher AP et al. (2020) Telepsychotherapy with children and families: Lessons gleaned from two decades of translational research. *Journal of Psychotherapy Integration* 30(2): 332–347. doi: 10.1037/int0000215.

Waite MC, Theodoros DG, Russell TG, Cahill LM (2010) Internet-based telehealth assessment of language using the CELF–4. *Language, Speech, and Hearing Services in Schools* 41: 445–458. doi: 10.1044/0161-1461(2009/08-0131).

Wechsler D (2003) *Wechsler Intelligence Scale for Children*, 4th edition. San Antonio, TX: Psychological Corporation.

CHAPTER 25

Feedback

Karen Postal

Presenting Concern

Natalie is an engaging 9-year-old girl with a history of asthma who was brought to my office by her mother, father, and maternal grandmother 6 months after a fall from a play structure resulted in a severe traumatic brain injury. The family recited the history with a palpable sense of disbelief at the frightening and stressful series of events they had navigated. Whilst they did so, Natalie proceeded to pick up every item on my desk and bookshelves before settling in at the light switch, turning it off and on repeatedly. Medical records sent by the referring paediatric neurologist catalogued a Glasgow Coma Scale score of 7, bilateral frontal subdural hematomas requiring emergent neurosurgical intervention, and evidence on magnetic resonance imaging of shear injury. After a 1-month acute hospital stay, and 3 months in a rehabilitation hospital, Natalie was back at school, and her elementary class was in an uproar. Within the first 2 weeks this previously well behaved, soft-spoken student had spent an average of 2 hours a day at the principal's office for infractions ranging from getting out of her seat during a test to pick up another student's paper, to yelling at her teacher, to bursting into uncontrollable, sustained tears on the playground.

With a history of a mild reading disorder, Natalie had academic and cognitive testing that was conducted by her school district prior to her injury to which we could compare her current function. Good preservation of average intellect with new onset problems in the area of sustained attention and verbal memory were apparent. Natalie had difficulty with rote memorisation, but her ability to recall information presented in a meaningful story form was average. Difficulties with frontal/executive self-monitoring and inhibition were clear both on formal testing and in my observations of Natalie finding the test instruments, my stopwatch, and anything not nailed down in the testing room irresistible. The testing was conducted over six short sessions due to her short attention span and low frustration tolerance.

During our initial family interview, we constructed a genogram (McGoldrick and Gerson 1985). I learned that Natalie's mother was second generation Korean American and her father was a fifth generation Italian American. Her maternal grandmother lived with the family, was a powerful stakeholder in Natalie's life, and was present during the assessment process.

THEORY

With neuropsychological *testing* we transform emotional experiences, behaviour, thinking abilities, and academic skills into numbers. With neuropsychological *assessment* we understand those numbers in the multilayered contexts of the child's developing brain, disease/injury processes, family system, cultural/linguistic heritage, and broader socio-economic community. With neuropsychological *feedback* our challenge is to partner with our patients and their families in constructing a shared understanding of the assessment that alters their lives. When feedback is done well, it is vivid, accessible, therapeutic, empowering, and one of the most difficult things we do.

Survey studies have clarified that most neuropsychologists conduct feedback sessions and that those sessions benefit even cognitively compromised patients and families with regards to improved knowledge and outcome (e.g. Farmer and Brazeal 1998; Pegg et al. 2005; Smith, Wiggins, and Gorske 2007; Postal et al. 2018; Austin et al. 2019). But because there had been little focus on the complex clinical process of feedback, Kira Armstrong and I embarked on a multi-year qualitative research project (Postal and Armstrong, 2013), inviting seasoned neuropsychologists to sit down with us for in-depth interviews, and share their understanding of the feedback process as well as their best analogies, metaphors, and stories for creating access to the language and assumptions of our field. Early on, we realised that the answer to the question 'How do we conduct effective feedback?' is as varied and complex as the assessment process itself. The rich data and multiple effective feedback pathways and strategies are presented in the book *Feedback That Sticks* (Postal and Armstrong 2013).

Constructing a shared understanding of paediatric neuropsychological assessments during feedback sessions presents unique challenges and requires a family systems focus (e.g. Griffin and Christie 2009). Just as paediatric neuropsychological *assessment* is not about a single brain and its behaviour, paediatric neuropsychological *feedback* necessarily involves at least one other person: the parent/caregiver. And, whether or not they are physically present during the feedback session, feedback most typically involves multiple parents/caregivers/family members and other stakeholders, each of whom brings a unique set of lived experiences, sociocultural contexts, hopes, fears, knowledge, and pre-existing theories about what is happening with the child to the feedback session. Creating a shared understanding of the neuropsychological status of the child and the necessary interventions to address that status during feedback involves acknowledging and navigating the multiple perspectives of those individuals.

In the same way that there is often no neuropsychological complaint for us to address were it not for the observations and distress of the child's family system, there are typically no recommended interventions that will be carried out without the assistance of the family. Beeler and colleagues (2020), for example, found that a critical variable in whether recommended educational supports for children with cognitive changes after central nervous system chemotherapy were carried out by schools was the family's ability to effectively harness social capital in their communities. That is whether a child actually receives one of our carefully thought out neuropsychological recommendations may depend on our ability to support family members during feedback sessions in navigating medical, school, and other broader systems.

An even more basic issue is whether a child's family agrees that they should implement the recommendations. Elias and colleagues (2021) found that only slightly more than half of all recommendations made by paediatric neuropsychologists to families were carried out and 33% of their sample implemented less than a third of the recommendations. Reasons reported by families for not carrying out recommendations included ambivalence about the need for the suggested intervention, lack of financial resources (socioeconomic status), and competing time requirements of other family obligations. Rather than framing the issue as 'resistance to recommendations', we can frame the problem as incomplete understanding of the multiple perspectives and factors that might become barriers to implementation.

WHERE DO WE BEGIN?

In the course of our research we heard over and over from seasoned clinicians that the best feedback sessions begin at the initial intake session. During the initial intake, as we invite the child and various family members to each share their goals for the assessment, their theories about what is going on, their fears about what the diagnosis might be, and family stories about the strengths and troubles of the child, we are not just engaging in history gathering to support our differential diagnosis. We are inviting the family to tell us how to successfully navigate the feedback session: to teach us the language *they* use to frame the problem and the family dynamics involved in the possible solutions.

In order to begin to understand the full complexity of the diverse perspectives each family member brings, we can ask the parents and child to share their goals for the assessment in a way that creates room for multiple and contradictory answers. I said to Natalie and her family:

> I always like to start with everyone's goals for the assessment. I am going to ask each of you, because sometimes everyone has exactly the same goals, but most often different family members have different goals and even different ideas about what is happening in the first place. And that's great. It really helps me to understand all the complexity of the situation better. (Looking at Natalie). I am going to start with your goals, because you are going to do all the work once we get started with the testing!

At this point in the session, Natalie stopped turning on and off the lights and told me that she wanted her teacher to love her again. As she shared this poignant goal, her mother, father, and grandmother visibly teared up. Natalie had given me a way to organise the clinical findings that she and her family could resonate with. What are the thinking, behavioural, and emotional changes from the traumatic brain injury that are making it difficult for Natalie to connect with her teacher and peers and follow the classroom structure as she once had? Will it get easier to do this over time as the recovery course continues, and how do we help Natalie's teacher and other adults understand how to help Natalie overcome those barriers to well-regulated behaviour?

Disrupting Traditional Academic Communication Patterns

When our goal from our very first interaction with the family is to learn the language of how they frame the problem, we are able to begin the feedback collaboration with the lived experience and language of our patients and their families. When we do this, we are necessarily *not* beginning feedback with the language and assumptions of neuropsychology.

This is an important distinction because, as professionals, we can easily forget that people outside of our field have never heard of our basic assumptions and jargon. Over the years, we use technical words and assessment concepts so often it is hard to even recognise that we are speaking in a language that people outside the field do not understand. When we communicate with other neuropsychologists, the names of tests and specific score values are rich and efficient sources of information. But the *name* of a specific test typically has no communication value at all for a family member, and specific test *scores* might mean something entirely different to a family member than the clinician intended.

But why begin with the language of neuropsychology in the first place? Our tests allow us to transform emotions, behaviour, thinking ability, and academic skills into numbers, so we can compare them to norms, but we often forget that it is equally our job to translate the numbers back into lived experience. Many seasoned clinicians conduct feedback sessions without talking about a single score. When scores are brought up, it is for specific emphasis or to address a particular issue rather than asking the family to listen as we share a laundry list of each test and each score during a feedback session.

Because Natalie had so poignantly identified her primary concern as 'I want my teacher to love me again', that's where our feedback began. When talking with Natalie and her family about why it might be so hard now to connect socially and behave the way she wants to, rather than focusing on reciting the results of specific tests or going through all the thinking domains one by one, I pulled out a brain model, pointed to the frontal lobe and said:

> This is the part of the brain that helps us do so much of what we need to do in school. Pay attention, solve problems, and stop one thing and shift to doing the

next thing. It even helps us stay calm when schoolwork or a friend is frustrating and helps us think through something first before we do it or say it. This is the part of your brain that is still healing. And while it does, it is harder for you to do all of those things! Have you guys all noticed that? What have you seen?

Notice that I did not give an abstract brain anatomy lesson, but rather brain anatomy was introduced in the context of the story of the change in Natalie's behaviour. The focus is the human experience; brain anatomy and test results are tools to advance the narrative.

Abandoning the language of neuropsychology as our starting point disrupts an academic communication style that has been taught to us from the earliest days of our training. This style values highly precise words ('gait' for 'walk', 'left lower extremity' for 'left leg', 'euthymic mood' for 'child is happy'), a 'journal article' style of presenting all the testing data first prior to eventually discussing the meaning of the data, an emphasis on erasing the perspective and emotions of the person speaking from the content, and a one-way 'download' of expert information from doctor to patient. We may actually graduate from our university programs with a diminished ability to communicate clearly and simply about the field we all love. Particularly, early career neuropsychologists and trainees may be convinced that formal, technical, highly precise academic language is the only pathway to establishing credibility with patients and families.

Use of vivid metaphors and analogies is another way to create access to neuropsychological concepts for patients and families, using common daily experiences as entry points. During the feedback session, as we were about to talk about how problems with executive function can impact her memory function, Natalie described her injury as, 'My brain was shook too hard.' I took that opportunity to adapt the 'tipped bookshelf' metaphor that one of our *Feedback That Sticks* interviewees, Michael Joschko, had shared with us.

> Your brain is like this really big bookshelf, with hundreds of thousands of books all about important information in your life. You told me you love soccer, so on the top shelf are books all about soccer, and on the next shelf you have books about your favourite ice cream, and song lyrics, and math facts …

> What happened with your accident, when your brain got all shook up is your bookshelf was tipping. And some of the books got scattered. As part of rehab, your bookshelf got straightened up. Most of the books got put back on the right shelf. But some of your books are upside down and sideways, or on the wrong shelf. That's why when you go to say your best friend's name you can't find it. It's on a different shelf. Or when you want a math fact, you have to really think … The books are all there, what you know is still there. But it's an access problem. It might take a little while to find that book. It's OK to take a breath

and give yourself time to answer – and I am going to make sure your teacher knows it's OK too!

Feedback as a Therapeutic Intervention

Seasoned clinicians we interviewed very frequently described feedback sessions as therapeutic. Consistent with this, Rosado and colleagues (2018) found that patients who receive neuropsychological feedback after assessments (as opposed to an assessment without feedback) reported not only a better understanding of their conditions but an improved quality of life and better ability to cope emotionally.

Inviting Emotions Into the Room

In most situations, the developmental disorders, learning disabilities, and medical and neurological conditions our patients and their families are coping with are highly emotional. But, in the fast-paced world of modern medicine, a family may have seen countless clinicians for relatively brief appointments while dealing with a catastrophic developmental or medical condition without any of the clinicians providing an opportunity for family members to talk about their emotional experience.

Ironically, our testing techniques often distance us from the emotions of our patients. For example a depression inventory breaks down painful emotional experiences into distinct symptoms, and then assigns each symptom numerical values that can be compared to norms and turned into standard scores. By the time we get to the 'T score of 90' on a child depression inventory, we are very far from the messy, overwhelming pain of the lived experience of the sadness. Our report writing patterns can also separate us emotionally from our patients' experiences. During our training, we are often taught to write reports without ever using the first person ('I observed', 'I experienced') and in extreme cases to refer to ourselves as 'this examiner'. Over time, our habit of taking our 'selves' and our emotions out of our writing may spill over into doing the same thing in our consulting rooms. When we disrupt these traditional academic communication patterns and instead allow ourselves to be present as a person in the clinical interaction and to express/reflect the emotions of the situation, our communication becomes vivid, immediate, warm, and 'real'. We are inviting every person in the room to be similarly emotionally present as well.

In the course of the *Feedback That Sticks* research, many seasoned neuropsychologists pointed out to us that the feedback session is an opportunity to give families permission to grieve, to cry, to express vulnerabilities, and to expand the focus to their own needs in addition to the needs of their child. The words to create those moments are often very simple, such as 'This has been hard …', 'It sounds like this is not the way you thought it would be …', 'Your child is not the only one suffering during the chemotherapy treatments …'.

While the words to invite families to grieve might be simple, the hard part for many of us as clinicians is to then stop talking. That is allowing a pause and not knowing what might emerge in the moment. One of our interviewees, Dr Hilary Shurtleff, told us,

> Giving parents space and your presence to grieve provides so much hope because it validates their feelings, validates them as people. Providing that presence, and not just rushing through data, was hard for me when I first started. Now I joke sometimes that I make mothers cry for a living!'

In my own practice, I frequently schedule two feedback sessions, one for the whole family and another for 'just adults', so we have an opportunity to talk about issues like parents' grief that might not be appropriate in front of the child.

In my own practice I continuously monitor the temperature of the emotions in the room as the family and I are navigating the feedback collaboration. Emotions may begin to run too high and interfere with participants' ability to collaborate. Emotions may also be minimised or ignored, and the absence of emotions may result in the stakeholders in the room disengaging.

As Natalie's parents and grandmother welled up with tears in our initial interview, I recognised their need to share their own emotional experience. In our 'just adults' feedback session, I opened up a space for them to share their emotional experience by saying, 'Natalie was not the only one hurt in the accident …'

We spent time processing the complicated emotions that arose. In the course of that session, I specifically asked each adult, 'In your culture, how do people generally show grief/hurt/regret?' Natalie's father brought up his tendency to freely, loudly, and frequently express his emotions and how puzzled he often is when others in the family perceive it as him being angry, regardless of what emotion he is experiencing. We processed the differences in showing emotions common in Korean versus Italian families and how Natalie's new difficulty regulating her emotions might be particularly hard for her family who might already be experiencing this as an area of tension.

Feedback in Our Diverse World

In order to meaningfully understand a child's developing brain in the context of their family system, we must also understand the impacts of larger cultural and linguistic systems on the child and family (e.g. Mindt et al. 2008). This understanding not only leads to competent normative interpretation of test data but also allows us to navigate complex dynamics in the feedback session. The dynamics can be multilayered in our ever-diversifying world, as roles within families and expectations of children that influence symptom reports vary considerably by culture, and also vary within those cultures based on levels of acculturation, blended cultures within families, and generational status among other things (e.g. Brickman et al. 2006; Mindt et al. 2008; Mindt et al.

2010; Postal 2018; also see Chapter 22, Culture). Multicultural competence in paediatric neuropsychology is therefore based in part on our willingness to ask questions like, 'How is this in your family?' and 'How does this go in your culture?' 'Do each of your extended families have different ideas about how much your children should be studying every day?' This is particularly relevant if the cultural or generational expectations conflict with the actual roles or expectations family members have adopted. One of our interviewees, Dr Tony Wong, put it this way,

> We don't need to walk into feedback sessions with complete a priori awareness of the cultural implications of our message: that would be impossible. Neuropsychologists are best able to pitch their message when they are open to engaging in a dialogue and asking questions about their patients' culture; it's important for someone from a different background to be OK with not knowing everything. So even if I suspect I know a different culture well, it's important to give the patient a chance to tell me. I will invite them to do so by directly asking, 'How's this in your culture?' Or, 'From your background, how do you deal with this?' When I am on their turf, I find out about their turf.

One of the benefits of drawing a family genogram at the initial interview is the ability to ask about cultural and language backgrounds. 'When did your family immigrate to this country?' 'What languages are spoken in your home?' 'In your family of origin's homes as you were growing up?' As we created their genogram I asked questions to Natalie's mother and grandmother like,

> How traditional were the parenting roles when you were a little girl? Were they based on traditional Korean family roles? Now that you are a grandmother, do you sometimes feel like your daughter is bringing in too much American parenting?

And questions to Natalie's father like,

> How do Italian American parenting strategies fit with Korean American tradition? When family members get sick, in your cultural tradition, what happens? How do roles change?

Empowering Patients and Families to Change Lives

When feedback sessions go well, neuropsychologists and families collaborate to create a shared understanding of the psychological, neurological, family, and greater cultural system interactions that together have produced the presenting complaint. And then what? Several studies have shown that parents' increased knowledge about their child's neuropsychological status does not necessarily automatically translate to an understanding of how to turn that knowledge into tangible change (e.g. Bodin et al. 2008; Austin et al. 2019). Perhaps one of the most important goals of feedback is using the shared understanding to develop plans for meaningful change. This is an inherently empowering process. One of our interviewees, Dr Mark Mahone, expressed it this way:

> It's my belief that we should try to change something about the family's and the child's lives with our exams. If we don't, our exams aren't really helping all that much. We change their lives by giving them new information, and helping them change the perspective they take when thinking about their child and their child's situation. We also change their lives by helping them to become empowered advocates. If we just give them good information and they walk out the door and nothing happens, then we didn't do our job. So it is our goal to do something dramatic with the assessment and the feedback session, so when they walk out the door, they will be inspired, empowered, and have access to new resources, so they can do something that can change their child's life.

Plans for change may involve parenting strategies, education settings and interventions, and access to a range of other professional's services such as speech therapy. Many neuropsychologists have expanded their concept of feedback sessions to include multiple visits for relatively short 'inhouse' interventions to address key barriers for the child's success. For example a chronically sleep deprived teenager might be invited back for two extra sessions for a cognitive behaviour therapy module to improve sleep hygiene.

It is important that paediatric neuropsychologists also recognise the value of the assessment in assisting other medical professionals to improve the effectiveness of their interventions (e.g. Lanca 2018). Natalie's medical course was complicated by lifelong asthma, and a review of her primary care notes tells us that she had two trips to the local hospital's emergency room following her accident due to asthma attacks. Where, prior to the brain injury, Natalie was conscientious about taking her daily asthma medication with breakfast and remembering her rescue inhalers when she went to friends' houses, following the injury she regularly forgot both, and given the new stress and chaos of the morning routine due to her difficulty focusing and poor frustration tolerance, her parents were forgetting the medication as well. One important outcome of the feedback session was the collaborative development of an 'asthma care plan', typed out for family members and the paediatrician, that included assigning Natalie's grandmother as the person in charge of ensuring she has taken her daily medicine and her rescue inhaler is packed in her sports bag that she takes to friends' houses.

SUMMARY

We are tremendously lucky to be involved in a field that allows us to work at the intersection of neuroscience and social science. By beginning with the language and perspectives of our patients and families from the first moments of our clinical interactions, disrupting rules of traditional academic communication with vivid, accessible language, and using our psychotherapeutic training to help families navigate complex and often contradictory expectations, we can conduct the type of collaborative feedback sessions that alter lives.

In this case, Natalie's primary concern, that she wanted her teacher to love her again, was embraced by the family as a meaningful way to organise the cognitive, behavioural, and emotional impacts of the severe traumatic brain injury. By saying 'Yes' to this way of framing the issue, the focus was shifted from ongoing tensions within the family fuelled by complex generational and cultural ideas about discipline and spoiling, to implementing strategies designed to assist Natalie's damaged frontal executive network system in modulating emotions, regulating behaviour, and connecting with others in a way that would help her meet her goals.

As Dr Byron Rourke was known to say (Postal and Armstrong 2013, p. 273),

> Neuropsychology is total psychology. Everything you have ever learned about child development, family therapy, psychopathology, testing, evaluation, communication skills, and life in general. There is nothing you have learned in your entire life that won't be important, and you will use it all at once. This is the coolest and most complicated thing you will ever do.

ACKNOWLEDGEMENT

Thank you to Dr Kira Armstrong for her assistance in reviewing the chapter and her ongoing collaboration.

REFERENCES

Austin C, Gerstle M, Baum KT et al. (2019) Evolution of parental knowledge and efficacy across the pediatric neuropsychological evaluation process. *The Clinical Neuropsychologist* 33(4): 743–759.

Beeler D, Paré-Blagoev EJ, Jacobson LA, Ruble K (2020) Educating childhood cancer survivors: A qualitative analysis of parents mobilizing social and cultural capital. *Journal of Cancer Education* 36(4): 819–825.

Bodin D, Beetar JT, Yeates KO, Boyer K, Colvin AN, Mangeot S (2008) A survey of parent satisfaction with pediatric neuropsychological evaluations. *The Clinical Neuropsychologist* 21: 884–898.

Brickman A, Cabo R, Manly J (2006) Ethical issues in cross-cultural neuropsychology. *Applied Neuropsychology* 13(2): 91–100.

Elias J, Zimak E, Sherwood A et al. (2021) Do parents implement pediatric neuropsychological report recommendations? *The Clinical Neuropsychologist* 36(6): 1117–1133.

Farmer S, Brazeal T (1998) Parent perceptions about the process and outcomes of child neuropsychological assessment. *Applied Neuropsychology* 5: 194–201.

Griffin A, Christie D (2009) Taking a systemic perspective on cognitive assessments and reports: Reflections of a paediatric and adolescent psychology service. *Clinical Child Psychology and Psychiatry* 13(2): 209–219.

Lanca M (2018) Integration of neuropsychology in primary care. *Archives of Clinical Neuropsychology* **33**(3): 269–279.

McGoldrick M, Gerson R (1985) *Genograms: Assessment and Intervention.* New York: W.W. Norton & Company.

Mindt M, Arentoft A, Kubo Germano K et al. (2008) Neuropsychological, cognitive, and theoretical considerations for evaluation of bilingual individuals. *Neuropsychological Review* **18**: 255–268.

Mindt, M, Byrd D, Manly J (2010) Increasing culturally competent neuropsychological services for ethnic minority populations: A call to action. *The Clinical Neuropsychologist* **24**(3): 429–453.

Pegg PO, Auerbach SM, Seel RT, Buenaver LF, Kiesler DJ, Plybon LE (2005) The impact of patient-centered information on patients' treatment satisfaction and outcomes in traumatic brain injury research. *Rehabilitation Psychology* **50**(4): 366–374.

Postal K (2018) The multigenerational family system in dementia assessment and management. In: Ravdin L, Katzen H, editors, *Handbook on the Neuropsychology of Aging and Dementia.* New York: Springer Publishing, pp. 131–145.

Postal K, Armstrong K (2013) *Feedback That Sticks: The Art of Effectively Communicating Neuropsychological Assessment Results.* New York: Oxford University Press.

Postal K, Chow C, Jung S, Erickson-Moreo K, Geier F, Lanca M (2018) The stakeholders' project in neuropsychological report writing: A survey of neuropsychologists' and referral sources' views of neuropsychological reports. *The Clinical Neuropsychologist* **32**(3): 326–344.

Rosado D, Buehler S, Botbol-Berman E et al. (2018) Neuropsychological feedback services improve quality of life and social adjustment. *The Clinical Neuropsychologist* **32**(3): 422–435.

Smith S, Wiggins C, Gorske T (2007) A survey of psychological assessment feedback practices. *Assessment* **14**(3): 310–319.

Measure Index

Domain	Measure	Reference	Chapter
Acculturation			
	Stephenson Multigroup Acculturation Scale (SMAS)	Stephenson M (2000) Development and validation of the Stephenson Multigroup Acculturation Scale (SMAS). *Psychological Assessment* **12**(1): 77–88.	22
Adaptive functioning			
	Adaptive Behavior Assessment System, Third Edition (ABAS-III)	Harrison P, Oakland T (2015) *Adaptive Behavior Assessment System for Children*, 3rd edition. Torrance, CA: Western Psychological Services.	3, 9, 20, 24
	Goal Oriented Assessment of Life Skills (GOAL)	Miller LJ, Oakland T, Herzberg DS (2013) *Goal-Oriented Assessment of Lifeskills (GOAL)*. Torrance, CA: WPS.	3
	Miller Function and Participation Scales (MFUN)	Miller LJ (2006) *The Miller Function and Participation Scales*. San Antonio, TX: Pearson.	3
	Scales of Independent Behavior, Revised (SIB-R)	Bruininks RK, Woodcock RW, Weatherman RF, Hill BK (1996) *Scales of Independent Behavior, Revised*. Itasca, IL: Riverside Publishing.	20
	Social and Occupational Functioning Scale (SOFAS)	Rybarczyk B (2011) Social and occupational functioning assessment scale (SOFAS). *LXIII, Encyclopedia of Clinical Neuropsychology* **1**: 2313.	24
	Vineland Adaptive Behavior Scales, Third Edition (Vineland-3)	Sparrow SS, Cicchetti DV, Saulnier CA (2016) *Vineland Adaptive Behavior Scales – Third Edition (Vineland-3)*. San Antonio, TX: Pearson.	3, 6, 20

(Continued)

Domain	Measure	Reference	Chapter
Attention			
	Conners' Continuous Performance Test, Third Edition (CPT-3)	Conners CK (2014) *Conners' Continuous Performance Test 3rd Edition Manual.* Canada: Multi-Health Systems Inc.	8, 9, 22
	D2 Test of Attention	Brickencamp R, Zillmer E (1998) *The d2 Test of Attention.* Seattle, WA: Hogrefe & Huber.	21
	Gordon Diagnostic System (GDS)	Gordon M (1986) *Instruction Manual for the Gordon Diagnostic System.* DeWitt, NY: Checkmate Plus.	8
	Integrated Variables of Attention (IVA)	Sanford JA, Turner A (2005) *Integrated Variables of Attention* [Computer software]. Richmond, VA: Braintrain Inc.	10
	Stroop Color-Word Test (SCWT)	Stroop JR (1935) Studies of interference in serial verbal reactions. *Journal of Experimental Psychology* **18**(6): 643.	8, 22
	Test of Everyday Attention for Children, Second Edition (TEA-Ch2)	Manly T, Anderson V, Crawford J, George M, Underbjerg M, Robertson I (2016) *Test of Everyday Attention for Children, TEA-Ch2,* 2nd edition. London: Pearson.	7, 8
	Test of Variables of Attention (TOVA)	Leark RA, Dupuy TR, Greenberg LM, Kindschi CL, Hughes SJ (2016) *TOVA Professional Manual: Test of Variables of Attention Continuous Performance Test.* Los Alamitos, CA: The TOVA Company.	8, 10
	Trail Making Test (TMT)	Reitan RM (1955) The relation of the Trail Making Test to organic brain damage. *Journal of Consulting Psychology* **19**(5): 393–394.	8, 21
Auditory processing			
	SCAN–3:A Tests for Auditory Processing Disorders in Children, Adolescents and Adults	Keith RW (2009) *SCAN-3 for Adolescents and Adults: Tests for Auditory Processing Disorders.* San Antonio, TX: Pearson.	10
	SCAN–3:C Tests for Auditory Processing Disorders for Children	Keith RW (2009) *SCAN-3 for Children: Tests for Auditory Processing Disorders.* San Antonio, TX: Pearson.	10

(Continued)

Domain	Measure	Reference	Chapter
Educational achievement/psychoeducational			
	Bracken Basic Concept Scale, Third Edition (Bracken-3)	Bracken BA (2006) *The Bracken Basic Concept Scale, Third Edition: Receptive.* San Antonio, TX: Harcourt Assessment.	20
	Neale Analysis of Reading Ability (NARA)	Greaney J, Hill E, Tobin M (1998) *Neale Analysis of Reading Ability: University of Birmingham, Users' Manual.* Peterborough: Royal National Institute for the Blind NFER/Nelson Publishing Company Ltd.	1
	Wechsler Individual Achievement Test, Third Edition (WIAT-III UK)	Wechsler D (2017) *Wechsler Individual Achievement Test – Third UK Edition.* London: Pearson.	9, 12, 17
	Wechsler Individual Achievement Test, Fourth Edition (WIAT-IV)	Wechsler D (2020) *Wechsler Individual Achievement Test,* Fourth edition. San Antonio, TX: NCS Pearson.	5
	Wechsler Test of Adult Reading (WTAR) (Wechsler 2001)	Wechsler D (2001) *Wechsler Test of Adult Reading.* San Antonio, TX: NCS Pearson.	24
	Woodcock-Johnson, Third Edition (WJ-III) Tests of Achievement	Woodcock RW, McGrew KS, Mather N (2007) *Woodcock Johnson III Tests of Achievement.* Rolling Meadows, IL: Riverside Publishing.	24
Executive function			
	Arrows and Colors Cognitive Test (ACCT)	Poletti B, Carelli L, Faini A et al. (2018) The Arrows and Colors Cognitive Test (ACCT): A new verbal-motor free cognitive measure for executive functions in ALS. *Plos One* **13**(8): 1–15.	21
	Behavioural Assessment of the Dysexecutive Syndrome for Children (BADS-C)	Emslie H, Wilson C, Burden V, Nimmo-Smith I, Wilson BA (2003) *Behavioural Assessment of the Dysexecutive Syndrome for Children.* Bury St Edmunds, UK: Thames Valley Test Company.	9, 11
	Behavior Rating Inventory of Executive Function, Second Edition (BRIEF-2)	Gioia GA, Isquith PK, Guy SC, Kenworthy L (2015) *Behavior Rating Inventory of Executive Function.* Odessa, FL: Psychological Assessment Resources.	2, 9, 11, 16, 18, 20, 24

(*Continued*)

Domain	Measure	Reference	Chapter
	Controlled Oral Word Association Test (COWAT)	Benton AL, Hamsher K, Sivan AB (1983) *Controlled Oral Word Association Test (COWAT) Multilingual Aphasia Examination*, 3rd edition. Iowa City, IA: AJA Associates.	24
	Corsi Block-Tapping Test	Corsi PM (1972) Human memory and the medial temporal region of the brain. *Dissertation Abstracts International* **34**(02): 819B.	21
	Delis-Kaplan Executive Function System (D-KEFS)	Delis DC, Kaplan E, Kramer JH (2001) *Delis-Kaplan Executive Function System*. San Antonio, TX: Pearson.	8, 9, 11, 18, 24
	Tasks of Executive Control (TEC)	Isquith PK, Roth RM, Gioia GA (2010) *Tasks of Executive Control (TEC)*. Lutz, FL: Psychological Assessment Resources, Inc.	11
	Tower of London	Culbertson WC, Zillmer EA (1999) *The Tower of London, Drexel University, Research Version: Examiner's Manual*. North Tonawanda, NY: Multi-Health Systems.	11, 24
	Wisconsin Card Sorting Test, computer version 4 (WCST: CV4)	Heaton RK (2004) *Wisconsin Card Sorting Test Computer Version 4, Research Edition*. Odessa, FL: Psychological Assessment Resources.	11
	Working Memory Rating Scale (WMRS)	Alloway TP, Gathercole SE, Kirkwood HJ (2008) *Working Memory Rating Scale*. London: Pearson.	2
Intelligence			
	Bayley Scales of Infant and Toddler Development, Fourth Edition (Bayley-4)	Bayley N, Aylward, GP (2019) *Bayley Scales of Infant and Toddler Development, Fourth Edition*. San Antonio, TX: Pearson Assessments.	4, 5, 20
	British Ability Scales, Third Edition (BAS-3)	Elliott CD, Smith P (2011) *British Ability Scales, Third Edition (BAS3)*. Swindon, UK: GL Assessment.	20
	Columbia Mental Maturity Scale (CMMS)	Reuter J, Mintz J (1970) Columbia Mental Maturity Scale as a test of concept formation. *Journal of Consulting and Clinical Psychology* **34**(3): 387–393. doi.org/10.1037/h0029272.	21

(*Continued*)

Domain	Measure	Reference	Chapter
	Comprehensive Test of Non-Verbal Intelligence, Second Edition (CTONI-2)	Hammill DD, Pearson NA, Wiederholt JL (2009) *Comprehensive Test of Nonverbal Intelligence*, 2nd edition. Austin, TX: Pro-Ed.	2
	Differential Ability Scale, Second Edition (DAS-II)	Elliot CD (2007) *Differential Ability Scales, Second Edition (DAS-II)*. New York, NY: Pearson Clinical Assessment.	20
	Intelligence Test for Visually Impaired Children (ITVIC)	Dekker R (1993) Visually impaired children and haptic intelligence test scores: Intelligence Test for Visually Impaired Children (ITVIC). *Developmental Medicine Child Neurology* **35**(6): 478–489.	1
	Kaufman Brief Intelligence Test, Second Edition (KBIT-2)	Kaufman AS, Kaufman NL (2004) *Kaufman Brief Intelligence Test*, 2nd Edition. Circle Pines, MN: American Guidance Service.	21
	Leiter International Performance Scale, Third Edition (Leiter-3)	Roid GH, Miller LJ, Pomplun M, Koch C (2013) *Leiter International Performance Scale-Third Edition*. Wood Dale, IL: Stoelting Company.	2, 20
	Mullen Scales of Early Learning (MSEL)	Mullen EM (1995) *Mullen Scales of Early Learning*. Circle Pines, MN: American Guidance Service Inc.	20
	Naglieri Nonverbal Ability Test, Third Edition (NNAT3)	Naglieri JA (2016) *Naglieri Nonverbal Ability Test*, 3rd edition. Bloomington, MN: Pearson.	2
	Panga Munthu Test (PMT)	Kathuria R, Serpell R (1998) Standardization of the Panga Munthu Test – A nonverbal cognitive test developed in Zambia. *Journal of Negro Education* **67**(3): 228–241.	22
	Raven's Progressive Matrices (RPM)	Raven J, Raven JC, Court JH (1998) *Manual for Raven's Progressive Matrices and Vocabulary Scales. Section 1: General Overview*. Oxford, UK: Oxford Psychologists Press; San Antonio, TX: The Psychological Corporation.	21

(Continued)

Domain	Measure	Reference	Chapter
	Reynell–Zinkin Developmental Scales for young children with visual impairments	Reynell J (1978) Developmental patterns of visually handicapped children. *Child: Care, Health and Development* **4**(5): 291–303.	1
	Snijders–Oomen Nonverbal Intelligence Test Revised (SON-R)	Snijders JT, Tellegen PJ, Laros JA (1989) *Snijders–Oomen Nonverbal Intelligence Test: SON-R 5½–17. Manual and Research Report.* Groningen, The Netherlands: Wolters-Noordhoff.	2
	Stanford-Binet, Fifth Edition (SB-5)	Roid GH (2003) *Stanford-Binet Intelligence Scales*, 5th edition. Itasca, IL: Riverside.	20
	Test of Nonverbal Intelligence, Fourth Edition (TONI-4)	Brown L, Sherbenou RJ, Johnsen SK (2010) *Test of Nonverbal Intelligence*, 4th edition. Austin, TX: Pro-Ed.	2
	Universal Nonverbal Intelligence Test, Second Edition (UNIT-2)	Bracken BA, McCallum RS (2016) *UNIT 2: Universal Nonverbal Intelligence Test.* Austin, TX: Pro-Ed.	2
	Wechsler Adult Intelligence Scale, Fourth Edition (WAIS-IV)	Wechsler D (2008) *WAIS-IV: Technical and Interpretive Manual.* Bloomington, MN: Pearson.	20, 24
	Wechsler Intelligence Scale for Children, Fifth Edition (WISC-V)	Wechsler D (2014) *WISC-V: Technical and Interpretive Manual.* Bloomington, MN: Pearson.	8, 9, 12, 17, 20, 22, 24
	Wechsler Intelligence Scale for Children, Fifth UK Edition, WISC-V[UK]	Wechsler D (2016) *Wechsler Intelligence Scale for Children*, 5th UK edition. London: Harcourt Assessment.	1, 2, 5, 6, 7, 24
	Wechsler Nonverbal Scale of Ability (WNV)	Wechsler D, Naglieri JA (2006) *Wechsler Nonverbal Scale of Ability: WNV.* San Antonio, TX: Pearson.	2
	Wechsler Preschool and Primary Scales of Intelligence, Fourth Edition (WPPSI-IV)	Wechsler D (2012) *WPPSI-IV: Technical and Interpretive Manual.* Bloomington, MN: Pearson.	20

(Continued)

Domain	Measure	Reference	Chapter
Memory			
	California Verbal Learning Test – Children's Version (CVLT-C)	Delis DC, Karmer JH, Kaplan E, Ober BA (1994) *California Verbal Learning Test – Children's Version.* San Antonio, TX: The Psychological Corporation.	9, 11, 24
	Child and Adolescent Memory Profile (ChAMP)	Sherman EMS, Brooks BL (2015a) *Child and Adolescent Memory Profile (ChAMP).* Lutz, FL: Psychological Assessment Resources, Inc.	9, 23
	Children's Auditory Verbal Learning Test, Second Edition (CAVLT-2)	Talley JL. (1993) *Children's Auditory Verbal Learning Test,* 2nd edition. Odessa, FL: Psychological Assessment Resources, Inc.	9
	Children's Memory Scale (CMS)	Cohen MJ (1997) *Children's Memory Scale.* San Antonio, TX: The Psychological Corporation.	9, 24
	Children's Test of Nonword Repetition (CN REP)	Gathercole S, Baddeley A (1996) *Children's Test of Nonword Repetition (CN REP).* London: Psychological Corporation.	9
	Everyday Memory Questionnaire, Revised (EMQ-R)	Royle J, Lincoln NB (2008) The Everyday Memory Questionnaire – revised: Development of a 13-item scale. *Disability and Rehabilitation* **30**(2): 114–121.	9
	Pyramids and Palm Trees (PPT)	Howard D, Patterson K (1992) *The Pyramids and Palm Trees Test: A Test for Semantic Access from Words and Pictures.* Bury St Edmunds: Thames Valley Test Company.	9
	Rivermead Behavioural Memory Test for Children (RBMT-C)	Wilson B, Ivani-Chalian R, Aldrich F (1991) *The Rivermead Behavioural Memory Test for Children Aged 5 to 10 Years.* Bury St Edmunds: Thames Valley Test Company.	9
	Self-Ordered Pointing Task (SOPT)	Petrides M, Milner B (1982) Deficits on subject-ordered tasks after frontal- and temporal-lobe lesions in man. *Neuropsychologia* **20**(3): 249–262.	9

(Continued)

Domain	Measure	Reference	Chapter
	Test of Memory and Learning, Second Edition (TOMAL-2)	Reynolds CR, Bigler ED (2007) *Test of Memory and Learning*, 2nd edition. Austin, TX: Pro-Ed.	9
	Wechsler Memory Scale, Fourth Edition (WMS-IV)	Wechsler D (2009) *Wechsler Memory Scale – Fourth Edition (WMS-IV) Technical and Interpretive Manual.* San Antonio, TX: Pearson.	24
	Wide Range Assessment of Memory and Learning, Third Edition (WRAML-3)	Sheslow D, Adams W (2021) *Wide Range Assessment of Memory and Learning*, 3rd edition. London: Pearson.	24
	Working Memory Test Battery for Children (WMTB-C)	Pickering S, Gathercole S (2001) *Working Memory Test Battery for Children* (now out of print). Hove: The Psychological Corporation.	9
Motor and sensory			
	Alberta Infant Motor Scale (AIMS)	Piper MC, Darrah J (1994) *Alberta Infant Motor Scale.* Alberta: Saunders.	4
	Assisting Hand Assessment (AHA)	Krumlinde-Sundholm L, Eliasson AC (2003) Development of the Assisting Hand Assessment: A Rasch-built measure intended for children with unilateral upper limb impairments. *Scandinavian Journal of Occupational Therapy* **10**(1): 16–26.	4
	Assisting Hand Assessment for Adolescents (Ad-AHA)	Louwers A, Beelen A, Holmefur M, Krumlinde-Sundholm L (2016) Development of the Assisting Hand Assessment for Adolescents (Ad-AHA) and validation of the AHA from 18 months to 18 years. *Dev Med Child Neurol* **58**(12): 1303–1309.	4
	Both Hands Assessment (BoHA)	Elvrum AKG, Zethraeus BM, Vik T, Krumlinde-Sundholm L (2018) Development and validation of the Both Hands Assessment for children with bilateral cerebral palsy. *Physical & Occupational Therapy in Pediatrics* **38**(2): 113–126.	4

(Continued)

Domain	Measure	Reference	Chapter
	Bruininks-Oseretsky Test of Motor Proficiency, Second Edition (BOT-2)	Bruininks RH, Bruininks BD (2005) *Bruininks-Oseretsky Test of Motor Proficiency*, 2nd edition. San Antonio, TX: Pearson Assessments.	4
	Clinical Observation of Motor and Posture Skills, Second Edition (COMPS-2)	Wilson B, Kaplan B, Pollock N, Law M (2000) *Clinical Observation of Motor and Postural Skills: Administration and Scoring Manual*, 2nd edition. Framingham, MA: Therapro, Inc.	4
	Detailed Assessment of Speed of Handwriting (DASH)	Barnett A, Henderson S, Scheib B, Schulz J (2007) *The Detailed Assessment of Speed of Handwriting (DASH)*. London: Pearson Assessment.	15
	Developmental Coordination Disorder Questionnaire 2007 (DCDQ-07)	Wilson BN, Crawford SG, Green D, Roberts G, Aylott A, Kaplan BJ (2009) Psychometric properties of the revised developmental coordination disorder questionnaire. *Physical & Occupational Therapy in Pediatrics* **29**(2): 184–204.	6
	Evaluation in Ayres Sensory Integration (EASI)®	Mailloux Z, Parham LD, Roley SS, Ruzzano L, Schaaf RC (2018) Introduction to the Evaluation in Ayres Sensory Integration® (EASI). *American Journal of Occupational Therapy* **72**: 7201195030.	3
	Gesture Imitation Test	Bergès J, Lézine I (1965) *The Imitation of Gestures: A Technique for Studying the Body Schema and Paxis of Children Three to Six Years of Age*. Translated by Arthur H. Parmelee. London: Spastics Society Medical Education and Information Unit with Heinemann Medical.	4
	Grooved Pegboard Test (GPT)	Lafayette Instrument Company (2014) *Grooved Pegboard User's Manual*. Lafayette, IN: Lafayette Instrument Company.	9
	Hand Assessment for Infants (HAI)	Krumlinde-Sundholm L, Ek L, Sicola E et al. (2017) Development of the Hand Assessment for Infants: evidence of internal scale validity. *Developmental Medicine & Child Neurology*, **59**(12): 1276-1283.	4

(Continued)

Domain	Measure	Reference	Chapter
	Handwriting Legibility Scale (HLS)	Barnett A, Prunty M, Rosenblum S (2018) Development of the Handwriting Legibility Scale (HLS): A preliminary examination of reliability and validity. *Research in Developmental Disabilities* **72**: 204–247.	15
	Jebsen Taylor Hand Function Test (JTHFT)	Jebsen RH, Taylor N, Trieschmann RB, Trotter MJ, Howard LA (1969) An objective and standardized test of hand function. *Archives of Physical Medicine and Rehabilitation* **50**: 311–319.	4
	Kids Assisting Hand Assessment (Kids-AHA)	Krumlinde-Sundholm L, Holmefur M, Eliasson A (2014). *Manual: Assisting Hand Assessment – Kids, 18 months to 12 years,* β-version 5.0, English. Stockholm: Karolinska Institutet.	4
	McCarron Assessment of Neuromuscular Development (MAND)	McCarron L (1997) *McCarron Assessment of Neuromuscular Development, Fine and Gross Motor Abilities.* Dallas, TX: McCarron-Dial Systems, Inc.	4
	Mini-Assisting Hand Assessment (Mini-AHA)	Greaves S, Imms C, Dodd K, Krumlinde-Sundholm L (2013) Development of the Mini-Assisting Hand Assessment: Evidence for content and internal scale validity. *Developmental Medicine & Child Neurology* **55**(11): 1030–1037.	4
	Movement Assessment Battery for Children, Second Edition (Movement ABC-2)	Henderson SE, Sugden DA, Barnett A (2007) *Movement ABC-2.* London: Pearson.	3, 4, 6
	Peabody Developmental Motor Scales, Second Edition (PDMS-2)	Folio MR, Fewell RR (2000) *Peabody Developmental Motor Scales,* 2nd edition. San Antonio, TX: Pearson Assessments.	4
	Purdue Pegboard Test (PPT)	Tiffin J, Asher EI (1948) The Purdue Pegboard: Norms and studies of reliability and validity. *Journal of Applied Psychology* **32**: 234–247.	4
	Sensory Integration and Praxis Test (SIPT)	Ayres AJ (1989) *Sensory Integration and Praxis Test.* Torrance, CA: WPS.	3

(Continued)

Domain	Measure	Reference	Chapter
	Sensory Processing Measure, 2nd Edition (SPM-2)	Parham LD, Ecker C, Kuhaneck H, Henry DA, Glennon TJ (2021) *Sensory Processing Measure*, 2nd edition (SPM-2). Torrance, CA: Western Psychological Services.	3
	Sensory Processing Three Dimensions Scale (SPD3)	Miller LJ, Schoen SA, Mulligan S (2020) *The Sensory Processing Three Dimensions Scale (SP3D: Research Edition)*. Torrance: Western Psychological Services.	3
	Sensory Profile-2 (SP2)	Dunn W (2014) *Sensory Profile-2*. San Antonio, TX: Pearson Assessments.	3
	Structured Observations of Sensory Integration-Motor (SOSI-M)	Blanche EI, Reinoso G, Kiefer DB (2019) *Structured Observations of Sensory Integration-Motor*. Novato, CA: Academic Therapy Publications.	3
	Test of Gross Motor Development, Third Edition (GMD-3)	Ulrich D (2000) *Test of Gross Motor Development, Examiner's Manual*. Austin, TX: Pro-Ed. Inc.	4
	Woods and Teuber Mirror Movements Scale	Woods BT, Teuber HL (1978) Mirror movements after childhood hemiparesis. *Neurology* **28**(11): 1152–1157.	4
Neuropsychological batteries			
	Comprehensive Vocational Evaluation System (CVES)	Dial JG, Mezger C, Gray S, Massey T, Chan F, Hull J (1990) *Manual: Comprehensive Vocational Evaluation System*. Dallas, TX: McCarron-Dial Systems, Inc.	1
	Mini Mental State Examination, Second Edition (MMSE-2)	Folstein MF, Folstein SE, White T, Messer MA (2010) *Mini-Mental State Examination – 2nd Edition (MMSE-2)*. Lutz, FL: Psychological Assessment Resources.	24
	A Developmental Neuropsychological Assessment, Second Edition (NEPSY-II)	Korkman M, Kirk U, Kemp SL (2007) *NEPSY-II*. San Antonio, TX: Pearson Assessment.	2, 8, 9, 11, 12, 21
	NIH Toolbox Cognition Battery	Gershon RC, Wagster MV, Hendrie HC, Fox NA, Cook KF, Nowinski CJ (2013) NIH Toolbox for assessment of neurological and behavioral function. *Neurology* **80**(11 Suppl 3): S2–S6.	21

(Continued)

Domain	Measure	Reference	Chapter
	Repeatable Battery for the Assessment of Neuropsychological Status (RBANS)	Randolph C, Tierney MC, Mohr E, Chase TN (1998) The Repeatable Battery for the Assessment of Neuropsychological Status (RBANS): Preliminary clinical validity. *Journal of Clinical and Experimental Neuropsychology* **20**(3): 310–319.	7, 24
Processing speed			
	Symbol Digit Modalities Test (SDMT) including oral version (SDMT-oral)	Smith A (1991) *Symbol Digit Modalities Test.* Los Angeles, CA: Western Psychological Services.	21, 24
Quality of life			
	Impact of Pediatric Epilepsy Scale (IPES)	Camfield C, Breau L, Camfield P (2001) Impact of pediatric epilepsy on the family: A new scale for clinical and research use. *Epilepsia* **42**(1): 104–112.	9
	Pediatric Quality of Life Inventory (PedsQL)	Varni JW, Seid M, Rode CA (1999) The PedsQL™: Measurement model for the pediatric quality of life inventory. *Medical Care* **37**(2): 126–139.	9
Social emotional and behavioural			
	Achenbach System of Empirically Based Assessment (ASEBA) including the Child Behaviour Checklist (CBCL)	Achenbach TM (2009) The Achenbach System of Empirically Based Assessment (ASEBA): Development, Findings, Theory, and Applications. Burlington, VT: University of Vermont Research Center for Children, Youth, & Families. https://aseba.org/	8, 13, 19
	Autism Diagnostic Interview-Revised (ADI-R)	Le Couteur A, Lord C, Rutter M (2003) *Autism Diagnostic Interview – Revised.* Los Angeles, CA: Western Psychological Services.	12
	Autism Diagnostic Observation Schedule, Second Edition (ADOS-2®)	Lord C, Rutter M, DiLavore PC et al. (2012) *Autism Diagnostic Observation Schedule*, 2nd edition. Torrance, CA: Western Psychological Services.	1, 12, 17, 20
	Autism Spectrum Screening Questionnaire (ASSQ)	Ehlers S, Gillberg C, Wing L. (1999) A screening questionnaire for Asperger syndrome and other high-functioning autism spectrum disorders in school age children. *Journal of Autism and Developmental Disorders* **29**(2): 129–141.	12

(Continued)

Domain	Measure	Reference	Chapter
	Awareness of Social Inference Test, Third Edition (TASIT)	McDonald S, Flanagan S, Rollins J (2017) *The Awareness of Social Inference Test*, 3rd edition. Sydney, Australia: ASSBI Resources.	12
	Behavior Assessment System for Children, Third Edition (BASC-3)	Reynolds CR, Kamphaus RW (2015) *Behavior Assessment System for Children*, 3rd edition. New York, NY: Pearson Clinical Assessment.	8, 13, 19, 20
	Brief Psychiatric Rating Scale (BPRS)	Overall JE, Gorham DR (1962) The brief psychiatric rating scale. *Psychological Reports* **10**(3): 799–812.	24
	Child Depression Inventory, Second Edition (CDI-2)	Kovacs M (2010) *Children's Depression Inventory*, 2nd edition. San Antonio, TX: Pearson.	19
	Child Problematic Traits Inventory (CPTI)	Colins OF, Andershed H, Frogner L, Lopez-Romero L, Veen V, Andershed AK (2014) A new measure to assess psychopathic personality in children: The Child Problematic Traits Inventory. *Journal of Psychopathology and Behavioral Assessment* **36**(1): 4–21.	13
	Childhood Autism Rating Scale, Second Edition (CARS-2)	Schopler E, van Bourgondien ME, Wellman GJ, Love SR (2010) *The Childhood Autism Rating Scale, Second Edition (CARS-2)*. Los Angeles, CA: Western Psychological Services.	12
	Children's Hope Scale (CHS)	Snyder CR, Hoza B, Pelham WE et al. (1997) The development and validation of the Children's Hope Scale. *Journal of Pediatric Psychology* **22**(3): 399–421.	4
	Conners-3; Conners Rating Scales	Conners CK (2008) *Conners 3rd Edition Manual*. Toronto, Ontario, Canada: Multi-Health Systems.	8, 9, 12, 13, 17
	Development and Well-Being Assessment (DAWBA)	Goodman R, Ford T, Richards H, Gatward R, Meltzer H (2000) The Development and Well-Being Assessment: Description and initial validation of an integrated assessment of child and adolescent psychopathology. *Journal of Child Psychology and Psychiatry, and Allied Disciplines* **41**(5): 645–655.	12, 19

(Continued)

Domain	Measure	Reference	Chapter
	Developmental, Dimensional, and Diagnostic Interview (3Di)	Skuse D, Warrington R, Bishop D, Chowdhury U, Lau J, Mandy W, Place M (2004). The developmental, dimensional and diagnostic interview (3di): a novel computerized assessment for autism spectrum disorders. *Journal of the American Academy of Child and Adolescent Psychiatry* **43**(5): 548–558.	12, 17
	Diagnostic Interview for Children and Adolescents (DICA)	Reich W (2000) Diagnostic interview for children and adolescents (DICA). *Journal of the American Academy of Child & Adolescent Psychiatry* **39**(1): 59–66.	13
	Diagnostic Interview for Social and Communication Disorders, 11th Edition (DISCO-11)	Wing L (2006) *Diagnostic Interview for Social and Communication Disorders*, 11th edition. Bromley, UK: Centre for Social and Communication Disorders.	12
	Diagnostic Interview Schedule for Children, Version IV (DISC-IV)	Shaffer D, Fisher P, Lucas CP, Dulcan MK, Schwab-Stone ME (2000) NIMH Diagnostic Interview Schedule for Children Version IV (NIMH DISC-IV): Description, differences from previous versions, and reliability of some common diagnoses. *Journal of the American Academy of Child & Adolescent Psychiatry* **39**(1): 28–38.	13
	Frith-Happé Animations Test	Abell F, Happe F, Frith U (2000) Do triangles play tricks? Attribution of mental states to animated shapes in normal and abnormal development. *Cognitive Development* **15**(1): 1–16. See http://sites.google.com/site/utafrith/research for examples of the stimuli.	12
	Gilliam Autism Rating Scale, Third Edition (GARS-3)	Gilliam JE (2013) *Gilliam Autism Rating Scale – Third Edition (GARS-3)*. Austin, TX: Pro-Ed.	12
	Inventory of Callous-Unemotional Traits (ICU)	Frick PJ (2003) *The Inventory of Callous-Unemotional Traits*. New Orleans, LA: University of New Orleans.	13
	Modified Checklist for Autism in Toddlers, Revised with Follow-Up (M-CHAT-R/F)	Robins DL, Fein D, Barton M (2009) The modified checklist for autism in toddlers, revised with follow-up (M-CHAT-R/F). *Pediatrics* **133**: 37–45.	12

(Continued)

Domain	Measure	Reference	Chapter
	Parenting Stress Index, Fourth Edition (PSI-4)	Abidin RR (2012) *Parenting Stress Index, Fourth Edition (PSI-4)*. Lutz, FL: Psychological Assessment Resources.	13
	Reading the Mind in the Eyes Test (Child)	Baron-Cohen S, Wheelwright S, Scahill V, Lawson J, Spong A (2001) Are intuitive physics and intuitive psychology independent? A test with children with Asperger syndrome. *Journal of Developmental and Learning Disorders* **5**: 47–78.	12
	Revised Children's Anxiety and Depression Scale (RCADS)	Chorpita BF, Moffitt CE, Gray J (2005) Psychometric properties of the Revised Child Anxiety and Depression Scale in a clinical sample. *Behaviour Research and Therapy* **43**(3): 309–322.	19
	Social Communication Questionnaire (SCQ)	Rutter M, Bailey A, Lord C (2003) *The Social Communication Questionnaire: Manual*. Los Angeles, CA: Western Psychological Services.	9, 12
	Social Responsiveness Scale, Second Edition (SRS-2)	Constantino JN, Gruber CP (2012) *Social Responsiveness Scale: SRS-2*. Torrance, CA: Western Psychological Services.	12
	Strange Stories	Happé FG (1994) An advanced test of theory of mind: Understanding of story characters' thoughts and feelings by able autistic, mentally handicapped, and normal children and adults. *Journal of Autism and Developmental Disorders* **24**(2): 129–154.	12
	Strengths and Difficulties Questionnaire (SDQ)	Goodman R (1999) The extended version of the Strengths and Difficulties Questionnaire as a guide to child psychiatric caseness and consequent burden. *The Journal of Child Psychology and Psychiatry and Allied Disciplines* **40**(5): 791–799.	2, 19, 24
	Theory of Mind Scale (ToM)	Wellman HM, Liu D (2004) Scaling of theory-of-mind tasks. *Child Development* **75**(2): 523–541.	12
	Theory of Mind Inventory, Second Edition (TOMI-2)	Hutchins TL, Prelock PA (2016) *Technical Manual for the Theory of Mind Inventory – 2*. Unpublished manuscript.	12

(Continued)

Domain	Measure	Reference	Chapter
	Theory of Mind Task Battery (ToMTB)	Hutchins TL, Prelock PA (2010) *Technical Manual for the Theory of Mind Task Battery.* Unpublished manuscript.	12
Speech and language			
	Boston Naming Test (BNT)	Kaplan E, Goodglass H, Weintraub S (1983) *Boston Naming Test.* Philadelphia, PA: Lee & Febiger.	24
	British Picture Vocabulary Scale, Third Edition (BPVS-III)	Dunn LM, Dunn DM, Styles B, Sewell J (2009) *The British Picture Vocabulary Scale III*, 3rd edition. London: GL Assessment.	5, 6, 9, 21
	Children's Communication Checklist, version 2 (CCC-2)	Bishop DVM (2003) *The Children's Communication Checklist, version 2 (CCC-2).* London: Pearson.	5, 6, 12, 13
	Clinical Evaluation of Language Fundamentals, Fifth Edition (CELF-5)	Wiig EH, Semel E, Secord WA (2013) *Clinical Evaluation of Language Fundamentals – Fifth Edition (CELF-5).* Bloomington, MN: NCS Pearson.	5, 6, 9, 12, 24
	Clinical Evaluation of Language Fundamentals Preschool-3 (CELF Preschool-3)	Wiig EH, Secord WA, Semel E (2020) *Clinical Evaluation of Language Fundamentals Preschool-3 (CELF Preschool-3).* San Antonio, TX: Pearson.	5
	Comprehensive Test of Phonological Processing, Second Edition (CTOPP-2)	Wagner RK, Torgesen JK, Rashotte CA, Pearson NA (2013) *Comprehensive Test of Phonological Processing – 2nd ed. (CTOPP-2).* Austin, TX: Pro-Ed.	17
	Diagnostic Evaluation of Articulation and Phonology (DEAP)	Dodd B, Hua Z, Crosbie S, Holm A, Ozanne A (2002) *Diagnostic Evaluation of Articulation and Phonology (DEAP).* London: Pearson.	6
	Expressive One-Word Picture Vocabulary Test, Fourth Edition (EOWPVT-4)	Martin NA, Brownell R (2010) *Expressive One-Word Picture Vocabulary Test*, 4th edition. Torrance, CA: Western Psychological Services.	9, 20
	Expressive Vocabulary Test, Third Edition (EVT-3)	Williams K (2018) *Expressive Vocabulary Test, 3rd ed. (EVT-3).* Toronto, Canada: Pearson.	5
	Goldman-Fristoe Test of Articulation, Third Edition (GFTA-3)	Goldman R, Fristoe M (2015) *Goldman-Fristoe Test of Articulation*, 3rd edition. London: Pearson.	6

(Continued)

Domain	Measure	Reference	Chapter
	Intelligibility in Context Scale (ICS)	McLeod S, Harrison LJ, McCormack J (2012) The Intelligibility in context scale: Validity and reliability of a subjective rating measure. *Journal of Speech, Language, and Hearing Research* **55**: 648–656.	6
	Khan-Lewis Phonological Analysis, Second Edition (KLPA-2)	Lewis NP, Khan LMK (2015) *Khan-Lewis Phonological Analysis*, 2nd edition. London: Pearson.	6
	Park Play	Patel R, Connaghan K (2014) Park Play: A picture description task for assessing childhood motor speech disorders. *International Journal of Speech-Language. Pathology* **16**(4): 337–343.	6
	Peabody Picture Vocabulary Test, Fourth Edition (PPVT-4)	Dunn LM, Dunn DM (2007) *Peabody Picture Vocabulary Test*, 4th edition. New York, NY: Pearson Clinical Assessment.	3, 6, 20, 21
	Preschool Language Scales, Fifth Edition (PLS5)	Zimmerman IL, Steiner VG, Pond RE (2011) *Preschool Language Scales – Fifth Edition (PLS-5)*. Bloomington, MN: Pearson.	5
	Receptive One-Word Picture Vocabulary Test, Fourth Edition (ROWPVT-4)	Martin NA, Brownell R (2011b) *Receptive OneWord Picture Vocabulary Test*, 4th edition. Novato, CA: Academic Therapy Publications.	6, 9
	Token Test	De Renzi A, Vignolo LA (1962) Token test: A sensitive test to detect receptive disturbances in aphasics. *Brain: A Journal of Neurology* **85**: 665–678.	21
Validity			
	Medical Symptom Validity Test (MSVT)	Green P (2004) *Medical Symptom Validity Test (MSVT) for Microsoft Windows: User's Manual.* Canada: Green's Publishing.	23
	Memory Validity Profile (MVP)	Sherman EMS, Brooks BL (2015b) *Memory Validity Profile (MVP)*. Lutz, FL: Psychological Assessment Resources, Inc.	23
	Test of Memory Malingering (TOMM)	Tombaugh TN (1996) *Test of Memory Malingering: TOMM*. Toronto, Canada: Multi-Health Systems.	19, 23

(Continued)

Domain	Measure	Reference	Chapter
Visuospatial			
	Beery-Buktenica Developmental Test of Visual Motor Integration, Sixth Edition (VMI-6)	Beery KE, Buktenica NA, Beery NA (2010) *Beery-Buktenica Developmental Test of Visual-Motor Integration*, 6th edition. Torrance, CA: Western Psychological Services.	9, 17, 20, 22, 24
	Children's Embedded Figures Task (CEFT)	Witkin HA, Otman PK, Raskin E, Karp S (1971) *A Manual for the Embedded Figures Test*. California: Consulting Psychologists Press.	7
	Clock-Drawing Test (CDT)	Agrell B, Dehlin O (1998) The clock-drawing test. *Age and Ageing* **27**(3): 399–403.	24
	Developmental Test of Visual Perception, Third Edition (DTVP-3)	Hammill DD, Pearson NA, Voress JK (2014) *Developmental Test of Visual Perception. Examiners Manual*, 3rd edition. Austin, TX: Pro-Ed.	7, 21
	Motor-Free Visual Perception Test-4 (MVPT-4)	Colarusso R, Hammill D (2015) *Motor-Free Visual Perception Test-4*. Novato, CA: Academic Therapy Publications, Inc.	21
	Rey Complex Figure Test and Recognition Trial (RCFT)	Meyers JE, Meyers KR (1995) *Rey Complex Figure Test and Recognition Trial (RCFT)*. Odessa, FL: Psychological Assessment Resources.	9, 18, 22, 24
	Test of Visual Perceptual Skills, Fourth Edition (TVPS-4)	Martin NA (2017) *Test of Visual Perceptual Skills*, 4th edition. Novato, CA: Academic Therapy Publications.	7

Index

Measures are listed in the Measures Index starting on page 331.

22q11 deletion syndrome, 249

A

academic achievement test, 268, 269
academic performance, 100
academic skills, 269
acculturation, child and family's degrees, 282
acquired brain injury (ABI), 149
adaptive behaviour, 246
    executive function, 134
    participation, parent-report measures
        of, 35
adversity, early
    assessment/formulation, 212–13
    Child and Adolescent Mental Health
        Service, 209
    clinical formulation, 213
    intervention/management
        anxiety intervention/parenting, 214
        developmental dyslexia, 214
        social/peer intervention, 214
    language and motor skills, 209
    maltreatment, 210–11
    neural adaptations confer latent
        vulnerability, 211
    neurocognitive profile, 211–12
    outcome, 215
alternative communication devices (AACs),
    255
American Academy of Audiology Clinical
    Practice Guidelines, The, 122
American Academy of Clinical
    Neuropsychology/National Academy of
    Neuropsychology, 263
American Association on Intellectual and
    Developmental Disabilities, 247
American Psychological Association, 291
Angelman syndrome, 249
anticipatory motor planning, 48

anti-N-methyl-D-aspartate receptor, 235
antiseizure medications (ASMs), 105, 233,
    301
anxiety disorders, 214
applied behaviour analysis (ABA), 254
    intellectual disability, 254
    speech/language therapy, 254
articulation disorders, 73
asphyxia, 108
assess intellectual/developmental
    functioning, 253
asthma care plan, 327
attention, 100
    assessment/formulation, 97
        broader neuropsychological
            assessments, 100
        individual assessments of, 99–100
        neuropsychological assessments, 98–9
        rating scales, 98
    cognitive neuroscience, 95
    definition of, 94
    disorders of, 96–7
    distinct attentional networks, 96
    education services, 93
    intervention/management, 100–1
    outcome, 101–2
    types of, 94–5
    working memory, 107
attention-deficit/hyperactivity disorder
    (ADHD), 93, 94, 96–8, 134, 150, 161,
    172, 213, 219, 250, 251, 262
    behavioural characteristics, 98
    clinical diagnosis, 221
    co-occurring diagnosis of, 302
    DSM-IV-TR and DSM-5 diagnosis, 98
    executive functioning, disorder of, 220
    meta-analysis, 98
    National Institute for Clinical Excellence,
        101
    parenting programmes, 164
    psychosocial interventions, 101

audiogram, 20, 21
  for hearing perception, 120
  sounds, 21
audiological assessment, 26
audiology, 22
auditory deprivation, 22, 27
Auditory Figure-Ground, 125
auditory processing disorder (APD), 22, 122
  assessment/formulation, 121–6
    behavioural symptoms, 122
    CANS functions, 124
    electrophysiological measures, 125
    pathognomonic sign, 121
  CANS functions, 124
  central auditory disruptions/decrements, 120
  cross-disciplinary consultation, 121
  definitions of, 123
  differential diagnosis of, 125–6
  electrophysiological measures, 125
  intervention/management, 126–7
  language and nonlanguage aspects of, 124
  learning disorders, 121
  multiple diagnostic tests, 123
  neuropsychological assessment, 119
  speech perception, 121
auditory processing functions, 122
auditory training interventions, 127
augmentative and alternative communication (AAC) device, 261
autism spectrum disorder (ASD), 11, 37, 82, 145, 213, 250, 262
Avon Longitudinal Study of Parents and Children (ALSPAC), 173

B

Batten disease, 303
behavioural neuropsychological approach, 283
behavioural outcomes, 32
behavioural symptoms, 125
behaviour modelling, 152
bias, medium-high risk of, 150
birth defects, 201
blurred vision, 6
brain
  abnormalities, 234
  computerised tomography, 289

magnetic resonance imaging, 110
medications, chemicals, and diseases impact, 198–9
brain computer interface (BCI), 262, 265
  choice-making, 266
  strategies, 265
brain injury psychoeducation, 89
brain lesions, 234
brain plasticity, 248
brainstem, bilateral foci of hypointensity, 71
British Psychological Society, 312
British Society of Audiology, 122

C

CANS functions, 123
case study
  auditory processing, 125
  literacy, 172
  mental health, 238–9, 241
  prenatal exposure, to medicines/chemicals, 202
  sensory integration, 37
  speech, assessment/formulation, 268–9
  teleneuropsychology, paediatric, 311–12
  visuo-spatial processing, 86
central auditory disruptions, 120
central auditory nervous system (CANS), 120
central auditory pathways, 21
central nervous system (CNS), 32, 248
cerebral palsy, 53
  brain injury, 137
  motor impairments, 43
  NIH Common Data Elements, 266
  task-focused interventions, 53
chemotherapy, 321
Chiari malformations, 121
Child and Adolescent Mental Health Service, 209
child-centred social narratives, 152
children
  neurological system, maturation of, 44
  sensory/motor impairments, 32
  task-focused interventions, 53
Circle of Security Parenting programme, 214
cochlear-auditory-nerve junction, 121
cochlear implants, 20, 28
Cogmed, 27

cognitive abilities, 278
cognitive behavioural therapy (CBT), 101
    approaches, 254
    childhood social anxiety disorders, 240
    depression, in adolescents, 240
cognitive complaints, neuropsychological
    evaluation, 290
cognitive deficits, 248
cognitive 'scaffolding,' 100
cognitive test, 219
College of Alberta Psychologists Practice
    Guideline, 291
communication. *see also* social
    communication
    disorder, 75
    interventions, 150
    school-age children, 64
Communication Trust's 'What Works,'
    The, 67
Community Living Skills, 251
Comprehension of Instructions test,
    267
comprehensive neuropsychological
    formulations, 238
computer-based/online social skills
    instruction, 151
concussion/mild traumatic brain injury,
    294
congenital disorders, 238, 241
    academic performance, 203
    mental health, 235, 236
    peripheral visual system, 7
    vision impairment, 6
conscious control, 132
constraint-induced movement therapy,
    53
continuous performance tests (CPTs),
    99
Coping with Uncertainty in Everyday
    Situations (CUES) approach, 153
COVID-19 pandemic, 301
    neuropsychologists, 302
    neurorehabilitation, 306
cranial electrotherapy stimulation, 137
cranial nerves, 73
cross-cultural assessments
    cultural knowledge base, 280
    neuropsychological assessments, 279
cultural humility, 281
cultural knowledge base, 280

culture
    assessment/formulation
        interview, 281–3
        preparation, 280–1
        test selection/interpretation, 283
    background, 278
    intervention/management
        belief systems, 284–5
        report/feedback, 283–4
    language development, 277
    languages, 280
    neuropsychological assessments, 278–9
    outcome, 285

D

deaf
    awareness training, 26
    hard-of-hearing child, 27
decibel meter, 119
degrees of freedom (DOF), 45
depression, CBT-based intervention, 241
developmental coordination disorder (DCD),
    183
    copy best task, 188
    handwriting, children, 187
    pauses, within words, 187
    size control, 187
developmental language disorder (DLD), 58,
    172
    English-speaking children, 61
    identification of, 59
    language disorder, 62
    language functioning, 60
    pragmatic language skills, 61
    vocabulary knowledge, 61
    working memory, 62
Diagnostic and Statistical Manual (DSM),
    97
Diagnostic and Statistical Manual of Mental
    Disorders, Fifth Edition (DSM-5), 145,
    161, 172, 247
Digits Sequencing Task, 267
Directions into Velocity of Articulators
    (DIVA) model, 74
DIR®/Floortime, 38
disruptive behaviour disorders, 160
    assessment/formulation, 162–4
    environmental influences, 162

executive function, 160–1
  frontal lobe brain injury, 160
  intervention/management, 164–5
  language/verbal abilities, 161–2
  limited prosocial emotions/callous-
    unemotional traits, 161
  outcome, 166
disruptive behaviour problems (DBP), 160
  callous-unemotional traits, 161
  executive dysfunction, 160
  parenting programmes, 164
  psychiatric conditions, 162
  psychostimulants, 165
distant vision progresses, 6
DIVA model, 74
dorsal language stream, 73
dorsal stream, 4
  deficit, 83
  vulnerability, 9
Down syndrome, 249
dysarthria, 73, 77
dysfunctional signal transmission, 121
dyslexia, 172, 183
  child's phonological deficit, 174
  developmental, 82, 211
  diagnosis of, 176
  family-risk of, 172
  fluent spelling, 186
  neural correlates, 173
  proximal cause of, 173

E

educational attainment testing, 178
educational neuropsychology assessment, 223
Education Plan, 245
education/school
  assessment/formulation, 223–5
  assessment/intervention, tiered approach,
    221–3
  attention-deficit/hyperactivity disorder
    (ADHD), 219
  cognitive test, 219
  developmental stage, 220–1
  executive function, 220
  intervention/management, 225–8
    environmental/instructional
      considerations, 226–7
    executive functioning coaching, 227

executive skills, training of, 227
    family work, 226
    functional behavioural assessment,
      226
    independent strategies, 227, 228
    individualised therapy, 227
    peer group support, 227
    precision teaching, 227
    psycho-education, 226, 227
    psychosocial/systemic foundations, 226
    skills, 226–7
    social skills training, 226
    token economy system, 228
  outcome, 228–9
  provisions, 221
  social inclusion, 220
electroencephalogram, 277
encephalitis, 236
environmental changes, 203
epilepsy, 112, 234, 241, 277
  mental health difficulties, in adolescents,
    234
  psycho-education sessions, 285
ethical implications, 265
euthymic mood, 323
event-related potential-based cognitive
  testing, 265
evidence-based practice
  language interventions, 67
  for teaching, 88
executive function
  actions/learning systems, 133
  adaptive behaviour, holistic view of,
    134
  assessment/formulation, 134–6
  coaching, 227
  development, 14
  ecological/ethological validity, 132
  education/school, 220
  intervention/management, 136–9
    neurologic music therapy, 136
    physiological interventions, 137
    school, 138
  neuropsychological evaluations, 132
  outcome, 138–9
  self-regulation/school refusal, 131–2
  skills, 132
eye-gaze technologies, 265
eye movement disorders, 10
eye structure, 5

F

face-to-face
  contact, 301
  video-teleconferencing, 304
facial expressions, 9
family-centred care, 254
family work, 226
feedback
  asthma, 319
  clinical findings, 321
  control system, 133
  disrupting traditional academic
    communication patterns, 322–4
  diversifying world, 325–6
  empowering patients, 326–7
  families, to change lives, 326–7
  initial intake, 321
  inviting emotions, into room,
    324–5
  neuropsychological testing, 320
  neuropsychologists, 254
  seasoned clinicians, 321
  sessions, 325–6
  therapeutic intervention, 324
Feedback That Sticks, 320, 323, 324
fetal alcohol spectrum disorder (FASD),
  196
  confounding factors, risk of, 197
  facial characteristics, 196
fetal brain development, symptoms/severity,
  197
fetal teratogen syndromes, 200
fetal valproate spectrum disorder, 202
floor effects, 65
Fragile X syndrome, 82, 249
functional behavioural assessment,
  226
function mapping, symptom, 106

G

GCSE level, 90
Glasgow Coma Scale, 159, 319
globalisation, 278
Goal Attainment Scaling, 36
Gross Motor Function Classification System
  (GMFCS), 43
group-based interventions, 151

H

handwriting, 184
  age-appropriate writing ability, 186
  assessment/formulation
    'allograph,' level of, 187
    size control/speed, level of, 187–9
    'spelling,' level of, 185–6
  children with DCD, 187
  developmental coordination disorder
    (DCD), 183
  intervention/management, 189–90
  learning of, 184
  letter formation, 190
  motor skill, 184
  neuroimaging studies, 184
  outcome, 191
  pen-on-paper practice, 190
  process modules, 185
  psychomotor model of, 185
  speed, 188, 189
  spelling, learning of, 184
  style of, 185
headache, treatment, 289
hearing impaired
  assessment/formulation, 23–6
  management
    educational strategies, 26–7
    intervention research, 27–8
  testing, 25
hearing loss
  bilateral sensorineural, 19
  congenital/prelingual sensorineural, 20
  permanent sensorineural, 20
  types of, 21, 23
hearing, permanent sensorineural hearing
  loss, 20
heightened verbal memory deficits, 115
Hickok model, 74
hippocampal-dependent memory, 109
hippocampal development, 109
hippocampus, 210

I

inferior frontal gyrus (IFG), 74
intellectual disability, 110, 246, 248–50
  adaptive functioning, 246
  assessment/formulation, 251–3

clinical characteristics, 247
common comorbidities, 250–1
genetic disorders, 249
idiopathic, 249
intervention/management, 253–6
  cognitive/behavioural interventions,
    254–5
  language difficulties, 255
  neuropsychological intervention,
    254
  pharmacological interventions, 255
  seizures, in children, 256
modern-day intelligence tests, 247
neuroanatomy, 248
outcome, 256
paediatric psychiatrist, 245
prenatal/early childhood factors, 249
prevalence/aetiology, 248–9
severity, clinical characteristics, 247
intelligence, definition of, 246
International Classification of Diseases,
  11th Revision (ICD-11), 196
International Classification of Diseases and
  Related Health Problems, 120
International Classification of Functioning,
  Disability and Health model, 47
International Statistical Classification of
  Diseases and Related Health Problems,
  10th Revision, 247
Internet-based Interacting Together
  Everyday, Recovery after Childhood TBI
  (I-InTERACT), 311
interpersonal communication, 246
IQ
  assessment, 76, 178
  scores, 247
  tests, 162

L

language
  abilities, 58, 280
  assessments/questionnaires, standardised,
    63
  behaviours, 65
  cortical regions/white matter pathways, 60
  development, 58, 174, 176
  difficulties, 174, 211
  phonological disorders, 72
    skills, 76
    therapy, 57
language disorders, 58, 67
  developmental/acquired, 65
  diagnosis of, 59
  flow chart illustrating pathways, 59
  Venn diagram of, 72
language encompasses multiple skills, 61
language impairments, 60
  aetiology of, 59–60
  assessment/formulation, 62, 65
    authentic assessment, 64–5
    communication history, 63
    communication sample, 64
    questionnaire, 64
    standardised assessment, 63–4
  classification of, 58–9
  cognitive domains, relationship, 62
  content, 61
  core components of, 61
  form of, 61
  intervention/management
    approaches, 65–6
    evidence-based practice, 67
  outcome, 67–8
  use, 61–2
learning
  deaf child's, 27
  difficulties, 71
  disorders, 126, 302
  errorless, 27, 88
  haptic/tactile means of, 7
  of magic tricks, 53
  and memory, 107
  multisensory, 13
LEGO® Therapy, 131, 151, 209
lifestyle choices, 196
linguistic processing, 60
literacy
  assessment/formulation, 174–6
  disorders, 178
  dyslexia, 172
  intervention/management, 176–8
  moderator variables, 178
  outcome, 178–9
  phonological deficit, 174
  reading comprehension, 173
  recommendation, 171
  skills/subskills, 175
literature, neuropsychological, 107

M

magic-themed bimanual training, 53
magnetic resonance imaging (MRI), 57, 73,
    105, 248, 278
magnocellular pathway, 4
maltreatment, 'latent' effect of, 211
Manual Ability Classification System (MACS),
    43
Medicines and Healthcare Products
    Regulatory Agency's Yellow Card scheme,
    204
memory
    assessment/formulation, 110–15
    attention/working, 107
    domain, 111–12
    epilepsy, 105
    episodic, 108
    function mapping, symptom, 106
    hippocampal-dependent, 109
    intervention/management, 115–16
        psychoeducation, 115
        scaffold memory/learning, 116
    learning, 107
    long-term, 108
    neuropsychological assessment, 113–15
    neuropsychological test, 114
    outcome, 115
    parental/self-report questionnaires, 113
    recall, 109
    recognition, 109
    semantic, 108–9
    standardised memory tests, 111–12
    verbal/nonverbal processing, 109–10
    well-validated, 111
mental health
    assessment/formulation, 236–8
    clinical application, 241
    cognitive difficulties, 235–6
    difficulties, 110, 237, 238
        neurological conditions, 234
        rates of, 234
    epilepsy, 233
    intervention/management, 240–1
    neurological underpinnings, 234–5
    neuropsychological difficulties, 234
    outcome, 241
    professional, 240
mental workload, 263
metabolism, genetic disorders of, 249

metacognitive processes, 174
mild dyslexia, 289
mobility/navigational skills, 9
Moderate Intellectual Disability, 253
morphosyntax, 61
motor coordination
    assessment/formulation, 47–8
    brain injury, 53–4
    development of, 44
    intervention/management, 48–53
    outcome, 53–4
    theoretical perspectives, 44–7
motor cortex (MC), 74
    bilateral foci of hypointensity, 71
    brain regions, 74
    inter-neuronal activity, 44
motor delay/motor disorders, 45, 46
motor impairments, 53
    assistive technology/cognitive load, 263
    physical limitations, 261
    psychometrics/validation, 263
motor learning theories, 53
motor skills, 48, 209, 251
    child's neurological system, 44
    organisation/difficulties, 43
motor speech disorders, 73
motor tests, standardised, 49–52
multi-component interventions, 165
multi-systemic therapy, 165

N

navigation tasks, 86
neural adaptations, 211
neural connections, comprehensive
    map/'wiring diagram' of, 21
neural maturation, 45
neurodevelopmental and mental health
    conditions, 32
neurodevelopmental disorders, 137, 211
neurofeedback, 137
neurological disorders, 235, 238, 240
    chronic, 234
    mental health, 234, 235
    psychiatric disorders, 235
neurological soft signs, 44–5
neurologic music therapy, 136
neuropsychological assessment, 14, 119, 200,
    201, 264

neuropsychological battery, 212, 305
neuropsychological deficits, in teratogen
    syndromes, 204
neuropsychological evaluations, 132
    follow-up, 256
    intervention and management, 283
    IQ testing, 247
    paediatric psychiatrist, 245
neuropsychological formulation, 112
neuropsychological literature, 107
neuropsychological tests, 113, 114
    auditory demands, 124
    behavioural, 283
    emotional experiences, 320
    feedback, 283
neuropsychologists, 278, 305
neuropsychology
    language of, 322
    literature, 290
neurorehabilitation site, map of, 88
neurosensory restoration, with cochlear
    implants, 22
neurotoxins, prenatal developmental, 200
NIH Common Data Elements, 266
noise-cancelling headphones, 126
noisy community environments, 125
noisy reafferent signals, 133
nonverbal assessments, 24
nonverbal skills, 23
non-Western assessments, 278

O

occupational performance, analysis of, 35
occupational therapy intervention, 38
ophthalmology assessment, 105
optic nerve hypoplasia, 3
optic radiation, axons of, 4
orientation-discrimination paradigm, 85

P

paediatric neurocognitive interventions (PNI)
    model, 222
    ADHD diagnosis, 225
    educational support, tiered system of,
        223
    psychosocial and systemic foundations, 223

paediatric neuropsychological assessments,
    320
paediatric psychiatrist, for neuropsychological
    evaluation, 245
parental questionnaires, 113
parent- or teacher-mediated techniques, 38
parent self-guided reading, 152
parieto-medial temporal pathway, 83
parieto-premotor pathway, 83
Parkinson disease, 136
patient scores, on assessment battery, 87
pattern recognition, 120
peer-to-peer communication, 302
performance validity tests (PVTs), 290
    catch liars, 291
    clinical decision-making, 292
    neuropsychological evaluation, 295
    paediatric neuropsychologists, 291
    paediatric neuropsychology, 290
peripheral visual system, congenital disorders
    of, 7
personal amplification systems, 126
Personal Living Skills, 251
phonological awareness, child's development
    of, 171
phonological deficit, 178
phonology, 61
Picture Exchange Communication System
    (PECS), 255
poor phonological processing, 211
Prader–Willi syndrome, 249
precision teaching, 227
premotor cortex (PMC), 74
prenatal developmental neurotoxins, 200
prenatal exposure, to medicines/chemicals
    area, advancing, 203–4
    assessment/formulation, 200–2
    clinical geneticist, 195
    fetal alcohol spectrum disorder, 196–7
    formulation, 202
    impact/development, 197–200
    intervention/management, 202–3
    outcome, 203
preview, question, read, state, test (PQRST),
    116
problem-solve occupational performance,
    39
problem-solving skills, 165
Prompts for Restructuring Oral Muscular
    Phonetic Targets (PROMPT) therapy, 77

psychiatric disorders, 235
psycho-education, 226
psychotropic medications, 255

R

Rapid Syllable Transitions Treatment,
    78
reading comprehension, 173
remote expert assessment, 304
remote method, 302
Response to Intervention (RTI), 222

S

SCAN battery, 127
school-based peer interventions, 151
self-monitoring function, 107
self-report questionnaires, 113
semantic memory, 108
sensorimotor interventions, 136
sensory integration
    assessment
        formulation, 34–6
        treatment of, 32
    framework, 38
    intervention/management, 37–9
    outcome, 39
    overview, 32–3
    processing, 32
sensory integration theory, 32, 33, 38
sensory integration therapy, 37
sensory motor behaviour, multiple primary
    deficits contribution, 46
sensory processing, disruption, 33–4
sensory systems, 74
Shape Coding, 67
Simple View of Writing model, 184
skill acquisition, 54
skilled motor behaviour
    maturational/ecological approaches,
        44
    neural developmentalists, 44
    neural functions, hierarchy of, 45
sleep difficulties, 236
social adjustment, 223
social brain, 144
social cognition, 144

social communication, 11, 146–8
    assessment, 143
    difficulties, 145
    parental/self-report questionnaires, 113
social functioning
    assessment, 145–9
    formulation, 149
    intervention/management, 149–52
        (*see also* social intervention)
    multifaceted process, 144
    outcome, 152–3
    Seamus's difficulties, 144
    social cognition, 144
    social communication assessment, 143
Social Interaction and Communication Skills,
    251
social intervention
    behaviour modelling, 152
    child-centred social narratives, 152
    child's interests, 151–2
    computer-based/online social skills, 151
    group-based interventions, 151
    joint attention, 150–1
    parent self-guided reading, 152
    school-based peer interventions, 151
    visual augmentative/alternative
        communication methods, 152
    visual materials, 152
social learning theory, 211
social mind, 144
social/pragmatic language difficulties, 162
social problem-solving, 144
social skills, 66
    coaching, 149
    computer-based/online, 151
    training, 226
socioeconomic disparities, 249
sociopolitical variables, 281
sodium valproate
    in neurodevelopmental difficulties, 195
    risks associated, 201, 202
sound-cancelling headphones, 124
spastic bilateral cerebral palsy, 261
spatial attention network, 96
speech
    assessment/formulation
        adapted assessment, literature review,
            264–5
        brain-computer interfaces, 265
        choice-making capabilities, 265–6

executive functions, 267
eye-gaze technologies, 265
prerequisites for testing, 265–6
processing speed, 267
receptive language, 266
selected domain-specific
    considerations, 266
visuospatial/perceptual reasoning,
    266–7
working memory, 267
assistive technology/cognitive load,
    263
childhood apraxia of, 73
impairments, 262
language difficulties, 174
and language therapy, 71
outcome, 269
physical limitations, 261
psychometrics/validation, 263
spastic bilateral cerebral palsy, 261
Venn diagram of, 72
speech and language therapist, 148
speech development, 72
speech disorders
    assessment/formulation, 75–7
        developmental history, via
            questionnaires, 75
        differential diagnosis of, 75–6
        intelligence assessment, 76
        language assessment, 76
        movement skills, 76
    classification of, 72–3
    intervention/management, 77–8
    outcome, 78
speech execution, 73
speech intelligibility ratings, 76
speech-language intervention, with school-aged
    children, 66
speech/language therapists, 28, 57
speech motor control, 75
    brain basis of, 73–4
    theoretical models of, 74–5
speech overlaps, 74
speech perception, in noise, 121
speech sound disorders, 72
speech therapy, 57
spelling, learning of, 184
spinal cord injury, 263, 267
Standards for Psychological and Educational
    Testing, 262, 264

stress
    brain networks, 210
    generation route, 211
    susceptibility, 211
stroop color and word test, 283
supplementary motor area (SMA), 74
supramarginal gyrus (SMG), 74
sustained attention, 99
symptoms/severity, variability of, 197
symptom validity tests (SVTs), 293, 295
Systematic Transition in Education Programme
    for ASD (STEP-ASD) resource, 153
systemic/skills-based interventions, 241

T

task-based assessments, 35
task-focussed evidenced-based intervention,
    54
teleneuropsychology, 301, 302, 305
teleneuropsychology, paediatric
    assessment/formulation, 306–8, 313
    clinician, in adjacent rooms, 303–4
    clinician, in clinic/home, 305
    within clinic-patient, 303–4
    confidentiality, 313
    consent/assent, 312
    COVID-19 pandemic, 302
    delivery models, 302
    ethical considerations, 312
    home-patient, at home, 305
    intervention/management, 308–11
    neurological/neurodevelopmental
        disorders, 301
    outcome, 313
    practical implications, 308
    remote-patient andclinician, in hospitals/
        clinics, 302–3
    security, 312
    test selection, 305–6
    video-teleconferencing (VTC) techniques,
        301
telerehabilitation, 301
temporal lobectomy/hippocampectomy, 115
temporal lobe epilepsy, 110
teratogen, concept of, 195
teratogen, physical effects of, 196
token economy system, 228
tools, for schools, 21

training
   executive skills, 227
   home-based tutor, 228
   peer group support, 227
   psycho-education, 227
transcutaneous vagus nerve stimulation, 137
traumatic brain injury, robust
   neuropsychological sequelae, 267

U

UK Teratology Information Service, 201
US-based Mother to Baby webpages, 201
Usher syndromes, 20

V

V5/MT, 4
*Validity Testing in Child and Adolescent
   Assessment: Evaluating Exaggeration,
   Feigning, and Noncredible Effort*, 293
validity testing, in paediatric evaluations
   assessment/formulation, 292–4
   cervical X-rays, 289
   cognitive complaints, 290
   ethics codes, 291
   intervention/management, 294–5
   lag, in routine validity test, 292
   literature, 290
   outcome, 295–6
validity tests, 292
verbal memory
   deficits, 115
   tests, 237
verbal/non-verbal reasoning abilities,
   14–15
vicious cycle, psychological formulation of,
   239
video communication, 302
video-teleconferencing (VTC) techniques,
   301, 303
   adult neurocognitive tests, 306
   face-to-face test scores, 304–6
   paediatric assessment, 309–11
   psychoeducation, 311
   remote assessment, 313
   remote home-based, 305
vision impairment, 3, 10

adaptive behaviour, 9
adaptive skills, 10–11
assessment measures, 12–13
assessment, preparation of, 10
attention/executive functions/memory,
   8–9
behaviour, 10–11
childhood, 6–7
children, 10
cognitive/attainment testing, issues of,
   11
congenital, 6
developmental challenge, 3–6, 8
formulation, 10
intellectual disability, 8
intervention/management, 13–14
language/social communication, 9
learning profiles, 8
self-determination, 14
sensitive periods of, 6
social relating, 10–11
spectrum of, 8
vision impairment-specific tests, 12
visual acuity, 6
   central visual processing, 122
   levels of, 7
   vision, measure of, 6
visual augmentative/alternative
   communication methods, 152
visual dysfunction, 6
visual materials, 152
visual-motor planning, 34
visual pathways, eye to visual cortex, 4
visual perceptual abilities, 278
visual-stream hypothesis, 89
visual system
   development of, 6
   dorsal/ventral pathways of, 5
   neuroplasticity of, 6
visuomotor skills, 9
visuo-spatial processing, 81–4, 88
   brain injury, 81
   cortical processing, 82
   diagnosis/treatment, 82, 83
   intervention/management, 88–9
   outcome, 89–90
   parieto-premotor pathway, 83
   patient scores, on assessment battery,
      87–8
   skills and graphomotor coordination, 102

visuo-spatial skills, 86, 87
visuo-spatial task battery, 83
visuospatial working memory tests, 267
vocabulary knowledge, 172

W

Western cultures, 278
'where' pathway, 4

Williams syndrome, 82, 249
wiring diagram, 21
Wolf-Hirschhorn syndrome, 245, 251
    clinical features, 251
    cognitive-behavioural profiles, 251
word recognition, 171
working memory
    assessment of, 267
    attention, 107
    deficits, 22
writing, theoretical models of, 184